W0106422

THE KIDNEY IN PLASMA CELL DYSCRASIAS

The kidney in plasma cell dyscrasias

edited by

LUIGI MINETTI
Ca'Granda Hospital, Milan

GIUSEPPE D'AMICO
San Carlo Hospital, Milan

CLAUDIO PONTICELLI
Maggiore Hospital, Milan

Kluwer Academic Publishers
DORDRECHT/BOSTON/LONDON

Library of Congress Cataloging in Publication Data

The Kidney in plasma cell dyscrasias.

(Developments in nephrology)
Includes index.
1. Plasma cell diseases--Complications and sequelae.
2. Kidneys--Diseases--Immunological aspects. 3. Multiple myeloma--Complications and sequelae. 4. Amyloidosis--Complications and sequelae. 5. Paraproteinemia--Complications and sequelae. I. Minetti, L. II. D'Amico, G. (Giuseppe) III. Ponticelli, C. (Claudio) IV. Series.
[DNLM: 1. Immunoglobulins, Light Chain. 2. Kidney.
3. Paraproteinemias. W1 DE998EB / WJ 300 K4528]
RC918.P55K53 1988 616.6'1 88-8913

ISBN-13: 978-94-010-7085-0 e-ISBN-13: 978-94-009-1315-8
DOI: 10.1007/978-94-009-1315-8

Published by Kluwer Academic Publishers,
P.O. Box 17, 3300 AA Dordrecht, The Netherlands

Kluwer Academic Publishers incorporates the publishing programmes of D. Reidel, Martinus Nijhoff, Dr W. Junk and MTP Press.

Sold and distributed in the U.S.A. and Canada
by Kluwer Academic Publishers,
101 Philip Drive, Norwell, MA 02061, U.S.A.

In all other countries, sold and distributed
by Kluwer Academic Publishers Group,
P.O. Box 322, 3300 AH Dordrecht, The Netherlands

Softcover reprint of the hardcover 1st edition 1988

Contents

Part IV. THE THERAPEUTIC APPROACH

Part V.

List of first authors

Raymond ALEXANIAN, University of Texas, M.D. Anderson Hospital and Tumor Institute, Houston, TX 77030 (USA)

Giovanni BANFI, Department of Nephrology, Maggiore Policlinico Hospital, Milan (Italy)

Bart BARLOGIE, Department of Hematology, M.D. Anderson Hospital and Tumor Institute, 1515 Holcombe Blvd. — Box 55, Houston, TX 77030 (USA)

Ghil BUSNACH, Department of Nephrology, Niguarda Ca'Granda Hospital, Milan (Italy)

J. Stewart CAMERON, Clinical Science Laboratories, Guy's Hospital, London Bridge, SE1 9RT (UK)

Arthur H. COHEN, Department of Pathology, Harbor-UCLA Medical Center, 1000 West Carson Street, Torrance, CA 90509 (USA)

Giuliano COLASANTI, Division of Nephrology, San Carlo Hospital, Milan (Italy)

Giacomo COLUSSI, Department of Nephrology, Niguarda Ca'Granda Hospital, Milan (Italy)

Edward H. COOPER, Unit for Cancer Research, University of Leeds and Department of Immunology, University of Birmingham (UK)

Gloria GALLO, Department of Pathology, New York University School of Medicine, NYU Medical Center, 560 First Avenue, New York, NY 10016 (USA)

Dominique GANEVAL, Department of Nephrology, Hôpital Necker, 161 Rue de Sèvres, F-75743 Paris Cedex 15 (France)

Robert A. KYLE, Mayo Clinic and Mayo Foundation, Rochester, MN 55905 (USA)

Netar P. MALLICK, Department of Renal Medicine, Central Manchester Health Authority, Manchester Royal Infirmary, Oxford Road, Manchester M13 9WL (UK)

Jacob B. NATVIG, Institute of Immunology and Rheumatology, Rikshospitalet, 0172 Oslo 1 (Norway)

Conrad L. PIRANI, College of Physicians and Surgeons of Columbia University, Department of Pathology, 630 West 168th Street, New York, NY 10032 (USA)

Jean-Louis PREUD'HOMME, Laboratory of Immunology and Immunopathology (CNRS VA 1172), Poitiers University Hospital, BP 577, 86021 Poitiers Cedex (France)

Pierre RONCO, Unité INSERM U.64 and Service de Néphrologie, Hôpital Tenon, 4, Rue de la Chine, F-75970 Paris Cedex 20 (France)

Paul W. SANDERS, Nephrology Research and Training Center, Division of Nephrology, Department of Medicine and Pathology, University of Alabama at Birmingham, Birmingham, AL 35294 (USA)

Tsuranobu SHIRAHAMA, The Arthritis Center, Boston University School of Medicine, and The Thorndike Memorial Laboratory and The Division of Medicine, Boston City Hospital, Boston, MA 02118 (USA)

Peter SMOLENS, Department of Medicine, University of Texas, Health Science Center at San Antonio, San Antonio, TX 78284 (USA)

Alan SOLOMON, University of Tennessee Medical Center at Knoxville. 1924 Alcoa Highway, Knoxville, TN 37920 (USA)

Pietro ZUCCHELLI, Division of Nephrology, M. Malpighi Hospital, Bologna (Italy)

Dorothea ZUCKER-FRANKLIN, University Hospital, Room 445, Department of Medicine, New York University Medical Center, 560 First Avenue, New York, NY 10016 (USA)

Part I. The plasma cell dyscrasias

1. A perspective of plasma cell dyscrasias: Clinical implications of monoclonal light chains in renal disease

ALAN SOLOMON & DEBORAH T. WEISS

Introduction

The term 'plasma cell dyscrasia' may be interpreted broadly as any type of anatomical, developmental, or functional alteration in the B cell or humoral system. Specifically, the diseases or syndromes associated with plasma cell dyscrasias result from under or over proliferation of the most differentiated cellular elements of this system, plasma cells and their immediate B lymphocyte precursors, or from immunoglobulin (Ig) molecules which are produced by these cells and function as antibody. The plasma cell dyscrasias include a spectrum of diseases. They may be inherited or acquired, reactive or neoplastic, but all are characterized by some type of Ig alteration (Table 1). In addition, these diseases may be

Table 1. Immunoglobulin aberrations in plasma cell and other B cell related dyscrasias.

- Hypogammaglobulinemia
  - Congenital/Acquired
- Hypergammaglobulinemia
  - Immune complex and chronic inflammatory diseases
- Multiple myeloma
- Waldenström's macroglobulinemia
- Amyloidosis AL
- Heavy chain diseases
  - Gamma, Alpha, Mu
- Lymphoma/CLL
- Miscellaneous gammopathies
  - Idiopathic (MGUS)
  - Aging
  - Autoantibodies
  - Cryoglobulins

Minetti et al. (eds.), The kidney in plasma cell dyscrasias. ISBN 978-94-010-7085-0

intrinsic to B cells only or may involve other types of cells or factors that control B cell growth and maturation.

Immunoglobulins and plasma cell dyscrasias

Quantitative and qualitative alterations in Ig synthesis are hallmarks or 'biomarkers' of the plasma cell dyscrasias. These changes, which are characterized by the under or over production of Ig, can involve any of the protein components that constitute the humoral immune system. Proliferative disorders that involve a particular B cell clone are typically manifested by the particular Ig product of that clone. These homogeneous Ig products are called monoclonal Igs or M-proteins. Monoclonal Igs occur as 'complete' (i.e., whole) Ig molecules, or as 'incomplete' (i.e., aberrant) components that are subunits, fragments, or atypical forms of the native protein (Table 2). The most common example of an Ig subunit is Bence Jones protein, which represents monoclonal light chains [1]. Alternatively, proliferative multiclonal B cell disorders are characterized by multiple Ig products. The term polyclonal Ig refers to the heterogeneous Ig products of this type of alteration.

The fact that Igs serve as indicators of plasma cell and other B cell related dyscrasias has considerable diagnostic import [2]. The widespread use of electrophoretic and other types of serological analyses [3] provides a ready means to detect and identify Ig abnormalities in serum and urine specimens (Fig. 1).

The monoclonal and polyclonal Igs associated with the plasma cell dyscrasias represent Ig constituents found in normal individuals, albeit at

Table 2. Monoclonal immunoglobulins associated with plasma cell dyscrasias.

Complete	• Myeloma proteins IgG, IgA, IgD, IgE • Waldenström macroglobulins IgM
Incomplete	• Light chains (Bence Jones proteins) Kappa, Lambda • Heavy chains Gamma, Alpha, Mu (Delta, Epsilon) • Half molecules Alpha-Kappa, etc.
Aberrant	• Abnormal size Polymers, insertions or deletions, etc.

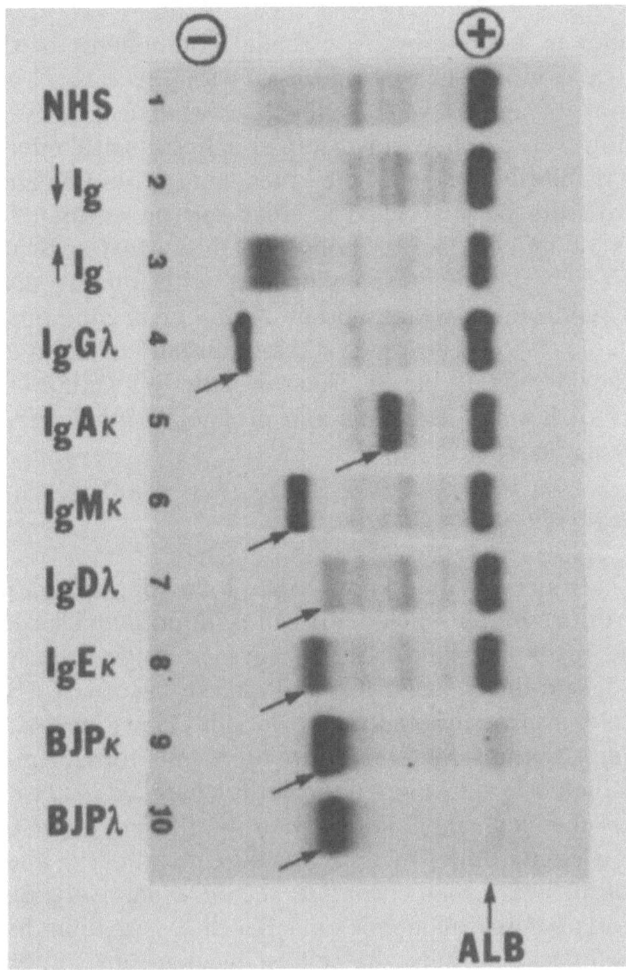

Fig. 1. Agarose gel electropherogram of specimens from patients with various types of plasma cell dyscrasias. Specimens 1—8, serum; 9, 10, urine. 1: normal human serum; 2: hypogammaglobulinemia (multiple myeloma); 3: polyclonal hypergammaglobulinemia (Sjögren's syndrome); 4: monoclonal IgGλ (multiple myeloma); 5: monoclonal IgAκ (multiple myeloma); 6: monoclonal IgMκ (Waldenström's macroglobulinemia); 7: monoclonal IgDλ (multiple myeloma); 8: monoclonal IgEκ (multiple myeloma); 9: Bence Jones protein κ (multiple myeloma); 10: Bence Jones protein λ (multiple myeloma). The heavy chain class and light chain type of monoclonal Igs were identified by immunoelectrophoresis [3]. The location of albumin (ALB) is as indicated and those of the monclonal components are shown by the *arrows* (Paragon® Electrophoresis System, Beckman).

greatly increased concentrations. The amount of these components found in serum and urine primarily reflects the degree of clonal proliferation and synthetic rates characteristic for each Ig class. The concentration of different forms of Igs in body fluids is also influenced by distinctive metabolic factors and by host factors such as renal function [4].

Ig molecules as antibodies are essential components of the humoral immune system and, as such, are necessary for life. Excess quantities or aberrant forms of Igs as well as those with unusual physicochemical properties, however, can have adverse pathophysiological effects. Many of the disease manifestations and the attendant morbidity and mortality associated with the plasma cell dyscrasias can be attributed directly to certain types of monoclonal or polyclonal Igs. Most striking are those proteins, chiefly IgM, that are associated with the hyperviscosity or cryoglobulin syndromes. Also important are other Ig components, such as IgA or Bence Jones protein, which interact directly or indirectly with the kidney or other organs (Table 3). Therefore, the recognition of pathophysiologic types of Ig has therapeutic and prognostic implications and is of obvious clinical importance.

Characterization of immunoglobulins

Remarkable advances in our knowledge of the human immune system have come from research on clonal B cell proliferative disorders, particularly multiple myeloma and Waldenström's macroglobulinemia [5]. The monoclonal Ig products associated with these disorders (Bence Jones proteins, myeloma proteins, and macroglobulins) have been an invaluable source of material for study since they represent normal Ig constituents and can be isolated in quantities sufficient for detailed analyses. Investigation into the chemical and biological properties of these proteins has provided knowledge of the structure, function, metabolism, and genetics of the family of proteins that constitute the Ig system [4]. Similarly, the availability for analyses of monoclonal B cell populations has also provided the means to determine the cellular mechanisms responsible for Ig synthesis.

Within the past 25 years much has been learned: The basic heavy and light polypeptide chain structure of Igs and the delineation of the five heavy chain classes (γ, α, μ, δ, and ε) and two light chain types (κ and λ)

Table 3. Pathophysiological consequences of monoclonal and polyclonal immunoglobulins.

- Hyperviscosity (IgM, IgG3)
- Cryoglobulins (Types I, II, and III)
- Autoantibodies (Rheumatoid factor, myelin, etc.)
- Organ Specificity (Bence Jones protein, IgA)
- Amyloidosis (Light chain and fragments)

have been elucidated. Amino acid sequence analyses have revealed the characteristic primary structure of the heavy and light chains (Fig. 2). Each chain is characterized by a series of ~ 110-amino acid residue, structurally homologous domains. The amino-terminal domains of the heavy and light chains vary in sequence and are thus designated the variable or V portion of the molecule. The carboxyl-terminal portion of each chain is relatively invariant in sequence and is thus designated the constant or C region. Immunochemical, affinity labeling, and X-ray crystallographic analyses have demonstrated the seminal role of the heavy and light chain V domains in conveying the individual properties associated with Ig molecules, namely, idiotypy and antibody specificity. Metabolic properties and other biological functions are associated with the C region domains [4].

Advances in recombinant DNA technology have revealed the extraordinary means by which Igs are synthesized. The heavy and light polypeptide chains of Igs are not encoded by a single gene but rather each chain is a product of multiple genes located on different chromosomes [5]. Within the germ line DNA are three gene families, V, D, and J, that encode the heavy chain V region, and two gene families, V and J, that encode the light chain V region. Similarly, the C regions of the heavy and light chains are

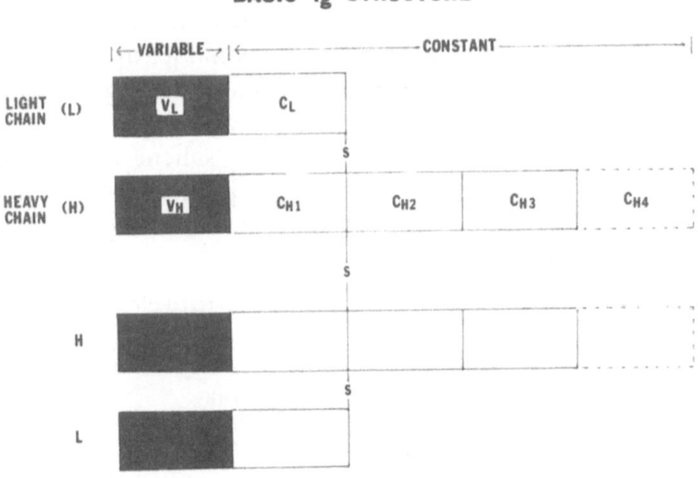

Fig. 2. Schematic diagram of the basic domain structure of the light (L) and heavy (H) polypeptide chains of immunoglobulins. The domains in the aminoterminal portion of each chain, the variable regions, are designated V_L and V_H for the light chain and heavy chain, respectively. The domains in the carboxyl-terminal portion of each chain, the constant regions, are designated C_L and C_H for the light chain and heavy chain, respectively; the three C_H domains are designated C_{H1}, C_{H2},C_{H3} (the C_H of immunoglobulins M and E contains an additional domain designated C_{H4}). The light and heavy chains are linked covalently by interchain disulfide bonds (—S—).

encoded by multiple forms of C genes. Remarkably, the process of B cell differentiation involves the translocation and recombination of selected germ line V, D, J, and C gene segments to form in somatic cell DNA a mRNA transcript that encodes the complete Ig molecule. This process also involves deletion or exclusion of unwanted Ig gene segments. Further, there are other genetic elements that promote or regulate Ig gene expression.

Thus, research on the plasma cell dyscrasias has led to the establishment of the chemical basis for antibody specificity and of the genetic and cellular events responsible for Ig synthesis.

Monoclonal immunoglobulins (Bence Jones proteins) in renal disease

The primary focus of this book, 'The Kidney in Plasma Cell Dyscrasias', involves the pathophysiological role of Igs in the renal syndromes associated with these diseases [6—11]. Virtually all types of monoclonal and polyclonal Igs, as well as subunits and fragments of Igs, have been implicated as being directly or indirectly responsible for glomerular or tubular dysfunction (Table 4). Among these components, monoclonal light chains (Bence Jones proteins) have long been associated with renal pathology. Monoclonal light chains and related fragments may be deposited as casts within the renal tubules (myeloma [cast] nephropathy), as nodules in basement membrane and mesangial tissue (light chain deposition disease), or as fibrils located in blood vessel walls and in tissues throughout the body (amyloidosis AL). The salient features of these diseases have been extensively reviewed [6—11]. These light chain deposits ultimately result in functional renal impairment and account for many of

Table 4. Immunoglobulins associated with renal disease.

- Bence Jones Proteins
  - Myeloma (cast) nephropathy
  - Light chain deposition disease
  - Amyloidosis AL
  - Fanconi syndrome
- IgA
- IgM
- Immune complexes
- Cryoglobulins
- Hypergammaglobulinemia

the disease manifestations and poor prognoses of patients with these disorders.

Bence Jones proteins

Bence Jones proteins represent synthetic products that are found in the urine of 60 to 80% of patients with multiple myeloma. They are less commonly found in other B cell related malignancies, and are rarely manifest as a monoclonal gammopathy of unknown significance. These components are the major protein constituent in the renal and systemic Ig deposits that characterize amyloidosis AL and light chain deposition disease. Often the clinical diagnosis of these diseases is first made by the detection of Bence Jones protein.

Many techniques have been used to identify Bence Jones proteins [11]. We have found immunofixation electrophoresis to be most useful for this purpose (Fig.3). This method is particularly helpful when urine specimens contain other Igs or proteins such as transferrin that can often obscure the

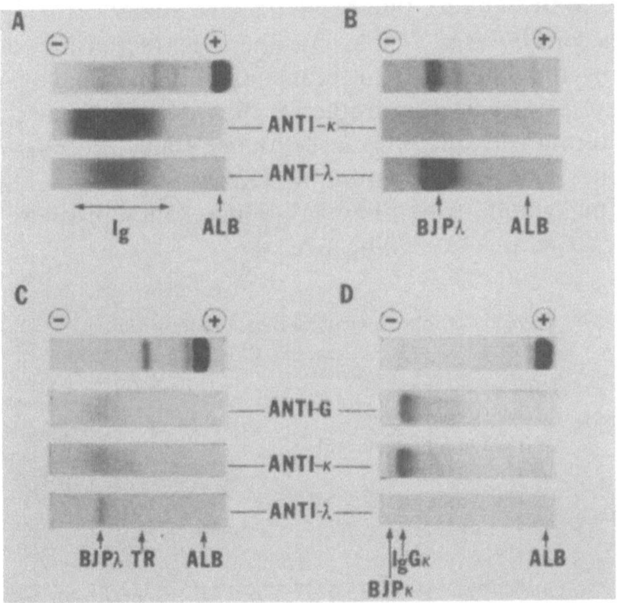

Fig. 3. Identification by immunofixation electrophoresis of Ig-related urinary components. After electrophoresis of urine specimens (protein concentrations, 50 mg/ml) on agarose gel, the membranes were stained for protein and with specific antisera as indicated. Depending on the antiserum employed, the specimens were diluted appropriately to obtain optimum precipitin reactions. *A*. Polyclonal Ig (κ and λ). *B*. Dimeric and monomeric Bence Jones proteins (λ). *C*. Bence Jones protein (λ) and polyclonal Ig. *D*. Bence Jones protein (κ) and monoclonal IgG (κ). The locations of transferrin (TR) and albumin (ALB) are also shown.

presence of Bence Jones proteinuria. For this type of analysis, urine specimens can be examined directly. However, in those cases where the amount of Bence Jones proteinuria is relatively low (i.e., <1 mg/ml), we have found it advisable to concentrate the urine specimen to at least 50 mg/ml. Because of the pathogenic role of Bence Jones proteins in the light chain-associated renal and systemic diseases, the recognition of these components and an awareness of their potential toxicities are of major clinical significance.

The quantity of Bence Jones proteins excreted depends on synthetic and catabolic factors which are determined primarily by tumor cell mass and renal function, respectively [12]. The kidney is the organ that filters, partially reabsorbs, and metabolizes these proteins [13, 14]. Thus, any factor that adversely affects renal function can reduce light chain catabolism and thereby potentiate the inherent nephrotoxicity of Bence Jones proteins. There is, however, no quantitative relationship between the amount of Bence Jones protein excreted and the presence or absence of tubular casts or other types of light chain deposition. Although a number of host factors may contribute to the renal damage observed in patients with Bence Jones proteinuria (Table 5), there is increasing evidence that differences in the chemical and functional properties of the proteins themselves are primarily responsible for their deposition as casts, nodules, or fibrils. Alternatively, in some cases, Bence Jones proteins, even in high concentrations, have no apparent ill effects [15]. Thus, the ability to distinguish “malignant” from “benign” Bence Jones proteins has obvious prognostic and therapeutic significance.

Table 5. Nephrotoxicity of Bence Jones proteins.

Host
- Dehydration
- Tubular transport
- Catabolism
- Synthesis
- Ancillary factors (Ca^{++}, anemia, etc.)
- Infections
- Radiographic contrast agents (IVP, CAT)

Protein
- Kappa vs Lambda
- Isoelectric point
- Solubility
- Molecular weight (monomer/dimer/tetramer; aberrant forms)
- Antibody

Malignant vs benign Bence Jones proteins

In an effort to elucidate why some proteins are nephrotoxic and others are not, several types of in vitro and in vivo models have been employed. In one such experimental model, described in 1976 by Koss, Pirani, and Osserman [16], a single 200 mg intraperitoneal injection of a human Bence Jones protein into a mouse resulted in its deposition as casts in the distal renal tubules of the recipient animal. Two other Bence Jones proteins tested in similar fashion did not form casts. Because the induced mouse nephropathy was similar to human myeloma (cast) nephropathy and because both species metabolize light chains similarly, we have further investigated the capability of the mouse model to reproduce this and other types of light chain-associated diseases in an effort to determine the clinical relevance of this experimental model.

Experimental production of human light chain-associated diseases. We first chose for study two κ Bence Jones proteins obtained from patients with multiple myeloma. One patient, who was excreting ~6 gm Bence Jones protein daily, had severely impaired renal function. The second patient, despite massive Bence Jones proteinuria (~40 gm/24 hr), had normal renal function. Injection of the first protein into the mouse resulted in deposition within the renal tubules of homogeneous, eosinophilic, PAS-negative casts. Immunohistochemical studies demonstrated that the casts in the mouse kidneys contained the injected human κ Bence Jones protein. The histologic appearance and Ig-nature of these casts in the mouse kidneys were identical to that found in the patient's kidney. The Bence Jones protein from the second patient produced no lesions in the mouse kidney. When other Bence Jones proteins were injected into mice, it was evident that only certain human proteins could induce the histopathologic alterations characteristic of myeloma (cast) nephropathy. In those patients in whom renal histologic data were available, there was complete concordance between the clinical and experimental findings.

The extent of cast formation was dose-dependent and was potentiated by dehydration of the mouse. Alternatively, vigorous hydration of the mouse reduced cast formation. The lesions were also reversible with time. In addition, the molecular portion of the light chain responsible for cast formation was localized to the V region. Injection of the variable portion (V_L) from a nephrotoxic Bence Jones protein produced identical pathology as did the intact protein. Conversely, no casts were formed when mice were injected with the constant portion (C_L) of the same protein (Table 6).

Another histologic alteration was seen in mice injected with certain clinically 'nephrotoxic' Bence Jones proteins. Rather than forming casts,

Table 6. Experimental model of myeloma (cast) nephropathy.

Correlation in mouse and man of histopathological, clinical, and laboratory parameters of Bence Jones protein-associated nephrotoxicity	
Histology:	• Characteristic renal tubular Bence Jones protein-containing casts (light-, electron-, and immunomicroscopy)
Pathophysiology:	• Renal dysfunction and cast formation (mouse) • Potentiation of lesions (dehydration) • Reversibility of lesions (hydration; time) • Non-toxicity of renal contrast agent • Pathogenic importance of V_L (vs C_L) • Identification of nephrotoxic Bence Jones proteins

these proteins were deposited in mouse glomeruli and renal tubular cells in a similar way to that noted in human light chain deposition disease (Table 7).

To date, we have studied in this experimental in vivo model 29 human Bence Jones proteins, 20 of which were obtained from patients with renal dysfunction (Table 8). Fifteen of these 'nephrotoxic' light chains were deposited as casts in the renal tubules of mice sacrificed 48 to 72 hr post-injection. No renal pathology was evident with the 9 clinically non-toxic Bence Jones proteins. Four of the other 5 'nephrotoxic' light chains were deposited within mouse glomeruli and renal tubular cells.

The light and electron microscopic studies of mouse kidneys and other organs obtained 3 to 7 days after a single injection of Bence Jones protein showed no evidence of amyloidosis. However, when mice were repeatedly injected over a 1- to 2-month period with Bence Jones proteins obtained from patients with amyloidosis AL, these human proteins were deposited as Congo-red positive, birefringent, fibrillar material within the blood

Table 7. Experimental model of light chain deposition disease.

Correlation in mouse and man of characteristic histopathological features of light chain-associated disease	
Histology:	• Characteristic glomerular and tubular light chain deposits (immunomicroscopy)
Pathophysiology:	• "Normal" vs "abnormal" light chains • Identification of "glomerular toxic" or "tubular toxic" light chains

Table 8. Nephrotoxicity of 29 human Bence Jones proteins.

Clinical (Renal functional status)	Experimental (Mouse renal pathology)		
	Normal	Casts	Glomerular/tubular deposits
Normal (9)	9	0	0
Abnormal[a] (20)	1	15	4

[a] BUN, > 30 mg/dl; creatinine, > 2 mg/dl.

vessel walls and interstitial tissue of the mouse kidney and other organs (Table 9).

Our studies demonstrate the predictive value of the experimental mouse model in identification of nephrotoxic or amyloidogenic light chains. The model provides a unique opportunity to learn more about the pathogenesis and treatment of the light chain-associated diseases.

Experimental data on nephrotoxic light chains. Because differences in V region sequence are responsible for the distinctive properties of light chains, we have also begun a systematic study to determine the chemical features that distinguish "benign" from "malignant" or "amyloidogenic" Bence Jones proteins. One V_L-related feature of Bence Jones proteins — their isoelectric point — has been implicated in the pathogenesis of certain light chain-associated renal diseases [11]. As shown in the agarose gel electropherogram (Fig. 4), there are marked differences in the electrophoretic mobility of Bence Jones proteins. Although it has been reported that the most cationic (electronegative) light chains are associated with myeloma cast nephropathy and the most anionic proteins (electropositive)

Table 9. Experimental model of amyloidosis (AL).

Correlation in mouse and man of histopathological features of light chain-associated amyloidosis	
Histology:	• Characteristic vascular and interstitial amyloid deposits (light-, electron-, and immunomicroscopy; Congo red ⊕-birefringent, thioflavin T ⊕-fluorescent, 7.5 nm-diameter, Bence Jones protein-containing fibrils)
Pathophysiology:	• Tissue and organ localization • Induction by λ and κ amyloid-associated Bence Jones proteins

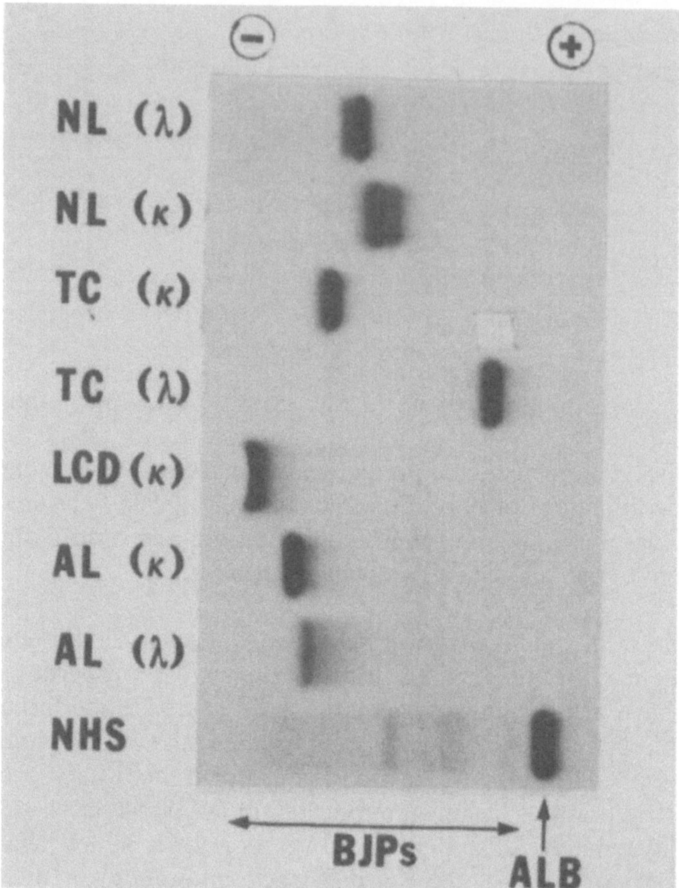

Fig. 4. Agarose gel electropherogram of monoclonal light chains isolated from urine specimens of patients with Bence Jones proteinuria. Samples (~ 10 mg/ml) were electrophoresed at 100 V for 25 min in 0.05 ionic strength barbital buffer, pH 8.6. Bence Jones proteins were obtained from patients with no evident renal disease (NL), tubular cast nephropathy (TC), light chain deposition disease (LCD), amyloidosis AL (AL). The light chain type κ or λ is as designated. BJPs, Bence Jones proteins, NHS, normal human serum; ALB, albumin.

with light chain deposition disease, we have not as yet found this relationship clinically or experimentally among our proteins. More detailed information on the structural properties of light chains is required to establish the features that render certain proteins nephrotoxic.

Another V_L-related feature of light chains is their susceptibility to proteolysis [3]. It is noteworthy that, with rare exception, the light chains isolated from amyloid deposits consist of fragments of the intact light polypeptide chain [9]. These fragments represent the entire V region or the V region plus ~ 50 residues of the C region (Fig. 5). "Amyloidogenic" Bence Jones proteins may be especially susceptible to enzymatic cleavage

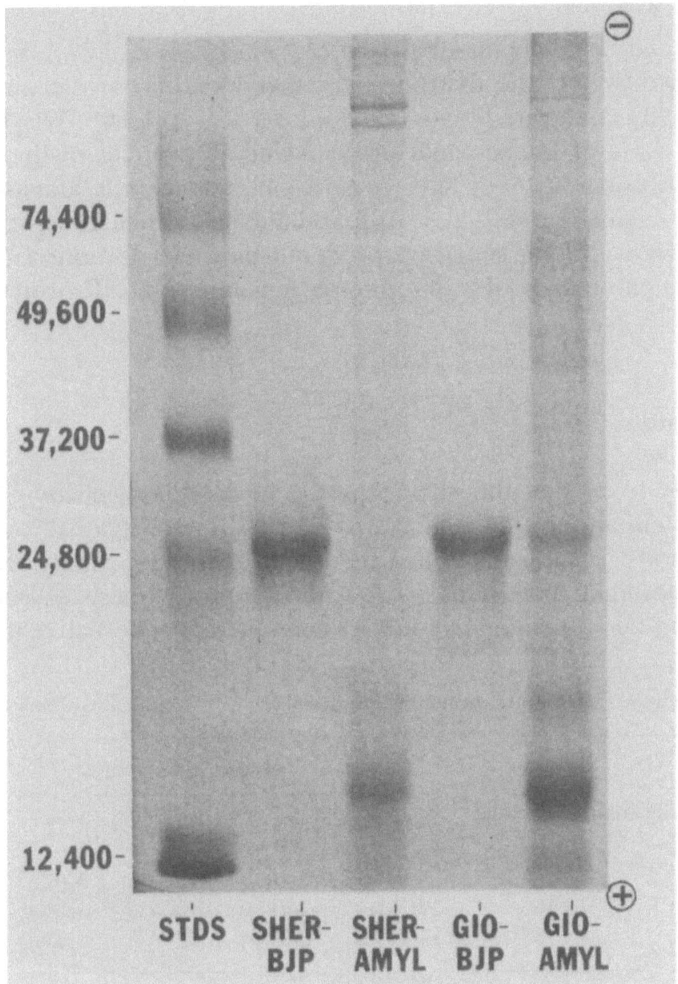

Fig. 5. SDS-polyacrylamide gel electropherogram of homologous Bence Jones proteins and amyloid fibril proteins. Samples were treated with 2-mercaptoethanol and electrophoresed in a 12% acrylamide gel. The Bence Jones proteins (BJP) isolated from urine specimens and fibril proteins (AMYL) isolated from amyloid deposits of patients GIO and SHER were electrophoresed with standard reference proteins (STDS). The molecular weights of the STDS are as indicated.

which could lead to the deposition of these light chain fragments as amyloid. Additionally, the role of host factors in generation of amyloidosis remains to be determined.

Human light chains are also characterized by multiple V region-related subgroups (and sub-subgroups) that have been defined chemically and serologically [3,17]. We have developed antisera in rabbits to human Bence Jones proteins that distinguish the four κ chain subgroups (κ_{I}, κ_{II},

κ_{III}, κ_{IV}) and six λ chain subgroups (λ_I, $\lambda_{II/V}$, λ_{III}, λ_{IV}, λ_{VI}). Using these antisera, we have found that one particular subgroup of λ chains, λVI, is preferentially associated with amyloidosis AL [11,18]. We have now identified 17 λVI Bence Jones proteins and all proteins of this relatively uncommon subgroup [19] have come from patients with amyloidosis AL (Table 10). Although we have not found among κ amyloid-associated light chains such a striking subgroup predominance, we do note a disproportionately high number of κII and a lower number of κIII proteins (Table 11).

Conclusions

The ability to predict the nephrotoxicity or amyloidogenicity of a Bence Jones protein and to understand what factors render it "toxic" will lead to new methods for more effective treatment of the potentially lethal complications of light chain deposition. Although the synthesis of Bence Jones protein can be reduced by cytotoxic chemotherapy, alternative methods of

Table 10. λ-type Bence Jones proteins from patients with or without amyloidosis AL.

		V_λ region subgroups [a]				
Patient classification	Number	$V_{\lambda I}$	$V_{\lambda II,V}$	$V_{\lambda III}$	$V_{\lambda IV}$	$V_{\lambda VI}$
Amyloid	34	5(15%)	7(20%)	5(15%)	0(0%)	17(50%)
Nonamyloid	103	29(28%)	43(42%)	28(27%)	3(3%)	0(0%)
Total	137	34(25%)	50(37%)	33(24%)	3(2%)	17(12%)

[a] Based on serological analyses with specific anti-λI, anti-λII, anti-λIII, anti-λIV, and anti-λVI antisera (proteins classified chemically as λV react with specific anti-λII antisera).

Table 11. κ-type Bence Jones proteins from patients with or without amyloidosis AL.

		V_κ region subgroups [2]			
Patient classification	Number	$V_{\kappa I}$	$V_{\kappa II}$	$V_{\kappa III}$	$V_{\kappa IV}$
Amyloid	15	10(67%)	4(27%)	1(6%)	(0%)
Nonamyloid	143	79(55%)	11(8%)	42(29%)	11(8%)
Total	158	89(56%)	15(10%)	43(27%)	11(7%)

[a] Based on serological analyses with specific anti-κI, anti-κII, anti-κIII, and anti-κIV antisera.

treatment may be given based on knowledge of why certain Bence Jones proteins are nephrotoxic, amyloidogenic, etc. Further information regarding the pathophysiological implications of these proteins and their diagnostic, therapeutic, and prognostic importance will be especially helpful for clinicians caring for patients with plasma cell dyscrasias.

Acknowledgements

We thank Meredith Patton for preparation of this manuscript and Teresa Williams and Mildred Conley for technical assistance.

This work was supported in part by research grants from the American Cancer Society (IM-430), the United States Public Health Service, National Cancer Institute (CA 10056), and the Stein Cancer Research Fund.

References

1. Edelman GM, Gally JA. The nature of Bence-Jones proteins. Chemical similarities to polypeptide chains of myeloma globulins and normal γ-globulins. J Exp Med 1962; 116: 207—27.
2. Solomon A. Monoclonal immunoglobulins as biomarkers of cancer. In: Sell S, ed. Cancer markers: developmental and diagnostic significance. Clifton, New Jersey: Humana Press 1980: 57—87.
3. Solomon A. Light chains of human immunoglobulins. Methods Enzymol 1985; 116: 101—21.
4. Solomon A. Current developments in immunoglobulins. In: Silber R, Gordon AS, LoBue J, Muggia FM, eds. Contemporary hematology/oncology, Vol 2. New York: Plenum Press, 1981: 399—465.
5. Yarbro JW, Bornstein RS, Mastrangelo MJ, eds. Semin oncol, Vol XIII(3). Orlando, Florida: Grune and Stratton, 1986.
6. Hill GS. Multiple myeloma, amyloidosis, Waldenström's macroglobulinemia, cryoglobulinemias, and benign monoclonal gammopathies. In: Heptinstall RH, ed. Pathology of the kidney, ed. 3. Boston: Little Brown & Co, 1983: 993—1067.
7. Gallo GR, Feiner HD, Buxbaum JN. The kidney in lymphoplasmacytic disorders. Pathol Annu 1982; 17: 291—317.
8. Pirani CL, Silva FG, Appel GB. Tubulo-interstitial disease in multiple myeloma and other nonrenal neoplasias. In: Cotran AS, ed. Tubulo-interstitial nephropathies, contemporary issues in nephrology, Vol 10. New York: Churchill-Livingstone, 1983: 287—334.
9. Glenner GG. Amyloid deposits and amyloidosis: the B-fibrilloses. N Engl J Med 1980; 302: 1283—92.
10. Fang LS. Light-chain nephropathy. Kidney Int 1985; 27: 882—92.
11. Solomon A. Clinical implications of monoclonal light chains. Semin Oncol 1986; 13: 341—49.
12. Solomon A. Bence-Jones proteins and light chains of immunoglobulins. N Engl J Med 1976; 294: 17—23; 91—98.

13. Wochner RD, Strober W, Waldman TA. The role of the kidney in the catabolism of Bence Jones proteins and immunoglobulin fragments. J Exp Med 1967; 126: 207—21.
14. Strober W, Waldmann TA. The role of the kidney in the metabolism of plasma proteins. Nephron 1974; 13: 35—66.
15. Solomon A. Bence Jones proteins: malignant or benign? (editorial). N Engl J Med 1982; 306: 605—7.
16. Koss MN, Pirani CL, Osserman EF. Experimental Bence Jones cast nephropathy. Lab Invest 1976; 34: 579—91.
17. Solomon A. Light chains of immunoglobulins: Structural-genetic correlates. Blood 1986; 68: 603—10.
18. Solomon A, Frangione B, Franklin EC. Bence Jones proteins and light chains of immunoglobulins. Preferential association of the $V_{\lambda VI}$ subgroup of human light chains with amyloidosis AL(λ). J Clinical Invest 1982; 70: 453—60.
19. Solomon A, Weiss DT. Serologically defined V region subgroups of human λ light chains. J Immunol 1987; 139: 824—30.

2. Genotypic and phenotypic diversity of plasma cell myeloma

BART BARLOGIE, JOSHUA EPSTEIN,
PETER SELVANAYAGAM & RAYMOND ALEXANIAN

Multiple myeloma is a neoplasm of monoclonal well differentiated B cells, and clinical symptoms result from bone destruction, anemia, hypercalcemia, renal failure and immunosuppression. Melphalan-prednisone has been the mainstay of therapy for 20 years, providing initial responses in at least half of the patients with few complete remissions, however, and a median survival time of only 2 to 3 years [1]. Patients presenting with low tumor mass and achieving marked cytoreduction account for the majority of the 5 to 10% of patients surviving up to 10 years, although they too ultimately succumb to progression of disease [2].

Studying the cellular biology of multiple myeloma should aid in the understanding of the heterogeneity in the clinical disease course and thus facilitate the selection of patients with poor prognosis for novel therapeutic strategies. Flow cytometry (FCM) is a convenient tool for quantitative tumor cell analysis. Using acridine orange for the combined analysis of cellular DNA and RNA content, 80% of patients exhibit *DNA aneuploidy* and a similar proportion of patients have a markedly *elevated RNA content* (Fig. 1) [3]. While the DNA abnormality is discrete with an excess in DNA content typically of 10 to 15%, there is considerable dispersion in RNA content with an average increase by 4 to 6 fold over that of normal hemopoietic cells. In more than 80% of patients, these DNA and RNA features remain stable throughout the disease course despite the development of drug resistance. About 1/3 of patients have *circulating aneuploid cells* in their blood (Table 1). Extramedullary plasmacytomas usually show DNA-RNA features that are concordant with those present in the bone marrow. The hallmark of plasma cells as terminally differentiated B cells is the presence of large amounts of *monoclonal cytoplasmic immunoglobulin* (cIg), which can be quantitated by FCM using appropriate Ig heavy and light chain antisera (Fig. 2) [4]. When examined in conjunction with cellular DNA content, monoclonal CIg light chain expression is usually confined to the aneuploid DNA stemline. In about 10% of patients, an additional

Minetti et al. (eds.), The kidney in plasma cell dyscrasias. ISBN 978-94-010-7085-0

diploid DNA stemline with concordant cIg expression can be observed. Likewise, 10 to 15% of patients demonstrate *dual light chain expression* by aneuploid tumor cells, all of whom had IgG lambda myeloma [4]. This is an important deviation from the widely accepted allelic exclusion dogma and the hierarchy of immunoglobulin gene rearrangement with an orderly succession from heavy to kappa and then lambda light chain genes [5]. DNA-cIg FCM can aid in detecting rare cases of non-secretory or

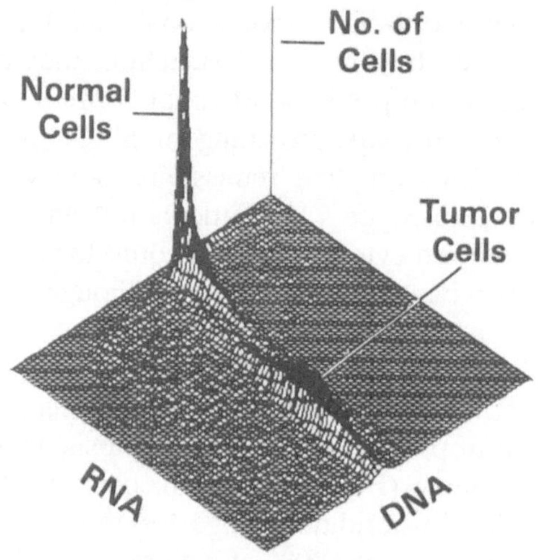

Fig. 1. Typical DNA-RNA distribution pattern of bone marrow cells from a patient with myeloma. Heparinized marrow was stained with acridine orange and subjected to flow cytometry. Compared to residual normal hemopoietic cells, myeloma plasma cells generally exhibit a discrete DNA excess of 10—15% and a markedly elevated RNA content (4 to 6-fold higher than that of normal lymphocytes) with considerable dispersion.

Table 1. DNA-RNA features in bone marrow and blood.

		Bone marrow	
Blood	N	Diploid-high RNA	Aneuploid
Normal	19	5	14
Diploid-high RNA	7	7	0
Aneuploid	15	0	15
Total	41	12	29

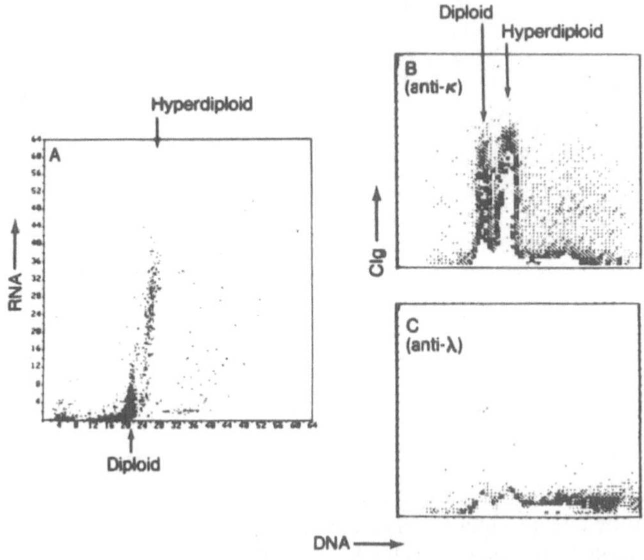

Fig. 2. DNA-cytoplasmic immunoglobulin (cIg) flow cytometry of hyperdiploid myeloma. Ethanol-fixed cells were reacted with anti-light chain reagents and counterstained with propidium iodide for nuclear DNA content. Note the monoclonal kappa expression by tumor cells with a hyperdiploid DNA content.

nonproducing myeloma [4]. Joint analysis of DNA, RNA and cIg affords an objective quantitation of marrow plasmacytosis in virtually all patients, identification of myeloma with low RNA index (with important prognostic implications, see below), recognition of DNA-biclonal disease and of unexpected dual light chain expression of yet unknown clinical relevance.

The nature of the myeloma stem cell has remained elusive, although recent reports have suggested the presence of a CALLA-antigen positive precursor population in the peripheral blood and bone marrow [6]. *Phenotype studies* have recently been conducted to determine the presence of tumor subpopulations with earlier B cell features such as B4, CALLA and B2 antigens using monoclonal antibody immunofluorescence and DNA counter-staining with FCM. Considerable heterogeneity in the expression of early, intermediate and mature B cell markers (CIg, R1-3) and beta-2-microglobulin (B2M) expression was noted, occasionally with differences in reactivity among aneuploid and diploid tumor subpopulations (Fig. 3). Among 44 patients studied to date, almost 90% expressed monoclonal cIg, R1-3 and B2M, 55% expressed the pre-B cell antigen CALLA, 23% had B4 and 17% expressed the B2 antigen [7]. CALLA was present together with monoclonal cIg either in the same or in different

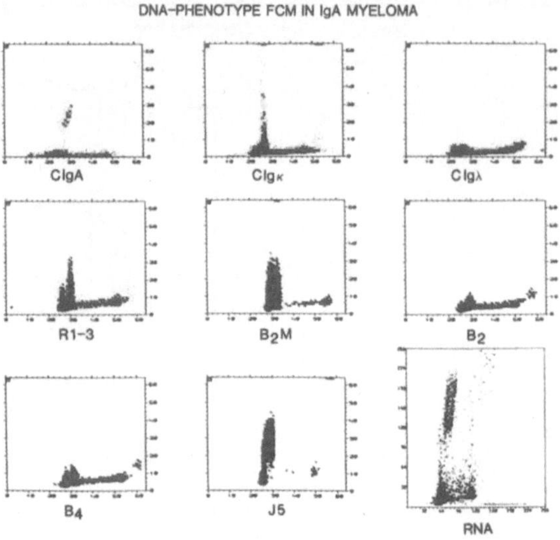

Fig. 3. DNA-phenotype analysis by flow cytometry. Surface and cytoplasmic properties were quantitated by direct or indirect immunofluorescence flow cytometry in relationship to nuclear DNA content (propidium iodide). Hyperdiploid tumor cells have a markedly elevated RNA content, expressed cIgA kappa, the mature plasma cell antigen R1-3, β_2-microglobulin (β_2M) and the pre-B cell antigen CALLA (J5). In addition, diploid cells also react with β_2M and J5 reagents, suggesting a diploid tumor stemline exhibiting only early B cell markers.

tumor cells, so that a model of myeloma ontogeny is proposed with a CALLA+/cIg-precursor compartment feeding into a novel CALLA+/cIg+phenotype without counterpart in normal B cell differentiation, that matures to the expected CALLA-/cIg+ plasma cell phenotype.

While DNA aneuploidy is a useful genotypic stigma for most patients with myeloma that is readily obtained regardless of tumor cell proliferative activity, profound knowledge of subtle genetic anomalies requires cytogenetic and molecular examination. In comparison with leukemias and lymphomas, there is limited information on *karyotype abnormalities* in plasma cell myeloma, due to technical difficulties in obtaining banded metaphase chromosomes of high quality in this typically slowly proliferating B cell disease with an average tritiated thymidine labelling index of 1 to 2% [8]. As a potential alternative to metaphase karyotyping, the technique of premature chromosome condensation (PCC) has been applied to patients with multiple myeloma to study the karyotype in interphase cells [9]. There was good agreement between ploidy levels assessed by DNA flow cytometry and modal chromosomal number derived from both metaphase and G1 PCC chromosomal studies (Fig. 4). The incidence of abnormal cytogenetics by standard metaphase karyotyping seemed independent of

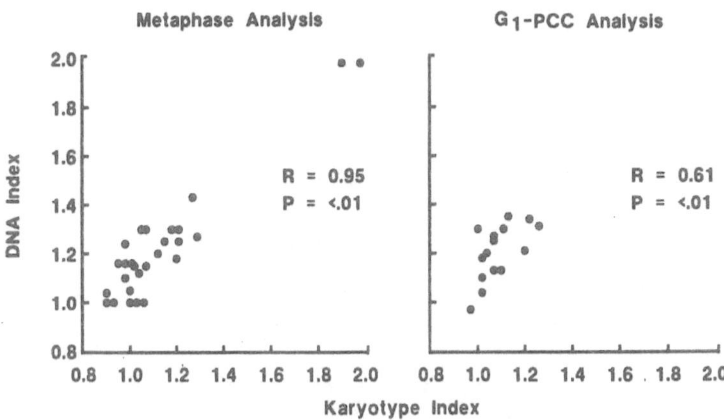

Fig. 4. Comparison of ploidy levels by DNA flow cytometry (DNA index) and karyotype index, derived either from standard metaphase (left) or G_1 interphase (G_1-PCC) cytogenetic analyses.

the degree of marrow plasmacytosis, but was higher in patients with drug-resistant than with previously untreated disease (60 vs 30%). Chromosomal aberrations were typically complex with marked numeric and structural aberrations. Chromosome gains involved preferentially chromosomes 3, 5, 7, 9, 11, and 15, whereas losses of chromosome 13 were most frequently encountered. Lymphoma-like translocations involved t(8; 14), t(11; 14) and t(14; 18) [10]. Chromosomal breakpoints clustered on chromosomes 1, 8, 11, and 14, whereas chromosomes 2, 18 and 22 were less frequently involved. Hypodiploid abnormalities were more frequently associated with light chain myeloma, whereas all t(8; 14) translocations had an IgA phenotype.

Molecular genetic studies were carried out to determine whether *cellular oncogenes* were altered in the process of chromosomal translocations has been reported in malignant lymphomas [11]. Over-expression of myc-RNA was noted in 25% of almost 50 patients studied, 3 of whom were associated with DNA rearrangement involving either typical gene sites like in endemic Burkitt's lymphoma or a novel site at the 3' flank of the gene [12]. Bcl-1 rearrangement was present in <10% of over 100 cases examined, and none of about 50 patients revealed bcl-2 rearrangement [13]. The frequent structural abnormalities of chromosome 1 prompted protein expression studies of the ras oncogene using FCM (Fig.5). Almost 80% of 20 patients with hyperdiploid myeloma showed high ras protein activity [14].

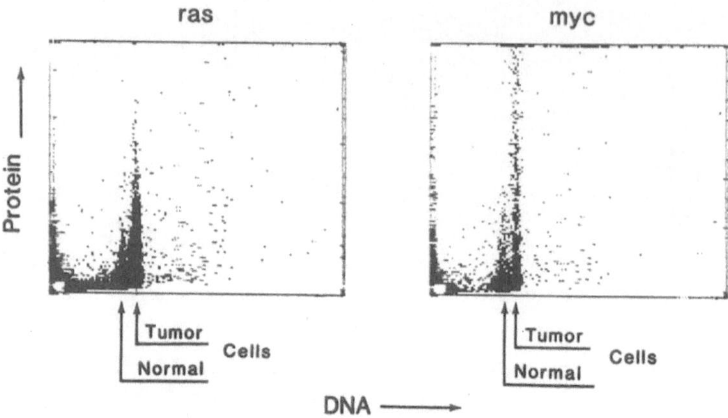

Fig. 5. DNA-oncogene protein flow cytometry in hyperdiploid myeloma. Ethanol-fixed cells were reacted with anti-ras (HAS-2) (left) or anti-myc (MYC-3) (right) antibodies and counterstained for DNA with propidium iodide. Preferential oncogene protein expression by hyperdiploid tumor cells compared to normal diploid hemopoietic cells.

Molecular genetic studies were also conducted to study the lymphoid differentiation and clonality of multiple myeloma. With the recently available *TcR-gamma* probe, single and multiple rearrangements were noted in 3 of 10 patients, together with rearrangements of the immunoglobulin heavy chain gene (J_H) [15]. Together with immunophenotype studies (see above) and lymphoma-like chromosomal translocations (occurring in the process of VDJ-joining during B cell commitment [16]), these molecular genetic observations (TcR-gamma rearrangement; alteration of c-myc and bcl-1) also indicate that myeloma may result from malignant transformation at the pre-B cell level.

Cytokinetic studies in myeloma using tritiated thymidine autoradiography have demonstrated a low proportion of cells in S phase (average of 1–2% at diagnosis, 5–7% at relapse). Higher proliferative activity at diagnosis was an adverse feature for survival, independent of tumor mass [8]. FCM has recently enabled a more convenient assessment of tumor cell proliferative activity using a bromodeoxyuridine (BUdR) monoclonal antibody to determine the proportion of cells that have incorporated BUdR during DNA synthesis (Fig. 6A) [17]. The Ki-67 antibody recognizes cells with proliferative potential, including those in G_1 and G_2 phases of the cell cycle and may thus provide a cytochemical means of growth fraction determination (Fig. 6B) [18].

A number of treatment-related cellular features have recently been examined, including *glucocorticoid receptor expression* by FCM using

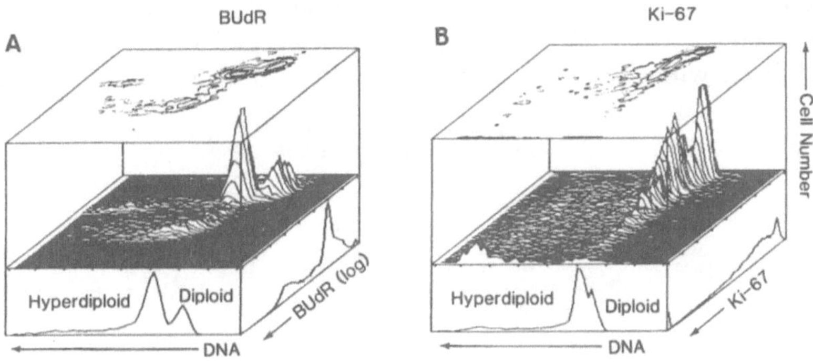

Fig. 6. Cytokinetic analysis in myeloma using flow cytometry: bone marrow cells were incubated with BUdR (20 μM) for 60 min at 37° and then fixed in 70% ethanol. Monoclonal antibody IU-4 was applied after DNA denaturation to determine the proportion of cells in S and their relative DNA synthetic activity (A). The use of Ki-67 monoclonal antibody permits identification of cells with a potential for proliferation, including cells in G_1 and G_2 (B). Counterstaining with propidium iodide allows the distinction between hyperdiploid tumor and diploid normal hemopoietic cells.

either FITC-conjugated cortisol as ligand or monoclonal antibody immunofluorescence assays (Figs 7A and B) [19]. The presence and intensity of reactivity are currently being examined as potential indicators for responsiveness to high doses of glucocorticoid [20]. The failure to control neoplastic disease has recently been attributed to the acquisition of *multi-drug resistance* usually to vinca alkaloid and anthracycline antibiotics [21]. A multi-drug resistant phenotype can now be defined by the presence of a p-glycoprotein of 170kd which can be conveniently measured by FCM using C-219 monoclonal antibody (Fig. 8) [22].

While a large body of cellular biologic, cytogenetic and molecular genetic data is being accumulated that will aid in the understanding of pathogenesis, disease manifestation and progression of multiple myeloma, practical usefulness for *prognosis* has already been derived from DNA ploidy and cellular RNA measurements [23]. Hypodiploid myeloma is completely refractory to standard melphalan-prednisone and VAD therapy (Table 2). Increasing plasma cell RNA index provides increasing sensitivity to chemotherapy, which is most evident among patients with IgG myeloma of low and intermediate tumor mass stage (Table 3). Multivariate analysis of pretreatment variables in newly diagnosed myeloma treated with VCAP or VCAD regimens demonstrated the strong adverse role of low plasma cell RNA content for response and of high tumor mass for survival [23]. Recent experience with high dose melphalan revealed that DNA hypodiploidy and low plasma cell RNA content were no longer prognostically important for response, so that this treatment seems to offer a true alternative for hitherto poor prognosis patients (Table 4) [24].

The biologic and clinical implications of nucleic acid and CIg FCM are summarized in Table 5. Genotypically, plasma cell myeloma is typically hyperdiploid with complex chromosome anomalies including lymphoma-

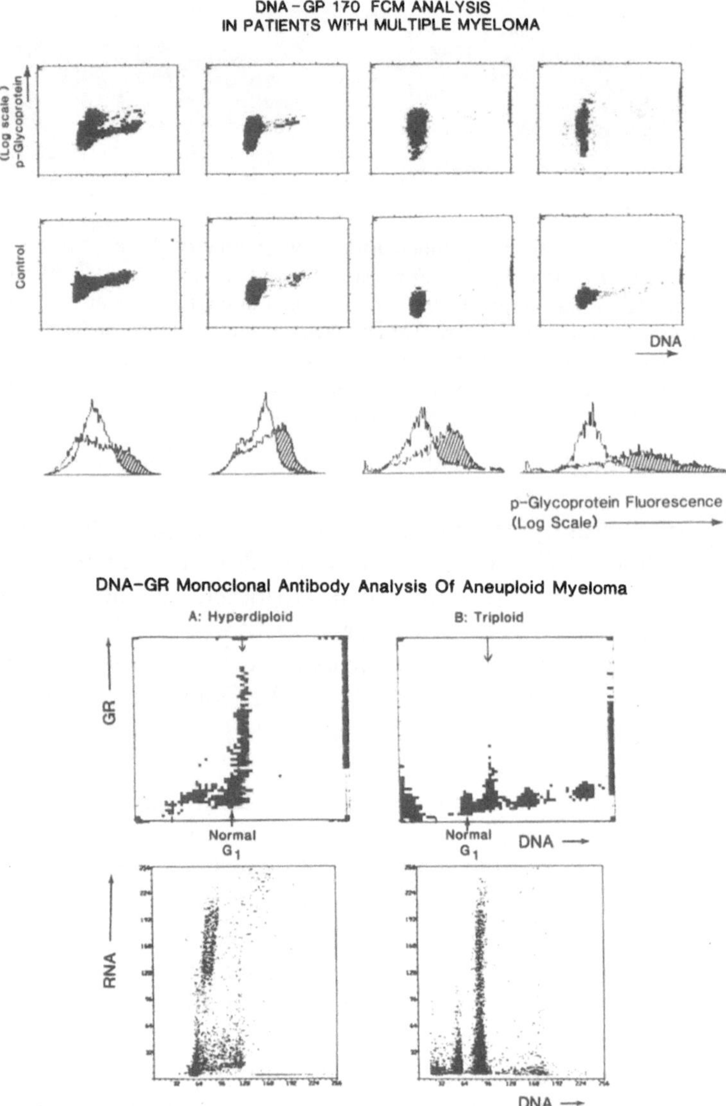

Fig. 7. Single cell glucocorticoid receptor analysis by flow cytometry using either FITC-conjugated cortisol (FC,A) or monoclonal antibody against the glucocorticoid receptor (GRMB, B). Counterstaining with propidium iodide for nuclear DNA content permits analysis of the glucocorticoid receptor in direct relationship to aneuploid tumor cells.

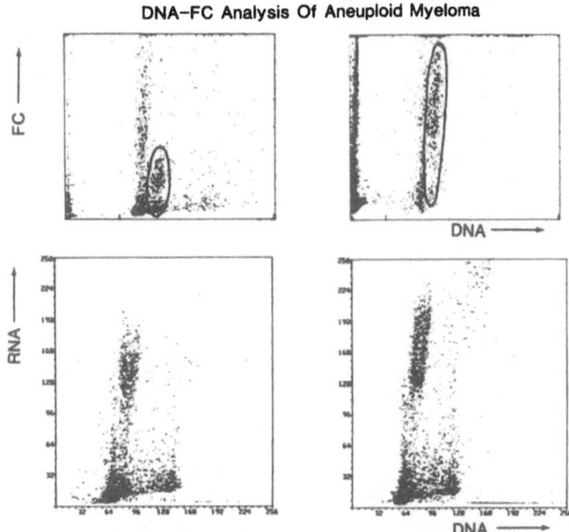

Fig. 8. Flow cytometric analysis of multi-drug resistant (MDR) phenotype using monoclonal antibody against gp 170 with counterstaining by propidium iodide for differential analysis of MDR expression by aneuploid tumor vs normal hemopoietic cells.

Table 2. Response in untreated myeloma according to DNA and RNA features.

		Percent patients responding with RNA index			
DNA Index	N	<4.0	4–6	6.1–8	>8
<1.0	12	0	0	33	–
1.0	28	43	64	71	100
1.01–1.20	60	25	53	92	81
>1.2	47	38	71	56	78
Total	147	29	54	71	81

Table 3. Response in untreated myeloma according to tumor mass, RNA index and Ig phenotype.

		Percent patients responding			
		IgG		non-IgG	
RNA Index	N	Low/int	High	Low/int	High
<4	28	25	43	30	14
4–6	41	60	83	54	14
6.1–8	31	82	67	75	0
>8	47	91	67	90	40
Total	147	76	64	61	18

Table 4. Response rate in untreated and refractory myeloma according to plasma cell DNA and RNA content.

	Untreated VCAP—VCAD		Treated DEXA—VAD		HDM	
Plasma cell feature	N	% Resp[a]	N	% Resp	N	% Resp
DNA-Ploidy						
Hypodiploid	12	8	2	0	5	60
Other	135	66	88	36	36	50
RNA Index						
<4.0	28	29	15	13	9	56
≥4.0	119	69	75	40	32	50
DNA and RNA Combined						
Adverse	35	26	15	13	11	55
Other	112	72	75	40	30	50

[a] % of patients responding

Table 5. Myeloma biology.

Genetics:	Frequently hyperdiploid (80%) Preferential but complex chromosome anomalies Lymphoma-type translocations associated with IgA Evidence for circulating tumor cells C-MYC and BCL-1 involvement
Phenotype:	Pre — B precursor cell? Co-expression of early and well differentiated B cell phenotypes
Systemic effects:	Bone lesions mediated by 'OAF's' (e.g. TNF-β) Cellular and humoral immune abnormalities

type translocations leading to alterations of c-myc and bcl-1. Phenotype, cytogenetic and molecular genetic studies suggest the possibility of a pre-B myeloma precursor cell and a novel co-expression of early and mature B cell markers. The systemic effects of myeloma such as bone lesions with hypercalcemia, anemia and renal failure, as well as immune abnormalities, probably result from tumor-derived cytokines, which have yet to be studied at the tumor cell level. It is furthermore anticipated that studies of B cell growth and differentiation factors and their receptors will help unravel the mechanisms of uncontrolled plasma cell growth (possibly linked to alterations of cellular oncogenes such as c-myc and bcl-1) and thus provide new targets for both cytotoxic and biologic therapy [25].

Acknowledgement

This work was supported by CA37161 and CA28771 from the National Cancer Institute, Bethesda, Md 20203.

References

1. Durie BMG, Salmon SE. A clinical staging system for multiple myeloma. Cancer 1981; 36: 842—54.
2. Alexanian R. Ten year survival in multiple myeloma. Arch Int Med 1985; 145: 2073.
3. Latreille J, Barlogie B, Dosik G, Johnston D, Drewinko B, Alexanian R. Cellular DNA content as a marker of human multiple myeloma. 1980; Blood 55: 403—8.
4. Barlogie B, Alexanian R, Pershouse M, Smallwood L, Smith L. Cytoplasmic immunoglobulin content in multiple myeloma. 1985; JCI 76: 765—9.
5. Korsmeyer SJ, Hieter JV, Ravetch DG, Poplack DG, Waldman TA, Leder P. Developmental hierarchy of immunoglobulin gene rearrangements in human leukemic pre-B-cells. Proc Natl Acad Sci USA 1981; 78: 7096—100.
6. Caligaris-Cappio F, Janossy G, Bergui L, Tesio L, Pizzolo G, Malavasi F, Chilosi M, Campana D, van Camp B, Gavosto F. Identification of malignant plasma cell precursors in the bone marrow of multiple myeloma. J Clin Invest 1985; 76: 1243—51.
7. Epstein J, Barlogie B, Alexanian R. Phenotype heterogeneity in multiple myeloma with aneuploid plasma cells. Proceedings ASCO 1987; Vol. 6, Abstr 756.
8. Latreille J, Barlogie B, Johnston D, Maxwell B, Drewinko B, Alexanian R. Ploidy and proliferative characteristics in monoclonal gammopathies. Blood 1982; 59: 43—51.
9. Hittelman WN, Barlogie B. Cytogenetic abnormalities in multiple myeloma detected in interphase cells using the premature chromosome condensation technique. Proceedings 1986; Vol. 27, 35, AACR, Asbtr #145.
10. Gould J, Goodacre A, Pathak S, Alexanian R, Barlogie B. Karyotype correlations with clinical features in multiple myeloma. Proceedings 1986; Vol. 68, Asbtr. 716, ASH.
11. Klein G, Klein E. Myc/Ig juxtaposition by chromosomal translocations: Some new insights, puzzles and paradoxes. Immunology Today 1985; G: 208—15.
12. Selvanayagam P, Blick M, Narni F, van Tuinen P, Ledbetter DH, Alexanian R, Saunders GF, Barlogie B. Alteration and abnormal expression of the c-myc oncogene in human multiple myeloma. Blood 1987; (in press).
13. Selvanayagam P, Goodacre A, Strong L, Saunders GF, Barlogie B. Alterations of bcl-1 oncogene in human multiple myeloma. Proceedings 1987; Vol. 28, Abstr #76, AACR.
14. Tsuchiya H, Epstein J, Dedman J, Barlogie B. Correlated flow cytometric analysis of p21 ras protein and nuclear DNA in multiple myeloma (MM). Proceedings 1987; Vol. 28, Abstr 77, AACR.
15. Lee MS, Selvanayagam P, Alexanian R, Stass Sa, Barlogie B. Rearrangement (REARR) of TcR-gamma chain gene in multiple myeloma. Proceedings 1987; Vol. 28 Abstr #706 AACR.

16. Showe LC, Croce CM. The role of chromosomal translocations in B- and T-cell neoplasia. Ann Rev Immunol Vol. 5, 1987; 253.
17. Gratzner H. Monoclonal antibody to 5-bromo- and 5-iododeoxyuridine: A new reagent for detection of DNA replication. Science 1982; 218: 474—5.
18. Gerdes J, Dallenbach F, Lennert K. Growth fraction in malignant non-Hodgkin's lymphomas (NHL) as determined in situ with the monoclonal antibody Ki-67. Hematol Oncol 1984; 2: 365.
19. Marchetti D, Van NT, Thompson EB, Barlogie B. Dual flow cytometric (FCM) analysis of glucocorticoid receptor (GR) expression in human leukemic cell lines using monoclonal antibody (MoAB) and fluoresceinated cortisol probes. Proceedings 1987; Vol. 28, Abstr. #965, AACR.
20. Barlogie B, Smith L, Alexanian R. Effective treatment of advanced multiple myeloma refractory to alkylating agents. NEJM 1984; 310: 1353.
21. Ling V. Drug Resistance and Neoplasia. Vol. 1. N. Bruchovsky and J. H. Goldie (eds). CRC Press, 1982; pp. 1.
22. Katner N, Evernden-Proelle D, Bradley G, Ling V. Detection of P-glycoprotein in multidrug-resistant cell lines by monoclonal antibodies. Nature 1985; 316: 820.
23. Barlogie B, Alexanian R, Dixon D, Smith L, Smallwood L, Delasalle K. Prognostic implications of tumor cell DNA and RNA content in multiple myeloma. Blood 1985; 66: 338.
24. Barlogie B, Zander A, Dicke K, Alexanian R. High dose melphalan with autologous bone marrow transplantation for multiple myeloma. Blood 1986; 67: 1298.
25. Quesada JR, Alexanian R, Hawkins M, Barlogie B, Borden E, Itri L, Gutterman JU. Treatment of multiple myeloma with recombinant alpha-interferon. Blood 1986; 67: 275—78.

3. Immunoglobulin synthesis in plasma cell dyscrasias with renal lesions

JEAN-LOUIS PREUD'HOMME

Abstract

Bone marrow cells from patients with light chain deposition disease (LCDD) or primary or myeloma amyloidosis were studied by immunofluorescence and biosynthesis experiments after incorporation of radioactive aminoacids. Monoclonal plasma cell populations were demonstrated even in patients without serum and urine monoclonal immunoglobulins and with a normal percentage of plasma cells. Structurally abnormal immunoglobulins were produced in several LCDD patients: abnormal light chains (by their short or large size, glycosylation and polymerization in vivo and in vitro) and abnormal (short) heavy chains. In other cases, light chains were normal sized and unglycosylated but they also showed a strong tendency to polymerize. The secretion of free light chains featured every amyloidosis case and the presence of light chain fragments almost all cases. Additional features in amyloidosis were synthesis of short γ chains (two cases), assembly block at the HL half molecule level of a monoclonal IgA (one case) and secretion of decameric enlarged κ chains (one case). This is in contrast with non-myelomatous secondary amyloidosis where the distribution of bone marrow plasma cells was normal by immunofluorescence and where normal sized immunoglobulins were synthesised, without free light chain secretion and fragments.

Introduction

The kidney involvement is a major manifestation of the various plasma cell dyscrasias, whatever their hematological presentation and 'benign' or overt malignant nature. Most kidney lesions certainly or probably relate to the secretion of monoclonal immunoglobulins (Ig). Myeloma kidney, macroglobulinemia and cryoglobulinemia kidneys are largely dealt with

Minetti et al. (eds.), The kidney in plasma cell dyscrasias. ISBN 978-94-010-7085-0

elsewhere in this volume and do not show any special Ig biosynthesis feature, except for excessive or exclusive light chain production in myeloma [1]. We will therefore focus on two diseases, namely light chain deposition disease (LCDD) and immunoglobulinic amyloidosis, in which abnormalities of Ig synthesis are probably directly relevant to the pathogenesis of tissue deposition.

Patients and methods

We studied 22 patients with LCDD who all had typical kidney lesions. They presented with the whole spectrum of plasma cell dyscrasias: multiple myeloma (14 cases), extra-osseous and solitary osseous plasmacytomas (one case each), Waldenström-like pleomorphic lymphoplasmocytic proliferation (1 case) and apparently benign monoclonal plasma cell dyscrasia even after prolonged follow-up (5 cases). No monoclonal Ig was detectable in the serum and urine in 7 cases but monoclonal plasma cell populations were easily identified by bone marrow immunofluorescence (IF) in every case (certain patients therefore had the so-called nonsecretory myeloma). By IF, tissue deposits contained κ chains in 17 cases and λ chains in 5, together with determinants of a heavy chain in 3 patients.

The present study also includes 14 patients with primary amyloidosis (in two of these patients, a diagnosis of myeloma was considered as probable later upon follow-up). No monoclonal Ig was detectable by electrophoretic and immunoelectrophoretic analysis of serum and concentrated urines in 4 cases, small amounts of urinary Bence-Jones protein (BJ) were found in 4 patients and the serum from 6 patients contained a monoclonal Ig in moderate concentrations (4 IgG, 1 IgA and 1 IgM). In 5 further primary amyloidosis patients, the bone marrow sample was poor and only Ig biosynthesis study was performed, but incorporated counts were too low for interpretable results. Two patients with myeloma and amyloidosis were also studied, one affected with 'nonsecretory' myeloma and one with BJ myeloma. Cells from 4 patients with secondary amyloidosis were studied as controls.

Bone marrow cells obtained by aspiration were studied by cytoplasmic immunofluorescence with monospecific conjugates against the various human heavy (H) and light (L) Ig chains. The method used to detect cellular Ig, the preparation, characteristics and specificity controls of the conjugated F(ab')2 fragments anti-human Ig were described in detail before [2]. When needed for an accurate counting (i.e. in primary and non-myelomatous secondary amyloidosis patients in whom the total percentage of bone marrow plasma cells was in the normal range), 5,000 to

10,000 bone marrow cells by IF slide were counted. Ig biosynthesis was studied as previously described [3—6]. Briefly, bone marrow cells were washed in spinner minimal essential medium lacking valine, threonine and leucine and incubated in the same medium for 1—3 hr, depending on the number of cells available, with ^{14}C or ^{3}H valine, threonine and leucine. Supernatants containing secreted proteins (sec.) were separated by centrifugation and cell pellets were lysed by the nonionic detergent NP40. Cytoplasmic extracts (cyto.) and sec. were immunoprecipitated using polyvalent anti-human Ig rabbit F(ab′)2 fragments and goat anti-rabbit Ig antibodies. Washed precipitates were dissolved in sodium dodecyl sulfate (SDS) and analysed by SDS-polyacrylamide gel electrophoresis (SDS-PAGE) at various gel concentrations. Internally labeled IgG, H and L chains from the murine plasmacytoma MPC 11 were used as molecular weight (Mw) markers. Monoclonal Ig purified from the serum of 3 patients with LCDD and the urinary BJ protein from a further LCDD patient were studied by classical immunochemical procedures.

Results

Since a large part of the data on LCDD were published previously [6—10], they will be only briefly mentioned whereas results in amyloidosis, that have not yet been published in detail, will be described in more length.

Light chain deposition disease

In every case, a monoclonal population of Ig-containing plasma cells was easily evidenced by IF in the bone marrow. Ig chain determinants found in the plasma cells matched those detected in tissue deposits except in 3 patients in whom plasma cells contained a monoclonal IgG whereas only monotypic L chains were detectable in tissues (Table 1). Biosynthesis experiments and immunochemical studies of purified serum or urine Ig allow to distinguish two groups of patients.

Patients with abnormal Ig biosynthesis. In 6 cases, biosynthesis studies displayed obviously abnormal results (Table 2). In 3 cases, only L chains were detectable and they were either abnormally large (2 cases) or small (1 case). They were secreted as covalent polymers. Patient Mo. was first affected with common IgA myeloma without renal lesions. He developed LCDD when relapsing after chemotherapy while the levels of his serum monoclonal IgA kept decreasing. Abnormally short κ and α (lacking one domain) chains were found in the plasma cells and not in the serum (the

Table 1. Ig chain determinants detected by IF in LCDD.

Number of cases	Tissue deposits	Plasma cells
13	κ	κ
2	κ	$\gamma\kappa$
2	$\alpha\kappa$	$\alpha\kappa$
3	λ	λ
1	λ	$\gamma\lambda$
1	$\gamma\lambda$	$\gamma\lambda$
22		

Table 2. LCDD patients with abnormal Ig synthesis.

Patient	Monoclonal Ig in serum and/or urine	IF Tissues	Plasma cells	Biosynthesis experiments Mw of Ig chains (kD) L Cyto	Sec	H	L chain polymerisation
Lau.	0	κ	κ	28	31	—	trimers
Cai.	0	κ	κ	30	31	—	160 kD
Ro.	0	κ	κ	12	20	—*	150 kD
Mo.	IgA κ**	$\alpha\kappa$	$\alpha\kappa$	20	23	43	?***
				23	25		
Ber.	IgG κ, no BJ	κ	$\gamma\kappa$	29	32	57	?***
An.	IgG κ, no BJ	κ	$\gamma\kappa$	29	31	50	+***

* Normal sized surface IgMκ and IgDκ.
** Normal sized IgA in decreasing amounts.
*** Hardly appreciable because of the presence of assembled molecules containing H and L chains.

serum IgA had normal sized H and L chains). This suggests the emergence of a mutant clone induced by alkylating agents, as documented in murine plasmocytomas [11]; this variant produces abnormal IgA molecules that are presumably responsible for tissue deposition [7]. In the last two patients (Ber. and An.), whose tissue deposits contained only κ chains, the cells secreted monoclonal IgG and free L chains, the latter being undetectable in serum and urines. The κ chains that were secreted as assembled molecules and as free L chains were abnormally large.

As a whole, these patients have in common the following abnormalities:

1. abnormal size of L chains,

2. L chain polymerization in vivo (biosynthesis experiments) and in vitro: monoclonal IgG were isolated from the serum of patients Ber. and An. and the κ chains were purified from these IgG. When these L chains were separated from the H chains, they polymerized as shown by gel filtration and SDS—PAGE.
3. glycosylation of L chains: this was suggested by the different apparent Mw of cytoplasmic and secreted L chains (Table 2) and confirmed in two cases by repeating the biosynthesis study in the presence of the inhibitor of N-glycosylation tunicamycine. In addition, PAS staining of PAGE-SDS of the serum L chains from patients Ber. and An. was strongly positive and the analysis of carbohydrates of these κ chains showed a content of 14.7 and 10.7%, respectively.
4. The abnormal L chains (and H chains in patient Mo.) were undetectable in the patient's serum and urine (whereas normal sized IgA and IgG from patient Mo., Ber. and An. gave serum peaks and were absent or probably absent in tissue deposits).

Patients without clearcut abnormalities of Ig chains. In two patients whose urines contained large amounts of BJ protein of the same type as the L chain determinants found by IF in tissue deposits, biosynthesis experiments showed the production of apparently non-glycosylated normal sized L chains that were secreted as monomers and dimers.

In a third similar patient, western blot analysis of SDS-PAGE of unreduced and reduced and alkylated serum and urines showed normal sized κ chains present as free monomers, dimers and several molecules of higher Mw. Fractionation of the urinary BJ protein on Sephadex G200 in non-dissociating conditions showed that the κ chains eluted in four fractions: F1 with a high Mw (in the void volume), F2 eluting at the position of IgG, F3 together with albumin and F4 lighter. SDS-PAGE of these fractions showed mostly L chain monomers and dimers in fraction F1 to F3 and monomers in F4. They were unstained by PAS. A 15 kD L chain fragment was also found in F3 and F4 but it was undetectable in the serum and hence likely represents a proteolytic product. Therefore, the situation in this patient differs from those with structurally abnormal L chains (normal size, no evidence for glycosylation) but shares a common feature, the strong tendency to polymerize by covalent and non-covalent bridges.

In a patient with deposited α and κ determinants, a monoclonal IgA was present in the serum. This component was purified. Its study showed no size abnormality of α and κ chains. Biosynthesis experiments could not be performed and we do not know whether the deposited IgA κ is the same as the serum monoclonal Ig or might correspond to a second clone whose secretion product is not detectable in the serum, as in patient Mo.

Amyloidosis

In the 4 studied patients with secondary amyloidosis, IF study of bone marrow cells showed a normal distribution of Ig containing cells both for H ($\gamma > \alpha > \mu > \delta$) and L ($\kappa > \lambda$) chains. The sum of H chain containing cells equalled that of L chain producing plasma cells (Table 3). Ig biosynthesis study showed the production of normal Ig molecules. Free L chains were found in cytoplasmic extracts, which is normal (there is normally a pool of cytoplasmic free L chains), but not in secretions.

In contrast, in primary (and myeloma) amyloidosis, IF study showed the presence of a monoclonal plasma cell population most often of the λ type in every case but two, even when the percentage of plasma cells amongst bone marrow cells was normal (Table 4). These data are summarized in Table 5. Interpretable results of biosynthesis experiments were available in 10 cases (Table 4). The secretion of large amounts of free L chains was a constant feature in all patients, including those without detectable urinary BJ protein and patient n° 6 in whom no monoclonal plasma cell population could be detected by IF. These L chains were secreted as monomers and, predominantly, dimers (except in case 10). The apparent Mw of λ chains was large (25—27 kD) in 5 cases. This is meaningless since it is well known that certain human λ chains have an abnormal behaviour in SDS-gels, leading to an erroneous appreciation of their Mw. The apparent Mw of the L chains was identical in cytoplasms and secretion in every case. One or two fragments of the size of about a half-L chain or slightly larger were present in cytoplasmic extracts from 9 of 10 patients but detectable in significant amounts in the secretion in only 3 cases. Interestingly, such fragments were the major cytoplasmic anti-Ig precipitable component in the two studied cases (n° 2 and 3) with no detectable monoclonal Ig or BJ in serum and urine.

Four primary amyloidosis patients had urinary BJ λ. In one case (n° 6) a huge excess of free L chain was found besides normal Ig molecules. In patients 7 and 8, only L chains and fragments were visible on the gels. In patient 9, in whom a monoclonal IgG λ was found by bone marrow IF, the cells secreted L chains, L chain dimers and fragments and assembled molecules. Upon reduction and alkylation, the major H chain component was abnormally short (apparent Mw 48 kD). Patient 10 had a BJ κ myeloma. His bone marrow plasma cells produced large (31 kD) κ chains that were secreted as a single covalent molecule of about 300 kD (probable decamer).

Results of biosynthesis experiment are available in 3 of the 6 primary amyloidosis patients whose serum contained a entire monoclonal Ig. As in the other cases, free L chains were secreted, mostly as dimers. One of

Table 3. Secondary amyloidosis.

Patient n°	Underlying disease	Monoclonal Ig in serum and/ or urine	Ig containing bone marrow cells (%) γ	α	μ	δ	κ	λ	ΣH	ΣL	Biosynthesis experiment
1	Portuguese amyloidosis	None	0.4*	0.1	0.1	0	0.4*	0.4*	1	1	Normal
2	Psoriasis, ankylosing spondylitis	None	0.64	0.44	0.14	0	0.64	0.45	1.22	1.09	?**
3	Behçet	None	0.56	0.33	0.30	0	0.78	0.33	1.19	1.11	Normal
4	Kidney carcinoma	None	0.74	0.34	0.11	0	0.79	0.33	1.19	1.12	Normal

* Accurate counting not possible due to the lack of a sufficient number of cells.

** Incorporated counts too low for an interpretable study.

Table 4. Primary amyloidosis and myeloma amyloidosis.

Patient n°.	Diagnosis	Monoclonal Ig in serum and/ or urine	Ig determinants in amyloid deposits by IF	Ig containing bone marrow cells (%) γ	α	μ	δ	κ	λ	ΣH	ΣL	Free L chain secretion	Mw*	Ig biosynthesis experiments Fragments cyto.	Mw	sec.	Comments
1	Primary amyloidosis	None	ND**	*6*	< 1	< 1	ND	1	*6*	*7*	*7*				ND		
2	Primary amyloidosis	None	ND	0.36	0.11	0.17	0.02	0.45	*1.0*	0.66	*1.75*	L2 > L	22	+++	11, 9	0	F as the major cytoplasmic Ig
3	Primary amyloidosis	None	All chains	0.07	0.13	0.10	0	0.39	*0.32*	0.30	*0.71*	L2 > L	22.5	+++	12	++	F as the major cytoplasmic Ig
4	Primary amyloidosis	None	ND	0.22	0.05	0.14	0.01	0.25	0.13	0.42	0.38				ND		
5	Myeloma	None	ND	< 1	*19*	< 1	ND	< 1	*19*	*19*	*19*				ND		
6	Primary amyloidosis	BJ λ	λ	0.18	0.07	0.04	0	0.17	0.09	0.29	0.26	L2 >> L	27	++	13	±	
7	Primary amyloidosis***	BJ λ	None	< 0.1	< 0.1	< 0.1	0	< 0.1	*3.5*	0.1	*3.5*	L2	27	+	12	0	No detectable H chains
8	Primary amyloidosis	BJ λ	ND	2	0.5	0.5	ND	2	*6*	3	*8*	L2	22.5	+	18, 11	0	No detectable H chains
9	Primary amyloidosis	BJ λ	ND	*3*	1	0.5	ND	1.5	*3*	*4.5*	*4.5*	L2 >> L	26	+	20, 17	++	Abnormally short H chains
10	Myeloma	BJ κ	ND	< 1	< 1	< 1	< 1	*30*	< 1	< 1	*30*	L10	31	+	15	0	Abnormally large κ chains secreted as a decamer
11	Primary amyloidosis	IgG λ	ND	*4*	< 0.1	< 0.1	0	< 0.1	*4*	*4*	*4*				ND		
12	Primary amyloidosis	IgG λ	λ				ND					L2	26	0		0	Abnormally short H chains
13	Primary amyloidosis	IgG κ	ND	*1*	0	0	0	*1*	0	*1*	*1*				Uninterpretable****		
14	Primary amyloidosis	IG κ	ND	0.23	0.09	0.06	0	*0.42*	0.07	0.38	*0.49*	L2 > L	22.5	++	12	+	
15	Primary amyloidosis***	IgA1 λ	None	0.86	*2.55*	0.10	0	0.40	*2.35*	3.5	2.75	L2 > L	25	++	13	0	Assembly block of IgA molecules
16	Primary amyloidosis	IgM λ	λ	0.5	1	9	ND	1.5	7	10.5	8.5				Uninterpretable****		

* Apparent Mw of the monomer on gels (kD).
** ND: not done.
*** Probable diagnosis of myeloma considered upon follow-up.
**** Incorporated counts too low.

Table 5. Monoclonal Ig in primary amyloidosis and myeloma amyloidosis.

Serum and/ or urine	Plasma cells	Number of cases
None	$\gamma\lambda$	1
None	$\alpha\lambda$	1
None	λ	2
None	None	1
BJ λ	None	1
BJ λ	λ	2
BJ λ	$\gamma\lambda$	1
BJ κ	κ	1
IgG λ	$\gamma\lambda$	1
IgG λ	ND*	1
IgG κ	$\gamma\kappa$	2
IgA λ	$\alpha\lambda$	1
IgM λ	$\mu\lambda$	1

$\kappa/\lambda = 3/12$
* ND: not determined

these patients (n° 12) is the only one in whom we did not detect L chain fragments. His monoclonal IgG was made of an abnormally short H chain (apparent Mw 47 kD). Patient 15's serum contained an IgA λ of the IgA1 subclass. His plasma cells synthesized normal size α chains (apparent Mw 60 kD) that assembled with L chains into a 84 kD molecule, with virtually no peak of the size of H2L2 molecules. This 84 kD molecule indeed contained H chains (since H chains were undetectable on unreduced gels) and it could not be a H2 dimer, which would have had a Mw of 120 kD. It contained L chains also, as shown by the comparison of the amount of L chains on reduced and unreduced gels. Therefore, this 84 kD molecule is a HL half molecule. Material was not available for biochemical study of the serum M component.

Discussion

The present study of a large number of LCDD patients clearly shows that this syndrome belongs to plasma cell dyscrasias since a monoclonal plasma cell population was found in every case, irrespective of the presence or absence (close to one third of cases) of serum and/or urine monoclonal Ig. The situation is the same in primary amyloidosis since evidences for monoclonal plasma cells were obtained by bone marrow IF in all patients but two, even in those with normal percentages of bone marrow plasma cells and without detectable monoclonal Ig in serum and urines. Furthermore, in the patient (n° 6) with a normal distribution of plasma cells by IF whose bone marrow cells could be studied for Ig biosynthesis, the amyloid substance stained for λ determinants, small amounts of BJ λ were present in urines and bone marrow cells secreted a huge excess of free L chains. These data confirm Osserman's concept that primary amyloidosis is a plasma cell dyscrasia [12]. It is worth noting that in both LCDD and amyloidosis certain patients presented with 'nonsecretory' myeloma or plasma cell dyscrasias or had a urinary BJ whereas their plasma cells produced both H and L chains. In such situations, we previously showed that the cells commonly produce structurally abnormal Ig chains that are indeed secreted but not detectable in serum and urines [5, 13—15]. The hypothesis that such abnormal Ig might be responsible for tissue deposition prompted us to perform biosynthesis experiments in LCDD and amyloidosis.

Such experiments allow to define a group of LCDD patients in whom grossly abnormal Ig chains were secreted. Abnormal H chains produced in a patient were short by about one domain whereas abnormal L chains displayed a triple abnormality: size (short or enlarged), glycosylation and polymerization. Glycosylation featured every such case, which is highly significant since glycosylated L chains are found in less than 15% of myeloma cases [16, 17]. Abnormally short H chains and L chain polymerization were also reported by others in individual cases [18, 19]. We have no direct evidence for the role of these abnormalities in tissue deposition but the correlation between in vivo (composition of the deposits by IF) and in vitro (biosynthesis experiments) findings is strongly suggestive. For instance, patient Mo. was free of renal disease before the emergence of a variant clone producing short α and κ chains and the deposits contained α and κ determinants; in patient Ber., whose plasma cells secreted abnormal free L chains and IgG molecules containing normal sized γ chains, only the former were found in tissues.

Conversely, in some patients as in a published case [20], normal sized L chains were secreted as free L chains and dimers, as in common myeloma without deposition, and they were found in urine as BJ proteins (in contrast to the patients discussed just above in whom the abnormal chains were undetected in serum and urines except for L chains when combined with normal sized H chains). The biochemical study of the free L chains in the serum and urines from one such further patient might provide a beginning of explanation: although normal sized and unglycosylated, these κ chains showed a very strong tendency to polymerize, as observed in vivo and in vitro in LCDD patients with abnormal Ig chains. Polymerization is hence perhaps the major factor involved in tissue deposition in LCDD. It has likely not a single mechanism.

In primary and myeloma amyloidosis, free L chain secretion was a constant feature. We also found L chain fragments in 9 of 10 cases. These results are in agreement with those recently published by Buxbaum [21]. The finding of fragments is special to amyloidosis since it is extremely unusual in common myeloma in our and others' experience [1, 21]. Whether fragments are synthetic products or result from the degradation of L chains, especially λ chains, synthesized as normal sized L chains is completely open. We rather favor the latter possibility since L chains from amyloidosis patients are especially susceptible to enzymatic degradation and since amyloid substance may be produced in vitro and probably in vivo by proteolysis of BJ proteins [22—26]. In the present study, the largest amounts of fragments were found in those patients in whom there was no BJ in urines, conceivably because of post-secretory degradation and this is in acordance with this hypothesis.

The probable mechanism of amyloidosis therefore usually involves proteolysis of L chains secreted as intact molecules and this contrasts with the structural abnormalities found in LCDD. However, certain patients affected with either of the diseases have similar features. As in LCDD, we found abnormally short H chains in two patients with primary amyloidosis, as reported in another case also [21]. In addition, in patient n° 15, an assembly block of a monoclonal IgA at the level of HL half molecules was observed. Although the apparent Mw of these α chains was normal, this suggests a structural abnormality. On the other hand, AL type amyloid substance is usually made of L chain fragments containing mostly the variable region and a variable segment of constant region. However, amyloid deposits in some patients include entire or even enlarged L chains [25]. We herein report one case where the plasma cells secrete decamers of enlarged κ chains. The synthesis of large κ chains and the secretion of tetrameric λ chains were also reported in one case each by Buxbaum [21, 27]. These various abnormalities of Ig synthesis could have been observed in LCDD as well. We therefore believe that LCDD and AL type amyloidosis are closely related diseases featuring tissue deposition of monoclonal Ig derived material. Their mechanisms appear to be different in "typical" cases but they are almost indistinguishable in certain patients. This led us to suggest the possibility of the association of both processes in the same patients [10], which was indeed observed in 3 recently reported cases [28].

Acknowledgements

We thank Drs. J. C. Brouet, D. Ganeval, J. P. Grünfeld, E. Mihaesco, L. Striker and G. Touchard for their participation in this study. The expert technical assistance of Mrs. S. Labaume and Mr. D. Thierry is gratefully acknowledged. This work was supported in part by Direction de la Recherche (Ministère de l'Education Nationale) and Fondation pour la Recherche Médicale.

References

1. Zolla S, Franklin EC, Scharff MD. Synthesis and assembly of immunoglobulins by malignant human plasmacytes. I. Myeloma producing γ-chains and light chains. J Exp Med 1970; 132: 148—57.
2. Preud'homme JL, Labaume S. Detection of surface immunoglobulins on human cells by direct immunofluorescence. In: Bloom BR, David JR, eds. In vitro Methods in Cell-Mediated and Tumor Immunity, New York: Academic Press, 1976; 155—169.
3. Preud'homme JL, Birshtein BK, Scharff MD. Variants of a mouse myeloma cell line that synthesize immunoglobulin heavy chains having an altered serotype. Proc Nat Acad Sci USA 1975; 72: 1427—30.
4. Preud'homme JL, Klein M, Labaume S, Seligmann M. Idiotype-bearing and antigen-binding receptors produced by blood T lymphocytes in a case of human myeloma. Europ J Immunol 1977; 7: 840—6.
5. Preud'homme JL, Labaume S, Praloran V. Synthesis of abnormal heavy chains in Bence Jones plasma cell leukemia with intracellular IgG. Blood 1980; 56: 1136—40.
6. Preud'homme JL, Morel-Maroger L, Brouet JC, Cerf M, Mignon F, Guglielmi P, Seligmann M. Synthesis of abnormal immunoglobulins in lymphoplasmacytic disorders with visceral light chain deposition. Amer J Med 1980; 69: 703—10.
7. Preud'homme JL, Morel-Maroger L, Brouet JC, Mihaesco E, Mery JP, Seligmann M. Synthesis of abnormal heavy and light chains in multiple myeloma with visceral deposition of monoclonal immunoglobulin. Clin Exp Immunol 1980; 42: 545—53.
8. Preud'homme JL, Mihaesco E, Gugliemi P, Morel-Maroger L, Ganeval D, Danon F, Brouet JC, Mihaesco C, Seligmann M. La maladie des dépôts de chaines légères ou d'immunoglobulines monoclonales: concepts physiopathogéniques, Nouv Presse Med 1982; 11: 3259—63.
9. Ganeval D, Mignon F, Preud'homme JL, Noel LH, Morel-Maroger L, Droz D, Brouet JC, Mery JP, Grunfeld JP. Visceral deposition of monoclonal light chains and immunoglobulins: a study of renal and immunopathologic abnormalities. In: Hamburger J, Crosnier J, Grünfeld JP, Maxwell MH, eds. Advances in Nephrology, Year Book Medical Publ 1982; 11: 25—63.
10. Ganeval D, Noel LH, Preud'homme JL, Droz D, Grunfeld JP. Light chain deposition disease. Its relation with AL-type amyloidosis. Kidney Internat 1984; 26: 1—9.
11. Preud'homme JL, Buxbaum J, Scharff MD. Mutagenesis of mouse myeloma cells with Melphalan. Nature 1973; 245: 320—2.
12. Osserman EF, Takatsuki K, Talal N. The pathogenesis of 'amyloidosis'. Studies on the role of abnormal gammaglobulin fragments of the Bence Jones (L-polypeptide) type in the pathogenesis of 'primary' and 'secondary amyloidosis' and the 'amyloidosis' associated with plasma cell myeloma. Semin Hematol 1964; 1: 33—85.
13. Preud'homme JL, Hurez D, Danon F, Brouet JC, Seligmann M. Intracytoplasmic and surface bound immunoglobulins in 'nonsecretory' and Bence-Jones myeloma. Clin Exp Immunol 1976; 25: 428—36.

14. Preud'homme JL, Danon F, Hurez D, Brouet JC, Seligmann M. Myélomes sans immunoglobuline monoclonale sérique ni urinaire (myélomes dits non excrétants). Actual Hématol 1977; 11: 213—9.
15. Preud'homme JL, Seligmann M. Human lymphoplasmacytic proliferations with production of structurally abnormal immunoglobulins. In: Dixon FJ, Miescher PA, eds. Immunopathology, VIIIth International Symposium. New York: Academic Press, 1982: 331—44.
16. Sox HC, Hood L. Attachment of carbohydrate to the variable region of myeloma immunoglobulin light chains. Proc Natl Acad Sci 1970; 66: 975—82.
17. Spiegelberg HL, Abel CA, Fishkin BG, Grey HM. Localization of the carbohydrate within the variable region of light and heavy chains of human γ G myeloma proteins. Biochemistry 1970; 9: 4217—23.
18. Solling K, Askjaer SA. Multiple myeloma with urinary excretion of heavy chain components of IgG and nodular glomerulosclerosis. Acta Med Scand 1973; 194: 23—9.
19. Gallo GR, Feiner HD, Buxbaum JN. The kidney in lymphoplasmocytic disorders. In: Sommers SC, Rosen PP, eds. Pathology Annual. Norwalk Connecticut: ACC (Appleton-Century-Crofts), 1982: 17 (part 1), 291—317.
20. Gallo GR, Feiner HD, Katz LA, Feldman GM, Correa E, Chuba JV, Buxbaum JN. Nodular glomerulopathy associated with non amyloidotic kappa light chain deposits and excess immunoglobulin light chain synthesis. Am J Pathol 1980; 99: 621—44.
21. Buxbaum J. Aberrant immunoglobulin synthesis in light chain amyloidosis. Free light chain and light chain fragment production by human bone marrow cells in short-term tissue culture. J Clin Invest 1986; 78: 798—806.
22. Glenner GG, Ein D, Eanes ED, Bladen HA, Terry W, Page DL. Creation of 'amyloid' fibrils from Bence Jones proteins in vitro. Science 1971; 174: 712—4.
23. Linke RP, Zucker-Franklin D, Franklin EC. The formation of amyloid-like fibrils in vitro from Bence-Jones proteins of the V λ 1 subclass. J Immunol 1973; 111: 24—6.
24. Epstein WV, Tan M, Wood IS. Formation of amyloid fibrils in vitro by action of human kidney lysosomal enzymes in Bence-Jones proteins. J Lab Clin Med 1974; 84: 107—10.
25. Glenner GG. Amyloid deposits and amyloidosis: the β-fibrillose. N Engl J Med 1980; 302: 1283—93, 1333—43.
26. Durie BGM, Persky B, Soehnlen BJ, Grogan TM, Salmon SE. Amyloid production in human myeloma stem-cell culture, with morphologic evidence of amyloid secretion by associated macrophages. N Engl J Med 1982; 307: 1689—92.
27. Buxbaum JN, Hurley ME, Chuba J, Spiro T. Amyloidosis of the AL type. Clinical, morphologic and biochemical aspects of the response to therapy with alkylating agents and prednisone. Am J Med 1979; 67: 867—78.
28. Jacquot C, Saint-André JP, Touchard G, Nochy D, D'Auzac de Lamartinie C, Oriol R, Druet P, Bariety J. Association of systemic light-chain deposition disease and amyloidosis: a report of three patients with renal involvement. Clin Nephrol 1985; 24: 93—8.

4. Renal amyloidosis: new perspectives

DOROTHEA ZUCKER-FRANKLIN

It has been recognized for more than 100 years that some forms of renal disease are associated with, or even due to, amyloidosis. Early papers merely described deposits of amorphous eosinophilic material. After Congo Red was introduced as a stain for amyloid, many reports appeared of the type exemplified by the publication of Heptinstall and Joekes [1] who, on studying the kidneys of patients with rheumatoid arthritis, were intrigued by finding amyloid primarily in the glomerular tufts and the basement membrane with little tubular involvement until late in disease. These descriptions were followed by the application of ultrastructural techniques and the discovery that amyloid is fibrillar [2—6]. In the kidney, such fibrils are seen in the region referred to as the mesangium, in close proximity to endo- and epithelial cells as well as within the basal lamina, particulary where they are thickened (Figs 1A and B). During the past two decades, when it became clear that amyloid may represent many different precursor proteins, it has even become possible to define the type of amyloid protein deposited in the kidney with the help of specific antisera which can be used on the light as well as on the electron microscopic level.

The theories attempting to account for amyloid formation usually revolve either around the abnormal or excessive synthesis of a particular protein or around the cells which are normally responsible for the synthesis or degradation of this protein. Some investigators maintain that an aberrant primary structure of a circulating protein is sufficient to result in the precipitation of an insoluble tissue deposit. Others hold that incomplete processing by cells of precursor molecules, which could be structurally normal or aberrant, would lead to peptide fragments not usually catabolized by the organism. Such peptides could self-assemble or become enzymatically crosslinked in the extracellular matrix. It is likely, that in some instances both mechanisms are operative. However, since most of our own work and that of the late Dr Edward C. Franklin has dealt with the latter aspect, this article will focus primarily on the defective

Minetti et al. (eds.), The kidney in plasma cell dyscrasias. ISBN 978-94-010-7085-0

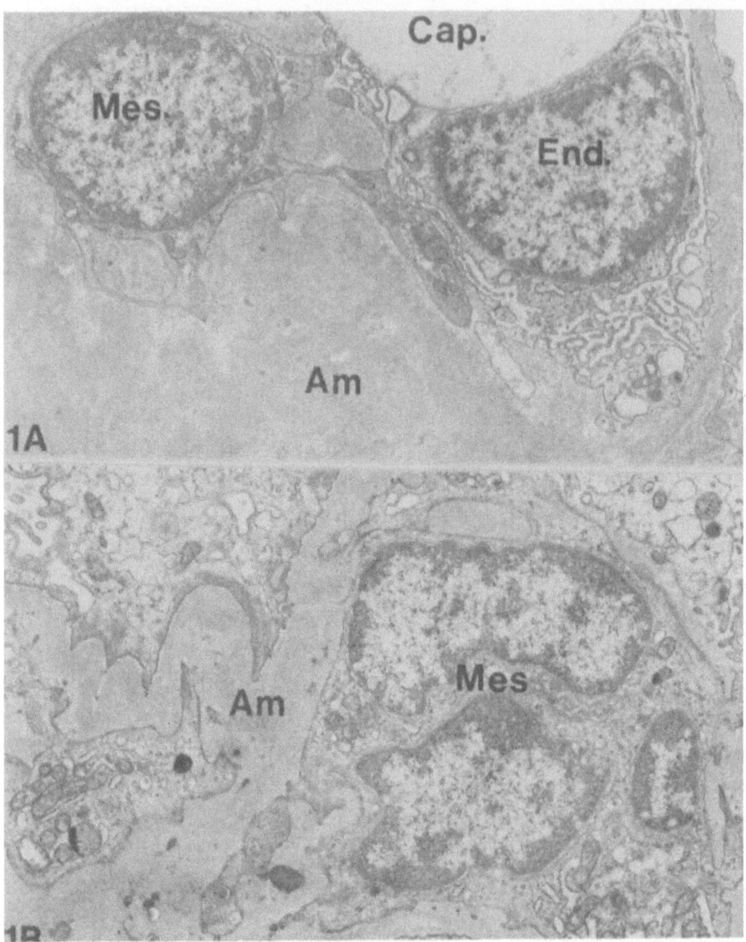

Fig. 1. Representative areas of renal biopsy specimens showing the relationship of mesangial cells (MES) to amyloid deposits (AM). (A) Endothelial cell (END) lines capillary lumen (CAP) whereas the mesangial cell (MES) occupies the matrix. Magnification × 6,400. (B) The morphologic resemblance of the mesangial cell (MES) to a macrophage is apparent. Amyloid fibrils (AM) are primarily seen in thickened basal lamina. Magnification × 8,000. (Illustrations were kindly provided by Dr Gloria Gallo, NYU Medical Center)

degradative function of the macrophage phagocytic system (MPS) in amyloid formation.

Precursor proteins

Historically, amyloidosis was thought to be related to the humoral immune response, for the condition was found in patients with hypergammaglobulinemia associated with chronic infections, as well as in patients with high immunoglobulin levels of the monoclonal type as seen with multiple myeloma and related diseases. Indeed, in 1971, Glenner et al demonstrated that in myeloma associated amyloidosis (now referred to as primary amyloidosis) the deposits are derived from fragments of the variable region of Ig light chains [7]. Although it has been recognized that lambda chains have a greater propensity for fibrillogenesis, kappa chains are also capable of amyloid formation [8]. It is not yet clear whether an anomaly in the primary structure of the Ig molecule is a prerequisite for amyloidogenesis or whether defective processing of normal light chains could also lead to fibril formation. It seems redundant to reiterate here that the Ig precusor of amyloid (AL) is synthesized in plasma cells and that it can precipitate locally, presumably when there is overproduction of immunoglobulin at poorly vascularized sites, e.g., in plasma cell tumors as well as at distant sites such as the kidney [9]. This will be covered by other contributors to this volume (pp. 57, 207).

An early clue to that fact that amyloid may not always consist of immunoglobulin was the observation that patients with the congenital form of agammaglobulinemia or individuals who were severely immunosuppressed could also develop amyloidosis [10]. The solubilization of amyloid fibrils deposited in organs of patients with chronic inflammatory diseases [2, 5] led to the biochemical definition of the amyloid A protein (AA) as the presumed derivative of the acute phase reactant serum amyloid A (SAA), a peptide which has nothing at all in common with Ig light chains [11, 12]. The AA protein is the second most commonly encountered amyloid found in the kidney. SAA, its presumed precursor, is primarily, though perhaps not exclusively, synthesized by hepatocytes where its synthesis is believed to be stimulated by IL-1.

The biochemical definition of other amyloids followed suit. By now amyloid has become a generic term describing a fibrillar protein with a marked affinity for the dye Congo Red which will render the fibrils green birefringent when viewed under polarized light. In most instances, but not always, its ultrastructure is also characteristic. The peptides capable of forming amyloid described to date are listed in Table 1. Since many of these are normal proteins, it is within the realm of possibility that a single individual can develop more than one type of amyloidosis. In fact, reactivity of renal amyloid with antisera to AL, as well as AA, is not uncommon [13] and the existence of 'mixed' amyloid deposits has been suggested by others [14]. Nevertheless, so far, only AL and AA have been described in renal biopsies. This may reflect limited sampling of the organ, or the possibility that the quantities of precursor molecules that filter through the kidney in some types of amyloidosis are too small to result in renal deposition. The author likes to draw attention, however, to the high

Table 1. Clinical and biochemical aspects of amyloidosis.

Clinical type	Chemical nature of fibrils	Precursor
Primary, myeloma-associated	Ig-L-chain or fragment	L-chain or variant
Secondary, inflammation-associated, some familial forms and experimental	AA (~8,000 D)	SAA (~12,500 D)
Senile brain, heart, pancreas	Pre-albumin	Pre-albumin (Transthyretin) and variants
Localized, endocrine organs	Various hormones	e.g., insulin, thyrocalcitonin, glucagon
Localized, carpal tunnel syndrome, bone, heart, synovium	β_2-microglobulin	β_2-microglobulin
Hereditary cerebral hemorrhage (Icelandic form)	Cystatin-c fragment	Cystatin-C variant
Alzheimer's disease, Down syndrome, etc.	Amyloid β-protein	Unidentified

levels of β_2-microglobulin in serum of patients with chronic diseases [15]. Recently, after an increased incidence of carpal tunnel syndrome had been reported in patients undergoing long-term hemodialysis, it was shown that the amyloid deposited in the perineural tissue of the median nerve of such patients was composed of β_2-microglobulin [16]. β_2-microglobulin is the invariant component of the Class I major histocompatibility antigen produced by many cells and shed into the circulation where it may reach high levels in disease. In patients on hemodialysis deposits of this protein have subsequently been found in many other tissues [17, 18]. Since β_2-microglobulin is normally excreted in the urine, it seems possible that the peptide could be deposited in fibrillar form within the renal mesangium under some conditions. Perhaps, it could account for some renal amyloid which does not react with antiserum to AA or AL.

Fibrillogenesis

As is true for other extracellular fibrillar proteins, their precursors are secreted in soluble form and polymerized subsequently. In the case of amyloid, continuity between extracellular and intracellular fibrils can sometimes be seen when the deposits are massive and have led to surface membane disruption (Fig. 2). Besides, amyloid fibrils are subject to phagocytosis [19]. Fibrils can be made in vitro from Ig light chains by a variety of manipulations, usually requiring acid hydrolysis with proteolytic enzymes [8, 20]. It is likely that such conditions also exist in vivo at sites where fibril deposition takes place, e.g., in the renal mesangium or in other micro environments with a low pH. Indeed, an early report from the laboratory of Dr Allen Cohen showed amyloid fibrils within a 'lysosome' [21] which in the light of current knowledge of cell biology may be interpreted to mean that an endocytotic vesicle containing the amyloid precursor protein had coalesced with a lysosome whose enzymes and pH provided the conditions necessary for fibril formation.

In the kidney, the region referred to as the mesangium, and perhaps even the surface of endo- and epithelial cells which are contiguous to, and

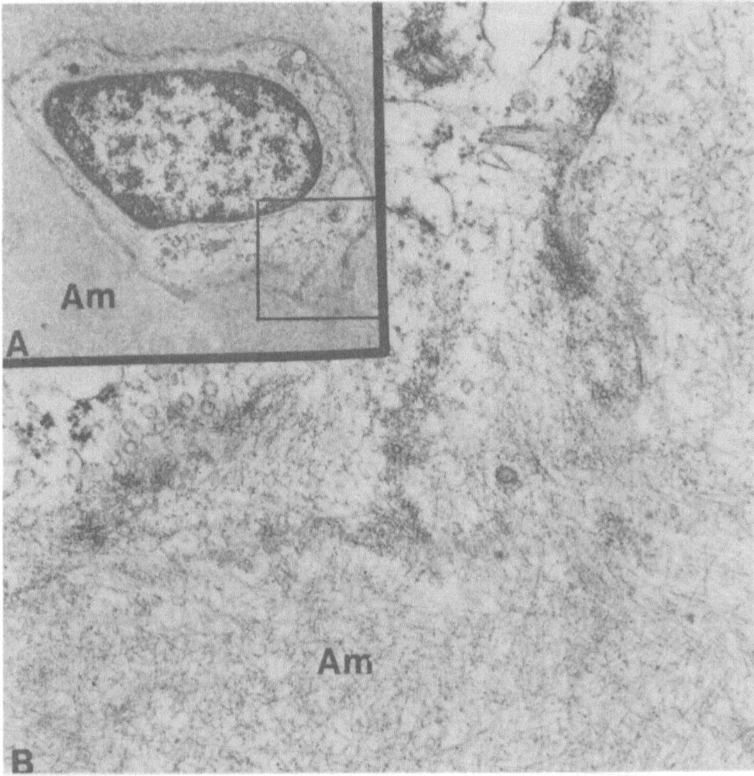

Fig. 2. (A) Mononuclear cell surrounded by amyloid fibrils from the specimen of a patient with myeloma-associated amyloidosis. The area within the rectangle is shown at higher magnification in B. Magnification × 6,800. (B) Higher magnification of the area within the rectangle in A reveals that the plasma membrane of this cell is disrupted and no longer provides a barrier between intra- and extracellular fibrils. Magnification × 36,800.

often in continuity with the basal lamina, may have the suitable conditions which lead to fibrillogenesis. In vitro fibrillogenesis has also been achieved with some of the hormone precursors and with synthetic peptides that have homology with fragments of amyloid precursor proteins [20, 22]. Attempts to polymerize fragments of SAA into fibrils have been less successful [23]. Most serum proteins are catabolized by the MPS and the reticulo-endothelial system has often been implicated in amyloid formation. In experimental amyloidosis, fibrils first appear around the MPS cells in the liver and spleen of animals, and monocytes bear serine proteinases on their surface which degrade SAA (see below). In the kidney, the MPS is represented by the mesangial cell [24]. Whether this cell is normally also involved in the catabolism of SAA is a moot point at the present time. The fact that these cells may become defective in the processing of SAA does not explain by what mechanism the remaining AA peptide polymerizes into insoluble fibrils. We have postulated that another enzyme or enzymes secreted by stimulated macrophages, perhaps enzymes akin to factor XIII which crosslinks soluble fibrin monomers into insoluble fibrin, may be involved. This still requires experimental proof.

Role of the Macrophage Phagocytic System (MPS)

The knowledge that the MPS is not only involved in the elimination of foreign materials and proteins, but also in the catabolism of normal blood components led to experiments which established that blood monocytes degrade SAA [25, 26]. In these studies, peripheral blood monocytes of normal individuals and from patients with amyloidosis were incubated in serum-free medium containing 500 μg/ml SAA purified as described [27]. Aliquots of the medium were collected after various time intervals and subjected to SDS-PAGE. In supernates of monocytes from most healthy individuals no SAA remained and no intermediate degradation product was seen — at least at the time intervals tested. Monocytes of the majority of patients with amyloidosis degraded SAA incompletely, showing an intermediate product of about 8,000 KD, which has antigenic cross-reactivity with AA. While it is known that monocytes secrete many proteinases following non-specific stimulation [28], SAA appears to be degraded by elastase-like enzymes located on the surface membrane of unstimulated cells [29]. No degrading activity was found in the extracellular medium. Treatment of the cells with DFP prevented degradation but did not interfere with SAA binding which could be demonstrated by immunofluorescence. Subsequently, the enzymes responsible for the degradation of SAA were localized and partially characterized in extracts of purified monocyte plasma membrane preparations [30].

To test the hypothesis that defective processing of SAA by the MPS may precede amyloid deposition required the analysis of experimentally induced amyloidosis. To this end, C57BL/6J mice were injected daily with 10% casein as described in detail elsewhere [23]. Under conditions of our protocol, the animals required a minimum of 18 injections to develop amyloidosis. Kuppfer cells (KC) were isolated from groups of mice which had received 0, 8, 13, 18, 20 and 30 injections of casein. The KC were incubated with SAA for 0, 4, 8, and 18 hours after which their supernatants were analyzed by SDS-PAGE to determine the amount of remaining SAA or to detect degradation products. The KC isolated from unstimulated mice degraded SAA completely with a reduction in the concentration of SAA to 33% of the original amount added, within 4 hrs. The KC from animals that had received as few as 8 injections of casein showed 50% residual SAA after 4 hrs. More importantly, in the latter case a band corresponding to the AA protein had appeared which was, however, degraded after overnight incubation. As can be seen in Figs 3 and 4, with increasing numbers of casein injections progessively larger amounts of residual SAA and AA were found in the supernates of KC cultures. It should be noted that the intermediate AA degradation product appeared in supernatants of KC cultures before any amyloid could be detected in the livers, spleens or kidneys of the animals from which the KC had been prepared.

Since the completion of the above studies, other evidence showed that stimulation of macrophages which increases the synthesis and secretion of many products may, at the same time, down-regulate others, such as lysozyme and cystatin-c [31]. As regards the kidney, it may be useful to

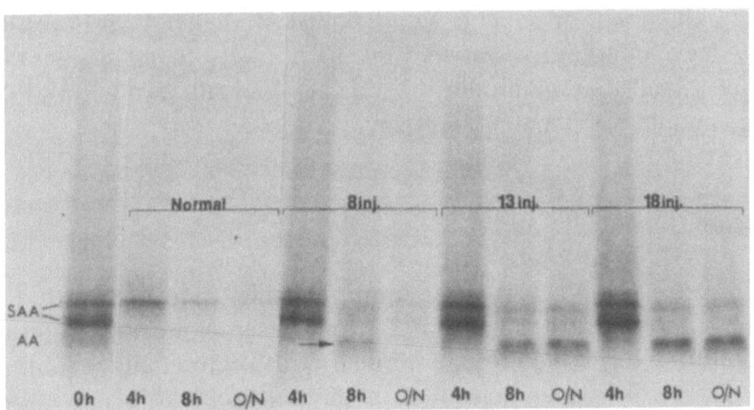

Fig. 3. SDS-PAGE profiles obtained with supernatants of Kupffer cell cultures prepared from the livers of mice that had received 0, 8, 13 or 18 injections of casein. The cells were incubated with SAA for 4h, 8h and overnight (O/N). Control shows the two SAA isotypes characteristic for mice. Arrow indicates AA band. (Reproduced from reference 23.)

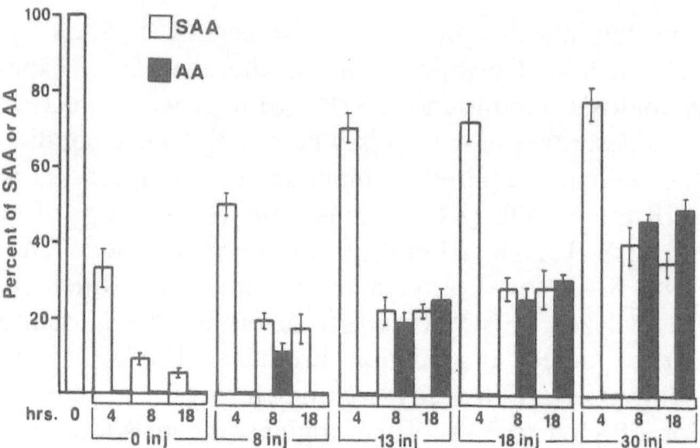

Fig. 4. Spectrophotometric quantitation of residual SAA and AA in supernatants of KC. The cells were derived from mice that had received 0, 8, 13, 18, or 30 injections of casein and were incubated for 4, 8, or 18 h with SAA. Larger amounts of residual SAA and increasing quantities of AA appeared during the amyloid induction period. When the animals had been given more than eight injections of the stimulant, their KC were no longer able to eliminate the AA intermediate product. (Reproduced from reference 23.)

determine the enzyme profiles of the mesangial cells during experimentally evolving amyloidosis to learn whether down-regulation may also pertain to this macrophage type. This could be done histo- or immunochemically.

When casein injections are discontinued for 6 weeks or more, normal KC function is restored. This seems in agreement with other evidence suggesting that amyloidosis can be arrested or even reversed when the inciting stimulus is removed. There are isolated reports indicating that even renal amyloidosis in man is to some extent reversible following removal or treatment of infectious foci [32, 33]. Although as yet unexplained, colchicine treatment of patients with Familial Mediterranean Fever (FMF) prevents development of amyloidosis to a large extent [34]. Whether colchicine permits elimination of existing amyloid still awaits serial studies on a large number of patients over many years.

Conclusion

Amyloid has become a generic term referring to proteins of diverse biochemical composition. To be designated as amyloid, the protein must have an affinity for Congo Red, a fibrillar ultrastructure, and insolubility in physiologic media when deposited in the extracellular matrix. Amyloid precursors are normally occurring peptides which may have a normal or aberrant primary structure. By in vitro manipulation or in disease states, when unusual microenvironmental conditions may exist, these peptides or their fragments self-assemble with or without the help of enzymatic crosslinking. In the case of AA amyloid, the participatory role of the MPS has been established. Down-regulation of some of its degradative function is concomitant with stimulation and precedent to amyloid formation. The mechanisms whereby the amino terminal end of SAA, the AA peptide, polymerizes into fibrils remains to be determined. It is not remote, however, to postulate that enyzmes induced by macrophage stimulation, such as the transglutamidases, may be instrumental. In renal amyloidosis, particularly of the AA type, the mesangial cell is a candidate for this role.

Acknowledgement

These studies were supported by National Institute of Health Grants AM12274 and AM01431.

References

1. Heptinstall RH, Joekes AM. Renal amyloid. Annals of Rheum Dis 1960; 19: 126—34.
2. Pras M, Zucker-Franklin D, Rimon A, Franklin EC. Physical, chemical and ultrastructural studies of water-soluble human amyloid fibrils. J Exp Med 1969; 130: 777—95.
3. Shirahama T, Cohen AS. High-resolution electron microscopic analysis of the amyloid fibril. J Cell Biol 1967; 33: 679—708.
4. Shirahama T, Cohen AS. Fine structure of the glomerulus in human and experimental renal amyloidosis. Am J Path 1967; 51: 869—911.
5. Pras M, Schubert M, Zucker-Franklin D, Rimon A, Franklin EC. The characterization of soluble amyloid prepared in water. J Clin Invest 1968; 47: 924—33.
6. Jao W, Pirani CL. Renal amyloidosis: Electron microscopic observations. Acta Path Microbiol Scand 80 Supplement 1972; 233: 217—27.
7. Glenner GG, Terry W, Harada M, Isersky C, Page D. Amyloid fibril proteins: Proof of homology wiht immunoglobulin light chains by sequence analysis. Science 1971; 172: 1150—1.
8. Linke RP, Zucker-Franklin D, Franklin EC. Morphologic, chemical and immunologic studies of amyloid-like fibrils formed from Bence-Jones proteins by proteolysis. J Immunol 1973; 111: 10—23.
9. Franklin EC, Zucker-Franklin D. Current concepts of amyloid. Advances in Immunol 1972; 15: 249—304.
10. Teilum G. Amyloidosis secondary to agammaglobulenemia. J Path Bact 1964; 88: 317—20.
11. Levin M, Franklin EC, Frangione B, Pras M. The amino acid sequence of a major non-immunoglobulin component of some amyloid fibrils. J Clin Invest 1972; 51: 2773—6.
12. Ericksen N, Ericksson LH, Pearsall N, Lagunoff D, Benditt EP. Mouse amyloid protein AA: Homology with non-immunoglobulin proteins of human and monkey amyloid substance. Proc Natl Acad of Sciences 1976; 73: 964—7.
13. Westermark P, Natvig JB, Anders RF, Sletten K, Husby G. Coexistence of protein AA

and immunoglobulin light-chain fragments in amyloid fibrils. Scan J of Immunol 1976; 5: 31—6.

14. Gallo GR, Feiner HD, Chuba JV, Beneck D, Marion P, Cohen DH. Characterization of tissue amyloid by immunoflorescence microscopy. Clin Immunol and Immunopath 1986; 39: 479—90.
15. Karlsson FA, Wibell L, Evrin PE. β_2-microglobulin in clinical medicine. Scan J Clin Lab Invest Supplement 154 1980; 40: 27—37.
16. Gejyo F, Yamada T, Odani S, Nakagawa Y, Arakawa M, Kunitomo T, Kastaoka H, Suzuki M, Hirasawa Y, Shirahama T, Cohen AS, Schmid K. A new form of amyloid associated with chronic hemodialysis was identified as β_2-microglobulin. Biochem and Biophys Res. Comm. 1985; 129: 701—6.
17. Shirahama T, Skinner M, Cohen AS, Gejyo F, Arakawa M, Suzuki M, Hirasawa Y. Histochemical and immunohistochemical characterization of amyloid associated with chronic hemodialysis as β_2-microglobulin. Lab Invest 1985; 53: 705—9.
18. Gorevic PD, Munoz PC, Casey TT, DiRaimondo CR, Stone WJ, Prelli FC, Rodrigues MM, Poulik MD, Frangione B. Polymerization of intact β_2-microglobulin in tissue causes amyloidosis in patients on chronic hemodialysis. Proc Natl Acad Sci USA 1986; 83: 7908—12.
19. Zucker-Franklin D. Immunophagocytosis of human amyloid fibrils by leukocytes. J Ultrastructure Res 1970; 32: 247—57.
20. Glenner GG, Eanes ED, Bladen HA, Linke RP, Thermine JD. β-pleated sheet fibrils: a comparison of native amyloid with synthetic protein fibrils. J Histochem and Cytochem 1974; 22: 1141—58.
21. Shirahama T, Cohen AS. Intralysosomal formation of amyloid fibrils. Am J Path 1975; 81: 101—16.
22. Castano EM, Ghiso J, Prelli F, Gorevic PD, Migheli A, Frangione B. In vitro formation of amyloid fibrils from synthetic peptides of different lengths homologous to Alzheimer's disease β-protein. Biochem Biophys Res Comm 1986; 141: 782—89.
23. Fuks A, Zucker-Franklin D. Impaired Kupffer cell function precedes development of secondary amyloidosis. J Exp Med 1985; 161: 1013—28.
24. Farquhar MG, Palade GE. Functional evidence for the existence of a third cell type in the renal glomerulus. J. Cell Biol 1962; 13: 55—87.
25. Lavie G, Zucker-Franklin D, Franklin EC. Degradation of serum amyloid A protein by surface-associated enzymes of human blood monocytes. J Exp Med 1978; 148: 1020—31.
26. Lavie G, Franklin EC, Zucker-Franklin D. Elastase-type proteases on the surface of human blood monocytes: Possible role in amyloid formation. J Immunol 1980; 125: 175—80.
27. Rosenthal CJ, Franklin EC, Frangione B, Greenspan J. Isolation and partial characterization of SAA — An amyloid related protein from human serum. J Immunol 1976; 116: 1415—8.
28. Cohn ZA. The activation of mononuclear phagocytes: Fact, fancy and future. J Immunol 1978; 121: 813—6.
29. Zucker-Franklin D, Lavie G, Franklin EC. Demonstration of membrane-bound proteolytic activity on the surface of mononuclear leukocytes. J of Histochem and Cytochem 1981; 29: 451—6.
30. Fuks A, Zucker-Franklin D, Franklin EC. Identification of elastases associated with purified plasma membranes isolated from human monocytes and lymphocytes. Biochimica et Biophysica Acta 1983; 755: 195—203.
31. Warfel AH, Zucker-Franklin D. Down-regulation of macrophage lysozyme by lipopolysaccharide and interferon. J Immunol 1986; 137: 651—5.

32. Lowenstein J, Gallo G. Remission of the nephrotic syndrome in renal amyloidosis. New Eng J Med 1970; 282: 128–32.
33. Dikman SH, Kahn T, Gribetz D, Churg J. Resolution of renal amyloidosis. Am J Med 1977; 63: 430–3.
34. Zemer D, Pras M, Sohar E, Modan M, Cabill S, Gafni J. Colchicine in the prevention and treatment of the amyloidosis of familial Mediterranean fever. New Engl J Med 1986; 314:1001–10.

5. Amyloidogenesis and light chains

TSURANOBU SHIRAHAMA

Introduction

The purpose of this article is to illustrate the modern concept of amyloidogenesis and the role that has been played by immunoglobulin light chains in the genesis of amyloid and in the development of the concept.

Definition of the endproduct: Amyloid

What is amyloid, anyway? If this question must be answered in one sentence, it would be described: amyloid is a group of chemically diverse proteinaceous substances found in animal tissues and defined upon the physicomorphologic characteristics shared commonly amongst them.

How diverse chemically are they, then? When amyloid deposits in tissues in an excessive amount, it creates a disease state called amyloidosis. It has long been known that amyloidosis takes clinically many different forms. As it has become apparent now, practically each different form of amyloidosis is created by deposition of different protein (Table 1). Looking back the history of amyloid research in this respect, a very significant discovery was reported from Dr Glenner's laboratory at National Institutes of Health in 1971. By amino acid sequence analysis, they found that the amyloid fibril proteins from 2 cases of amyloidosis had a homology in their N-terminal sequence with immunoglobulin light chains [1]. This study not only established definitive chemical identity of amyloid protein for the first time in history, but also opened the gate for a flood of sequence studies of amyloid proteins which eventually disclosed chemical diversity of amyloid [2—5].

When these chemically diverse proteins once deposited in tissues as amyloid, however, they take a physically uniform structure. Three physical criteria are commonly used to define amyloid. The first is its characteristic

Minetti et al. (eds.), The kidney in plasma cell dyscrasias. ISBN 978-94-010-7085-0

Table 1. Classification of amyloid.

Clinicopathological form	Amyloid protein	Related protein (precursor?)
Systemic Forms		
Primary Myeloma-associated	AL	Light chains (kappa or lambda)
Secondary	AA	SAA
Heredofamilial (FAP)	$A_{prealbumin}$	Prealbumin (variant) (Transthyretin)
Hemodialysis-associated	$A_{beta\text{-}2\text{-}microglobulin}$	Beta-2 microglobulin
Localized Forms		
Alzheimer's dementia Down's syndrome	β-protein (4 kd protein)	?
Icelandic hereditary cerebral angiopathy	$A_{gamma\ trace}$	Gamma trace (Cystatin C)
Medullary carcinoma of thyroid	$A_{calcitonin}$ (procalcitonin fragment)	Calcitonin
Cardiac	$A_{prealbumin}$	Prealbumin

tinctorial property. Amyloid stains with a variety of so-called amyloid stains in characteristic ways. The most commonly used is Congo red staining. With this stain, amyloid is colored pink, and demonstrates a characteristic green birefringence when viewed under polarized light [6, 7]. The second criterion is the unique fibrillar ultrastructure [8—10]. In ultrathin tissue sections, amyloid shows distinct fibrillar structures; rigid, nonbranching, about 10 nm in width and of indeterminate length. Their ultrastructural details have been delineated by high resolution electron microscopy after isolation of the fibrils and shadow-casting or negative staining preparation. The third is the cross-beta crystallographic configuration [11, 12].

Precursors and their sources

As the isolation and characterization of amyloid fibril proteins progressed, antibodies to individual types of amyloid fibril proteins were developed. This further led to identification of proteins which shared chemical and immunologic identities with the amyloid fibril proteins in serum and other parts of the body. They were usually normal components of serum, and regarded as precursors to the amyloid fibril proteins (Table 1). This development made it easier for us to locate the sources of the amyloid fibril proteins. The sources of some amyloid protein precursors, for instance immunoglobulin light chains as AL protein precursors, had already been known. The sources of other proteins were also determined rather quickly. For example, the major constituent of the secondary amyloid fibrils was identified as AA protein which has an unique amino acid sequence. Antibodies to AA revealed the presence of a serum counterpart of the protein which was termed SAA. SAA was subsequently defined as an acute phase reactant, and it became possible to predictably induce its synthesis under experimental conditions [13, 14]. Using this nature, immunochemical, immunohistological and molecular biological studies identified the liver as the major source of SAA [15—23]. Very recently, we have localized SAA mRNA to the hepatocytes in the liver sections from a mouse that had been stimulated to increase the synthesis of SAA by an in situ hybridization technique using tritiated SAA cDNA, identifying the hepatocytes as the cells that possess the facility to synthesize SAA [24].

What character does make a protein amyloidogenic?

Cleavage of precursor proteins

Up to this point, the chemical structures of amyloid proteins have been defined, their putative precursors have been identified, and the origins of the proteins have been disclosed. The next logical question may be as to how these soluble precursor proteins transform into insoluble amyloid proteins and eventually polymerize into the fibrillar form.

One of the important findings regarding this mechanism was published again from Dr Glenner's laboratory in 1971 [25]. Because the AL proteins they had first analysed were smaller than whole light chain molecules, they attempted if they could create amyloid fibril proteins by enzymatic cleavage of light chains, and indeed were successful. This was subsequently confirmed in several different laboratories [26—28]. In our own experiment [28], when Bence-Jones proteins were subjected to peptic digestion, they were first cleaved into C-terminal and N-terminal portions. As the digestion progressed, the band in an agarose electrophoresis, that represented the C-terminal portion disappeared probably due to further degradation, but the N-terminal band remained. We stopped the digestion procedure at this point and precipitated the N-terminal portions. With this procedure we obtained precipitates which bore the characteristics of amyloid, in 3 out of 13 Bence-Jones proteins tested. These observations suggest us that cleavage of the precursor protein could be an essential mechanism involved in the precursor-to-endproduct transformation in amyloidogenesis.

The same concept is probably applicable to AA amyloidogenesis where the putative precursor SAA of reported molecular weight of 11,000 to 14,000 is larger than the amyloid fibril protein AA of 5,000 to 13,000 molecular weight [2—5].

This concept fits very well to the theory developed from morphologic observations that the reticuloendothelial cells play a key role in amyloid formation [6]. In a mouse AA amyloidosis model where we can pinpoint the stage of amyloid deposition, for example, initial amyloid deposits are usually seen very close to the reticuloendothelial cells. By electron microscopy of such amyloid deposits, amyloid fibrils are well oriented and positioned very closely to the reticuloendothelial cells, often in their cytoplasmic invaginations. This kind structural relationship was postulated in 1963 by Drs Gueft and Gidney [29] as the site of amyloid fibril formation, and has been generally accepted by others. Furthermore, when you observe more closely such sites in extremely rapidly produced amyloid model, you may find well oriented amyloid fibrils in single membrane bound cytoplasmic bodies that often demonstrate the characteristics of lysosomes, such as containing acid phosphatase activity [30].

The concept of the involvement of proteolytic cleavage in amyloid formation has been supported by a number of other studies as well. For example, studies from the laboratory of Drs Franklin and Zucker-Franklin documented the presence of proteolytic enzyme on the surface of monocytes that was capable of cleaving SAA [31, 32].

Primary structure and amyloidogenecity

At the time the above concept was developed in the mid 1970s, it was felt that it might be applied for the genesis of all forms of amyloid. However, it has soon become apparent that it is not necessarily true. The first such evidence emerged from the analysis of the amyloid fibril protein of heredofamilial amyloidotic polyneuropathy. This amyloid protein of prealbumin nature was found to have the same size as the monomer of serum prealbumin molecule, and it was eventually confirmed by sequencing the entire amino acid [4, 5]. Secondly, AL proteins in some cases were disclosed to be composed of whole light chain molecules [4, 5]. Furthermore, more recently, the amyloid fibril protein of beta-2 microglobulin nature which is often associated with chronic hemodialysis was also proven to be same size as intact beta-2 microglobulin [33—36]. Indeed, we have found that intact beta-2 microglobulins readily form a substance that bears morphologic characteristics of amyloid [37].

These findings suggest that the enzymatic cleavage of the precursor proteins is not the necessary process in amyloid fibril formation, although it may be the mechanism for some forms of amyloidogenesis. In 1980s, as the complete amino acid sequences of the amyloid proteins of prealbumin nature were being determined, very important fact came into light. It was revealed that the amino acid sequence of the amyloid fibril protein of the type 1 familial amyloid polyneuropathy had an amino acid substitution of a methionine for a valine at position 30 when compared with normal prealbumin [38—41]. Subsequent studies of different types and families of familial amyloid polyneuropathy revealed amino acid substitutions at other positions; isoleucine for phenylalanine at position 33 [42], alanine for threonine at position 60 [43], and serine for isoleucine at position 84 [44]. Further studies using antibodies and cDNA probes that specifically recognize the variant prealbumins and their gene products have established the close correlationship between possession of such genes and development of amyloidotic polyneuropathy [45, 46]. These findings strongly suggest that the amyloidogenecity of a protein can be dependent upon its primary structure.

Similar observation was also developed with AA amyloidosis. Recent studies indicate that SAA is encoded by a family of three genes [47—50]. SAA1 and SAA2 are synthesized mainly in liver and are found in circulation in nearly equal quantities. Drs Hoffman and Meek and others in Dr Benditt's laboratory reported that murine AA amyloid protein had N-terminal amino acid sequence identity only with SAA2, and SAA2 was selectedly removed from circulation during active amyloid deposition [51, 52].

The evidence for the primary structure dependent amyloidogenecity has also been sought extensively in the relationship between light chains and AL proteins by a number of investigators such as Dr Solomon of USA and Dr Sletten of Norway to name just a few. Some interesting observations have been published. Lambda light chains are more frequent source of AL than kappa chains by more than 2:1 ratio. Some subgroups, VλVI in particular, appear to be more amyloidogenic than the rests. However, no solid evidence has so far developed to relate certain specific primary structure to the amyloidogenecity [4, 53, 54].

Amyloid enhancing factor

So far this article has covered, though very superficially, the chemical and physical aspects of amyloidogenesis. There is an another important aspect of amyloidogenesis, that is the biological aspect.

About 2 decades ago, so-called the two phase theory of amyloidogenesis was brought forward by Dr Teilum of Denmark [55]. With some modifications, this theory seems to be applicable to the contemporary concept of amyloidogenesis. The first phase represents the process of synthesis of amyloid proteins in the forms of precursors. The second phase is the process transforming the precursors into the amyloid proteins that eventually polymerize into amyloid fibrils. One of mysterious phenomena in amyloidogenesis is that a considerable lag time is required between these two phases. For example, in a routine casein-induced murine amyloid model, synthesis and serum level of SAA can be elevated by 100s to 1000s folds in a matter of hours by a single injection of casein, yet about 20 daily casein injections are required to induce amyloid deposition. Such a lag time is observed practically in every form of clinical amyloidosis as well. Unfortunately, no clear explanation has yet been found to answer the question as to why the lag time is required or what factor initiates the second phase of amyloidogenesis. However, there is a concept which potentially will be able to answer the questions. That is the concept of amyloid enhancing factor.

AA amyloidosis can be induced in a variety of animal species by prolonged antigenic or inflammatory stimulus. One of the most widely used induction regimens, that is daily subcutaneous injections with 0.5 ml of 10% casein in CBA/J mice, results in splenic amyloid in 3 to 4 weeks. The induction time can be drastically shortened if the mouse is pre-treated with amyloidotic or pre-amyloidotic donor tissue homogenate or extract. This phenomenon was first reported by Werdelin and Ranlov in 1966 [56] and confirmed by many other investigators [57—60]. The active component is currently called amyloid enhancing factor (AEF).

In 1969, we reported that similar accelerated amyloid induction can be achieved in mice by injection of splenic homogenates from patients with secondary, primary and myeloma-associated amyloidosis [61]. This system that we called ‘heterologous transfer of amyloid’ was reproduced by Dr Keizman and his coworkers using extracts from amyloidotic human spleens [62]. Recently, we re-examined this heterologous amyloid transfer phenomenon [63]. We treated mice with the tissue homogenate or the ‘AEF extract’ of spleens from patients with AA amyloidosis, AL amyloidosis and type 1 familial amyloidotic polyneuropathy, followed by 4 daily subcutaneous casein injections, and found that amyloidosis was induced in these mice in an accelerated fashion. Our immunohistochemical study indicated that the resultant amyloid deposits in mice had strongly positive reactions with anti-mouse AA, and negative reaction with anti-human AA or anti-human prealbumin. The results support the idea that the accelerated amyloid induction in the recipient mice is unlikely to be due to transfer of human amyloid substance, but rather to formation of ‘native’ murine amyloid under the influence of a human amyloid enhancing factor.

Now, we have here a biologically active substance called amyloid enhancing factor. It presents in preamyloidotic and amyloidotic spleen and other tissues with a variety of amyloidosis forms. Its activity crosses species, and accelerates the induction of amyloid of the recipient's own kind. Despite the striking physical uniformity, definitive distinctions in the chemical and immunologic characteristics occur between the different forms of amyloid. No common factor involved in the genesis of the different forms of amyloidosis has so far been identified. The characteristics of amyloid enhancing factor so far disclosed suggest that it might be such an universal factor — a common denominator playing a key role in the second phase of amyloidogenesis in the different forms of amyloid.

Unfortunately, despite its potential significance and extensive efforts made by a number of investigators, the amyloid enhancing factor has so far eluded definitive characterization of its chemical and immunologic nature. It is pursued actively in many investigators all over the world, to name a few Dr Bob Kisilevsky of Canada, Dr Gruys of Holland, Dr Pepys of England and our group in USA.

Acknowledgement

This work was supported by grants from the United States Public Health Service, National Institute of Arthritis, Diabetes, Digestive and Kidney Disease (AM-04599, AM-07014, and AM-35337), National Institutes of Health Multipurpose Arthritis Center (AM-20613), the General Clinical Research Centers Branch of the Division of Research Resources, National Institutes of Health (RR—533) and the Arthritis Foundation.

References

1. Glenner GG, Terry W, Harada M, Isersky C, Page D. Amyloid fibril proteins: Proof of homology with immunoglobulin light chains by sequence analysis. Science 1971; 172: 1150—1.
2. Cohen AS, Shirahama T, Sipe JD, Skinner M. Amyloid proteins, precursors, mediator, and enhancer. Lab Invest 1983; 48: 1—4.
3. Glenner GG. Amyloid deposits and amyloidosis. The β-fibrillosis. New Engl J Med 1980; 302: 1283—92, 1333—43.
4. Husby G, Sletten K. Amyloid proteins. In: Marrink J, van Rijswijk MH, eds. Amyloidosis. Dordrecht: Martinus Nijhoff, 1986: 23—34.
5. Shirahama T, Cohen AS, Skinner M. Immunohistochemistry of amyloid. In: DeLellis RA, ed. Advances in immunohistochemistry. New York: Masson Publishing, 1984: 277—302

6. Cohen AS. The constitution and genesis of amyloid. Int Rev Exp Pathol 1965; 4: 159—243.
7. Puchtler H, Sweat F, Levine M. On the binding of Congo red by amyloid. J Histochem Cytochem 1962; 10: 355—64.
8. Cohen AS, Calkins E. Electron microscopic observations on a fibrous component in amyloid of diverse origins. Nature 1959; 183: 1202—3.
9. Cohen AS, Shirahama T, Skinner M. Electron microscopy of amyloid. In: Harries JR, ed. Electron Microscopy of Proteins, Vol. 3. London: Academic Press, 1982: 165—205.
10. Shirahama T, Cohen AS. High-resolution electron-microscopic analysis of the amyloid fibril. J Cell Biol 1967; 33: 679—708.
11. Bonar L, Cohen AS, Skinner M. Characterization of the amyloid fibril as a cross-β protein. Proc Soc Exp Biol Med 1969; 131: 1373—5
12. Eanes ED, Glenner GG. X-ray diffraction studies of amyloid filaments. J Histochem Cytochem 1968; 16: 673—7.
13. Benson MD, Scheinberg MA, Shirahama T, Cathcart ES, Skinner M. Kinetics of serum amyloid protein A in casein-induced murine amyloidosis. J Clin Invest 1977; 59: 412—7.
14. Sipe JD, Vogel SN, Sztein MB, Skinner M, Cohen AS. The role of interleukin 1 in acute phase serum amyloid A (SAA) and serum amyloid P (SAP) biosynthesis. Ann NY Acad Sci 1982; 389: 137—50.
15. Benson MD, Kleiner E. Synthesis and secretion of serum amyloid protein (SAA) by hepatocytes in mice treated with casein. J Immunol 1980; 124: 495—9.
16. Hoffman JS, Benditt EP. Secretion of serum amyloid protein and assembly of serum amyloid protein-rich high density lipoprotein in primary mouse hepatocyte culture. J Biol Chem 1982; 257: 10518—22.
17. Miura K, Takahashi Y, Shirasawa H. Immunohistochemical detection of serum amyloid A protein in liver and the kidney after casein injection. Lab Invest 1988; 53: 453—63.
18. Morrow JF, Stearman RS, Peltzman CG, Potter DA. Induction of hepatic synthesis of serum amyloid A protein and actin (mRNA/recombinant DNA/acute phase serum protein). Proc Natl Acad Sci USA 1981; 78: 4718—22.
19. Shirahama T, Skinner M, Cohen AS. Heterogeneous participation of the hepatocyte population in amyloid protein AA synthesis. Cell Biol Int Reports 1984; 8: 849—56.
20. Shirahama T, Cohen AS. Immunocytochemical study of hepatocyte synthesis of amyloid AA. Demonstration of usual site of synthesis and intracellular pathways but unusual retention on the surface membrane. Am J Pathol 1985; 118: 108—15.
21. Sipe J, Rokita H, Shirahama T, Cohen AS, Koj A. Analysis of SAA gene expression in rat and mouse during acute inflammation and accelerated amyloidosis. Coll Prot Biol Fluids 1986; 34: 331—4.
22. Takahashi M, Yokota T, Yamashita Y, Ishihara T, Uchino F. Ultrastructural evidence for the synthesis of serum amyloid A protein by murine hepatocytes. Lab Invest 1985; 52: 220—3.
23. Tatsuta E, Sipe JD, Shirahama T, Skinner M, Cohen AS. Different regulatory mechanisms for serum amyloid A and serum amyloid P synthesis by cultured mouse hepatocytes. J Biol Chem 1983; 258: 5414—8.
24. Shirahama T, Sipe JD, Rodgers OG, Cohen AS. Localization of amyloid SAA gene expression in mouse liver by in situ hybridization. Submitted for publication.
25. Glenner GG, Ein D, Eanes ED, Bladen HA, Terry W, Page DL. Creation of 'amyloid' fibrils from Bence-Jones proteins in vitro. Science 1971; 174: 712—4.
26. Epstein WV, Tan M, Wood IS. Formation of 'amyloid' fibrils in vitro by action of human kidney lysosomal enzymes of Bence-Jones proteins. J Lab Clin Med 1974; 84: 107—10.
27. Linke RP, Zucker-Franklin D, Franklin EC. Morphologic, chemical, and immunologic

studies of amyloid-like fibrils formed from Bence-Jones proteins by proteolysis. J Immunol 1973; 111: 10-23.

28. Shirahama T, Benson MD, Cohen AS, Tanaka A. Fibrillar assemblage of variable segments of immunoglobulin light chains: An electron microscopic study. J Immunol 1973; 110: 21—30.
29. Gueft B, Ghidoni JJ. The site of formation and ultrastructure of amyloid. Am J Pathol 1963; 43: 837—54.
30. Shirahama T, Cohen AS. Intralysosomal formation of amyloid fibrils. Am J Pathol 1975; 81: 101—16.
31. Lavie J, Zucker-Franklin D, Franklin EC. Degradation of serum amyloid A protein by surface-associated enzymes of human blood monocytes. J Exp Med 1978; 148: 1020—31.
32. Lavie G, Zucker-Franklin D, Franklin EC. Elastase-type proteases on the surface of human blood monocytes: Possible role in amyloid formation. J Immunol 1980; 125: 175—80.
33. Gejyo F, Yamada T, Odani S, Nakagawa Y, Arakawa M, Kunitomo T, Kataoka H, Suzuki M, Hirasawa Y, Shirahama T, Cohen AS, Schmid K. A new form of amyloid protein associated with chronic hemodialysis was identified as β_2-microglobulin. Biochem Biophys Res Commun 1985; 129: 701—6.
34. Gorevic PD, Casey TT, Stone WJ, DiRaimondo CR, Prelli FC, Frangione B. Beta-2 microglobulin is an amyloidogenic protein in man. J Clin Invest 1985; 76: 2424—9.
35. Gorevic PD, Munoz PC, Casey TT, DiRaimondo CR, Stone WJ, Prelli FC, Rodrigues MM, Poulik MD, Frangione B. Polymerization of intact β_2-microglobulin in tissue causes amyloidosis in patients on chronic hemodialysis. Proc Natl Acad Sci USA 1986; 83: 7908—12.
36. Shirahama T, Skinner M, Cohen AS, Gejyo F, Arakawa M, Suzuki M, Hirasawa Y. Histochemical and immunohistochemical characterization of amyloid associated with chronic hemodialysis as β_2-microglobulin. Lab Invest 1985; 53: 705—9.
37. Connors LH, Shirahama T, Skinner M, Fenves A, Cohen AS. In vitro formation of amyloid fibrils from intact β_2-microglobulin. Biochem Biophys Res Commun 1985; 131: 1063—8.
38. Dwulet FE, Benson MD. Primary structure of an amyloid prealbumin and its plasma precursor in a heredofamilial polyneuropathy of Swedish origin. Proc Natl Acad Sci USA 1984; 81: 694—8.
39. Kametani F, Tonoike H, Hoshi A, Shinoda T, Kito S. A variant prealbumin-related low molecular weight amyloid fibril protein in familial amyloid polyneuropathy of Japanese origin. Biochem Biophys Res Commun 1984; 125: 622—8.
40. Saraiva MJM, Birken S, Costa PP, Goodman DS. Amyloid fibril protein in familial amyloidotic polyneuropathy Portuguese type. J Clin Invest 1984; 74: 104—19.
41. Tawara S, Nakazato M, Kangawa K, Matsuo H, Araki S. Identification of amyloid prealbumin variant in familial amyloidotic polyneuropathy (Japanese type). Biochem Biophys Res Commun 1983; 116: 880—8.
42. Nakazato M, Kangawa K, Minamino N, Tawara S, Matsuo H, Araki S. Revised analysis of amino acid replacement in a prealbumin variant (SKO-III) associated with familial amyloidotic polyneuropathy of Jewish origin. Biochem Biophys Res Commun 1984; 123: 921—8.
43. Wallace MR, Dwulet FE, Conneally PM, Benson MD. Biochemical and molecular genetic characterization of a new variant prealbumin associated with hereditary amyloidosis. J Clin Invest 1986; 78: 6—12.
44. Benson MD, Dwulet FE. Identification of a new amino acid substitution in plasma prealbumin associated with hereditary amyloidosis. Clin Res 1985; 33: 590a.
45. Nakazato M, Kangawa K, Minamino N, Tawara S, Matsuo H, Araki S. Radioimmu-

noassay for detecting abnormal prealbumin in the serum for diagnosis of familial amyloidotic polyneuropathy (Japanese type). Biochem Biophys Res Commun 1984; 122: 719–25.

46. Sasaki H, Sakaki Y, Matsuo H, Goto I, Kuroiwa Y, Sahashi I, Takahashi A, Shinoda T, Isobe T, Takagi Y. Diagnosis of familial amyloidotic polyneuropathy by recombinant DNA techniques. Biochem Biophys Res Commun 1984; 125:636–42.
47. Lowell CA, Potter DA, Stearman RS, Morrow JF. Structure of the murine serum amyloid A gene family. Gene conversion. J Biol Chem 1986; 261: 8442–52.
48. Lowell CA, Stearman RS, Morrow JF. Transcriptional regulation of serum amyloid A gene expression. J Biol Chem 1986; 261: 8453–61.
49. Rokita H, Shirahama T, Cohen AS, Meek RL, Benditt EP, Sipe JD. Differential expression of the amyloid SAA 3 gene in liver and peritoneal macrophages of mice undergoing dissimilar inflammatory episodes. J Immunol 1987; in press.
50. Yamamoto K, Migita S. Complete primary structures of two major murine serum amyloid A proteins deduced from cDNA sequences. Proc Natl Acad Sci USA 1985; 82: 2915–9.
51. Hoffmen JS, Ericsson LH, Eriksen N, Walsh KA, Benditt EP. Murine tissue amyloid protein AA. NH-terminal sequence identity with only one of two serum amyloid protein (apoSAA) gene products. J Exp Med 1984; 159: 641–6.
52. Meek RL, Hoffman JS, Benditt EP. Amyloidogenesis. One serum amyloid A isotype is selectively removed from the circulation. J Exp Med 1986; 163: 499–510.
53. Sletten K, Westermark P, Husby G. Structural studies of the variable region of immunoglobulin light-chain-type amyloid fibril proteins. In: Glenner GG, Osserman EF, Benditt EP, Calkins E, Cohen AS, Zucker-Franklin D, eds. Amyloidosis. New York: Plenum Press, 1986: 463–75.
54. Solomon A, Kyle RA, Frangione B. Light chain variable region subgroups of monoclonal immunoglobulins in amyloidosis AL. In: Glenner GG, Osserman EF, Benditt EP, Calkins E, Cohen AS, Zucker-Franklin D, eds. Amyloidosis. New York: Plenum Press, 1986: 449–62.
55. Teilum G. Pathogenesis of amyloidosis. The two-phase cellular theory of local secretion. Acta Pathol Microbiol Scand 1964; 61: 21–45.
56. Werdelin O, Ranlov P. Amyloidosis in mice produced by transplantation of spleen cells from casein-treated mice. Acta Pathol Microbiol Scand 1966; 68: 1–18.
57. Axelrad MA, Kisilevsky R, Willmer J, Chen SJ, Skinner M. Further characterization of amyloid-enhancing factor. Lab Invest 1980; 47: 139–46.
58. Hardt F, Ranlov P. Transfer amyloidosis. Int Rev Exp Pathol 1976; 16: 273–334.
59. Hol PR, van Andel ACJ, van Ederen AM, Draayer J, Gruys E. Amyloid enhancing factor in hamster. Br J Exp Pathol 1985; 66: 689–97.
60. Kisilevsky R, Boudreau L. Kinetics of amyloid deposition. 1. The effects of amyloid-enhancing factor and splenectomy. Lab Invest 1983; 48: 53–9.
61. Shirahama T, Lawless OJ, Cohen AS. Heterologous transfer of amyloid – human to mouse. Proc Soc Exp Biol Med 1969; 130: 516–9.
62. Keizman I, Rimon A, Sohar E, Gafni J. Amyloid accelerating factor. Purification of a substance from human amyloidotic spleen that accelerates the formation of casein-induced murine amyloid. Acta Pathol Microbiol Scand Section A 80, Suppl 1972; 233: 172–7.
63. Varga J, Flinn MSM, Shirahama T, Rodgers OG, Cohen AS. The induction of accelerated murine amyloid with human splenic extract. Probable role of amyloid enhancing factor. Virchows Arch B (Cell Pathol) 1986; 51: 177–85.

6. Physiopathological aspects of plasma cell dyscrasias: A forum

B. BARLOGIE, R. A. COWARD, A. SOLOMON, J. N. BUXBAUM, R. ALEXANIAN, G. GALLO, J. L. PREUD'HOMME, J. B. NATVIG, D. ZUCKER-FRANKLIN, G. D'AMICO, A. H. COHEN, R. A. KYLE

BARLOGIE: High RNA content is associated with immunoglobulin production and perhaps one might speculate the high RNA reflects more differentiated plasma cells. On the other hand, CALLA is considered to be a very early B-cell marker. One could speculate on why a primitive marker is preserved in a more differentiated plasma cell and what that means. There is however a wide dispersion in plasma cell RNA content differing in the individual patient by factor as high as 20-fold. We suspected that a considerable RNA bioeterogeneity would also be expressed otherwise, i.e. we are looking for means to relate to each other the RNA and phenotype expression. We speculate that RNA as an indicator merely of potential protein synthesis would be fairly low in myeloma progenitor cells. Thus, CALLA-positive cells, not co-expressing cytoplasmic immunoglobulin, probably have low RNA content. But I've no good idea why the CALLA antigen is maintained and is not shut off as cells progress down the differentiation pathway.

COWARD: I would like to comment about polymerization: we have also found differences between SDS gels and column chromatography in the light chains, particularly with kappa chains. The kappa being readily dissociated into monomers with the unphysiological environment of SDS gel, yet appear as dimers only, with column chromatography.

I would like to raise the very important question, what is the physiological molecular state of light chain and what pathological significance it has? The molecular size in the serum must also be relevant to the light chain filtration through the glomerulus and have the potential for tubular absorption and catabolism.

SOLOMON: In collaboration with Shiffer and Stevens, we reported several years ago that there was a tremendous difference in the association constant among light chains up to a four log difference (10^{-3} to 10^{-7} KD). This difference may account for the ability of certain proteins to aggregate or polymerize more readily than others.

Minetti et al. (eds.), The kidney in plasma cell dyscrasias. ISBN 978-94-010-7085-0

BUXBAUM: We have looked at this for a number of years now and it's very clear that some light chains that polymerize must have an available sulfhydryl group. A number of them occur as tetramers or bigger molecules that are covalently bound and can only be found as the monomer by reduction. Normally, there is a tendency of lambda light chains to dimerize more than kappa light chains. If you look inside the cell in many of these patients you find lambda as dimers and you find kappa as monomers, when you look outside the cell you always find lambda as a dimer, unless it is missing an N terminal cysteine. There is usually more kappa dimer outside than inside. What Dr Preud'Homme has described and we have seen as well, is that in some of these proteins, usually of the lambda type, polymerization is covalent and may relate to the presence of an additional cysteine available to polymerize. As far as I know no one has looked at particular polymerizing chains and enumerated those cysteines. The other L-chain molecules that non-covalently polymerize may be glycosylated but there is very little data bearing on that issue.

BARLOGIE: About changes in phenotype markers with treatment we did a preliminary investigation, that I really cannot yet comment on. There are patients with very bizarre presentations at diagnosis that express early B-cell markers and have tremendously complex cytogenetic anomalies. I think that we will observe in longitudinal studies clonal and phenotypic progression. During the very late stages of disease, particularly after relapse from very aggressive therapy, we have already observed progressive dedifferentiation, where complete immunoglobulin production ceases, where Bence Jones proteinuria develops, with subsequent beta-2M, and sometimes only LDH production. In a recent group of some 40 patients treated with very high doses of melphalan, 10 had LDH values above 500, up to 3000—4000 μ/l.

ALEXANIAN: There are other phenotype markers you must interpret cautiously. We followed 30 patients with benign monoclonal gammopathy, or monoclonal gammopathy of undetermined significance, who were studied for nucleic acid analysis, and half of such patients had an aneuploid DNA stemline. None of these patients has shown disease progression. Thus, we are dealing with a scenario where a malignancy associated marker does not imply anything about the speed of disease progression. In other words, a malignant marker for a benign disease.

GALLO: Dr Barlogie reported that he had seen a number of bone marrows in which the plasma cells expressed both kappa and lambda light chains. Do you see it only in patients with myeloma or plasma cell dyscrasias, or in normal patients as well? When you prepare smears, is this a double-labelled technique on the same smear and have you compared the number of labelled cells in separately stained bone marrow smears?

BARLOGIE: The initial observation was flow cytometry or cell suspensions. We of course were very concerned about some artefact and used different reagents and performed competition studies with light chain reagents. All of these patients turned out to have an IgG lambda myeloma. One may postulate that kappa expression was retained during the process of Ig gene recombination.

PREUD'HOMME: We observed kappa and lambda L-chain reaction in the same cells, but we are sure of the artefact (pinocytosis) as shown by the disappearance of double staining after overnight culture in vitro, whereas these cells became single-staining.

BUXBAUM: In the cells expressing both kappa and lambda you must look at the molecular nature of the proteins. The argument has been made that one of the signals for lambda rearrangement at the gene level, is the absence of the functional kappa product. Some investigators have argued very strongly that the signal of the early B cell to turn on light chain rearrangement, is the presence of a functionally rearranged and a functionally expressed heavy chain gene product. They have also suggested that the reason the lambda locus gets activated is because there is no functional kappa protein to interact with some other signal unknown to terminate L-chain gene rearrangement. Recently, it has been reported that kappa and lambda are expressed at a distinct stage of normal B cell differentiation.

SOLOMON: We found that uropepsin which is contained in normal urine can cleave the light chain into variable and constant fragments. We have also studied the turnover (catabolism) of radio-labelled human Bence-Jones proteins and found no relationship between the rate of catabolism and the type of renal disease. Normally, these proteins have an exceedingly short half-life, but in presence of renal disease catabolism proceeds much more slowly and also the protein excreted intact is increased dramatically.

NATVIG: In some of the light chain diseases, with nephrotic syndrome, you can also find the other type, the secondary type of amyloid and the precursor SAA. We have seen it in a few patients which had very clear amyloidosis; in their serum there was an elevation of the secondary amyloid proteins because of the inflammatory process. In collaboration with Dr Westermark we have eluted the fibrils from some amyloid tissues with both AA and AL in the amyloid fibrils from the same patients. This has been published so one should be aware of patients with mixed type of amyloid fibrils also in the kidney amyloidosis.

GALLO: The cases that I have seen both AA amyloid and immunoglobulin were actually drug addicts who had what I believe to be immunocomplex deposits, superimposed on AA amyloid. So, I am not sure that the amyloid fiber deposits stained for the immunoglobulin light chain, as the staining patterns differed for Ig and for AA: staining for AA amyloid was more homogeneous and staining for light chains was very discrete like immune complexes, so I thought really they were staining different sites.

COWARD: We have all seen in patients amyloid deposition can affect different organs and even within a particular organ for various structures; for instance some patients have glomerular amyloid while others only have renal vessel involvement. Does this organ selection occur because of different amyloid protein structure or because of the metabolism of the putatively deposits of amyloid that varies between organs?

ZUCKER-FRANKLIN: I think they are patients with different diseases; if you go along with my hypothesis, then you can almost explain amyloid anywhere, because you would have to have the microenvironmental conditions necessary to assemble the fibrils and you would have to have a high concentration of the precursor protein locally, in that particular area. So, I could see this happening in different disease conditions in different organs.

D'AMICO: According to fascinating hypothesis of Dr Zucker-Franklin, chronic stimulation of mesangial cells and/or monocytes, invading in the capillary lumen, should down regulate some of the ectoelastases as well as some other enzymes, and then promote amyloidosis. However we don't find amyloidosis in long lasting mesangial activation as in glomerulonephritis or lupus nephritis, where we have at the same time activation of mesangium and of monocytes involving the glomerular capillaries.

COHEN: I assume that when you talk about mesangial cells dysfunction favouring amyloid deposition, you are referring to the type II mesangial cells, or bone marrow derived elements, which really represent at best 2—3% of the total population of mesangial cells. The others are smooth muscle derived which may or may not have the phagocytic properties that have been ascribed to them; therefore I assume that you are suggesting that there is dysfunction of only a very small % of mesangial cells. If this be the case, should patients who have amyloidosis have increased number of mesangial monocytes or a decreased number of these cells? Increased because they are present to perhaps degrade the amyloid fibres, or decreased because they are not performing their function.

ZUCKER-FRANKLIN: The mesangial cells of the kidney, to my knowledge, have some of the enzymes that are seen in monocytes, they have Fc receptors, they are phagocytic, but they may have many other monocyte properties, which need to be examined especially now there is the availability of monoclonal antibodies that allow us to define monocyte lineage. I am wondering whether in glomerulonephritis there is a migration of new monocytes into the kidney which are then able to perform the function of the depleted monocytes or down regulated population.

SOLOMON: About the seminal role of protein in amyloid deposition particularly the light chain, a unique structure would account for amyloidogenicity of lambda-VI light chains: lambda-VI proteins are unique in that the variable region of lambda-VI proteins is characterized by a 2-residue insertion between position 68 + 69. One of these two insertions is a highly acidic aspartic acid. Also most lambda-VI proteins have a basic residue at the beginning of the variable region. This particular combination of acid + basic residues can promote aggregation and possibly amyloid formation. We have identified 17 lambda-VI light chains (either as Bence Jones proteins or as intact monoclonal immunoglobulin: IgM, IgA, IgG, etc.), and all of these have come from patients with proven amyloidosis. In fact, in two of our cases with identified proteins that were lambda-VI the diagnosis of amyloidosis was made retrospectively via reconsideration by the pathologist of bone marrow or other tissue specimens. Among other amyloid-associated light chains, we have not found as yet characteristic primary structure that would characterize them amyloidogenic. But I would like to caution that sequence data alone will provide the necessary informations to deduce the tertiary structure. This information requires X-Ray crystallographic analysis. Unfortunately, such data on human light chains is quite limited; however from the information available, it is apparent there can be considerable differences on the tertiary structure of light chains. About selective organ deposition it should be noted that light chain have structural features of antibodies. Conceivably certain 'amyloidogenic' Bence Jones proteins function as antibodies and bind to specific tissue antigens.

KYLE: Dr Zucker-Franklin has called our attention to a very important aspect of amyloidosis: the role of the catabolism of the amyloid fibrils in the pathogenesis of the disease. Other groups have demonstrated the importance of the elastases associated with monocytes in patients with AA amyloid. Now, most of our therapeutic approaches have been directed in AL amyloid against the production of monoclonal light chains by the plasma cells. We have really not paid much attention to the degradation or catabolism of the amyloid fibrils in AL.

I suspect that degradation plays an important role in pathogenesis of amyloidosis as the production of light chains: I wonder if you could speculate upon possible therapeutic approaches to degradation of amyloid light chains in patients with AL.

ZUCKER-FRANKLIN: I think that the same holds true for AL. I think healthy monocytes would be able to remove AL amyloid when myeloma is successfully treated. However, our treatment for myeloma at this point, is fairly drastic and I am not aware of anybody having studied the function of monocytes of patients on chemotherapy. Now if monocytes/macrophages are functionally impaired because of the chemotherapy or radiation used, then it might be worthwhile to replace monocytes but I think that is a long way into the future.

SOLOMON: Lambda chains, which occur perhaps more commonly in amyloidosis AL, are relatively difficult to cleave enzymatically as compared to kappa chains which usually are quite susceptible to proteolysis. The host factors be very important. Nevertheless, certain types of light chains because of their tertiary structure, when present in a high concentration, will be deposited as amyloid or as tubular casts or glomerular deposits.

KYLE: You must look very carefully at the serum and the urine for evidence of a monoclonal light chain in patients with amyloidosis. I would like to emphasize that it is true and that not all patients who appear to have amyloidosis of the AL type do so. We have had occasional patients who appeared to have primary amyloidosis but as time passed another family member developed amyloidosis. Consequently one must stain the tissue with prealbumin antisera to detect those with familial amyloidosis. In addition those with a familial type do not always fit the typical clinical picture of the Portuguese, Swedish, Japanese amyloid cases. I would also point out the fact that we have recently recognized patients with congestive heart failure whose amyloid consisted in senile amyloid.

BUXBAUM: As far as the absence of light chains from the serum and urine of some patients who have AL disease, we must examine the quantitative relationships between cell number and the amount of L-chain present.

One way to think about the problem is to consider the relationship of primary amyloid and multiple myeloma as equivalent to that of an endocrine adenoma relative to an endocrine adenocarcinoma. What we are seeing in these limited monoclonal proliferations is the production of small numbers of L-chain related molecules, by relatively small monoclonal populations. The amounts of material in the serum and the urine are also small, but must have high tissue affinity. What determines tissue binding is probably very important in the pathogenesis of the disease, because it probably allows the molecules to by-pass excretory pathways and results in little or no L-chain protein in either the serum or the urine. My conception is that cells make these molecules, which make a quick pass through the circulation and bind to whatever they are going to bind. Vascular deposition is very prominent in many if not all cases of amyloid. So that the system that Dr Zucker-Franklin is talking about is, in fact, intrinsic to the blood vessel wall. Perhaps it is a function of vascular endothelial cells, which when activated have many of the markers of the macrophage/monocyte system. It may be that the high affinity coupled with such an intrinsic vascular wall mechanism may be one of the reasons why we see few circulating molecules and a lot of vascular disease.

This is not the whole answer, but I think it is one way conceptually to deal with a molecule which is not present in large amounts at any given moment, but over time a substantial quantity of this material is deposited throughout the body. There are many molecules deposited throughout the body because they are put down a little at a time. Eventually there is organ compromise, and perhaps the pathogenesis of this disease takes place over a much longer period of time than we really know. We look very late. We have no assay for total body amyloid load. We see the patients when they are already compromised. Consequently, even if we can stop the production of the precursor, the damage is already done. Resolution is very slow if it occurs at all. Biologically, we are left with patients who have damaged organs. We may be able to prevent further damage but what is already damaged is not going to be recover very much.

Part II. Light chain nephrotoxicity

1. Glomerular and associated tubular injury by light chains. The spectrum of damage and effect of treatment

N. P. MALLICK & G. WILLIAMS

Immunoglobulin light chains are physically and electrically heterogeneous. The distinctive amino-acid sequence of its variable region must account for the solubility, iso-electric point and affinity for other proteins of a given light chain and for its ability or otherwise to form aggregates, or to damage particular aspects of renal tubular metabolism.

In health immunoglobulin light chain production is proportional to that of heavy chains and little escapes free. Most of what does so is absorbed in the renal tubules where degradation occurs by lysosomal peptides. Tubular resorptive capacity varies according to the characteristics of the light chains present in glomerular filtrate but probably does not exceed 10 g/day.

Monoclonal B cell production occurs in a number of conditions, listed in Table 1. It may be transient, stable or expanding. It may secrete only an intact immunoglobulin, only immunoglobulin fragments, or both. Its secretion pattern may vary, and its kinetics are unique to it.

Although a light chain has a molecular weight of about 22000 daltons, free monoclonal lambda light chains usually circulate as covalently linked dimers, molecular weight about 44000 daltons; kappa light chains circulate as monomers or as non-covalent dimers; the effects in-vivo of 'free' light chains may differ from those described in vitro for purified monomer

Table 1. The secretion of free light chains which damage the nephron has been documented in all of the above diseases.

Monoclonal gammopathy
Myeloma
Macroglobulinaemia
Heavy chain disease
Lymphoma
Leukaemia

Minetti et al. (eds.), The kidney in plasma cell dyscrasias. ISBN 978-94-010-7085-0

preparations. Further, a given monoclone may secrete light chain fragments which are sufficiently complete to be biochemically active, yet not possess the immunological identity of the parent, be difficult to detect, yet responsible for renal damage.

The capacity of a given B cell product to react within the glomerulus or to pass freely into the urine is influenced by its size, shape and charge; proximal tubular cells have a considerable capacity to resorb filtered B cell products but the ways in which only some monoclonal light chains cause tubular cell damage remain elusive. The evidence that such damage occurs is summarised in a later paper (p. 85).

Typically, in the kidney the primary damage by free light chains or other fragments is to proximal more than to distal tubular cells. By light microscopy cells show vacuolation and swelling and by electron microscopy lysosomal damage; concurrently the urine contains tubular lysosomal enzymes such as N-acetyl B-D-glucosaminidase (NAG) [1, 2] and those low molecular weight proteins which a healthy tubular system would resorb. With time, there is tubular atrophy, rupture and interstitial reaction and associated nephron loss. There is cast formation, sometimes florid. Additional, rarer features are light chain crystallisation in tubular cells, glomeruli and interstitium, and amyloid formation. There is also a variety of glomerular pathology. This spectrum of damage is summarised in Table 2, with the presentations and the light chain characteristics which might cause the lesions.

The spectrum of light chain involvement points to a parallel range of

Table 2. The spectrum of nephron damage caused by free monoclonal light chains. The characteristics of the light chains vary and determine the different forms and sites of damage.

Presentation	Damage	Characteristic
Albuminuria Nephrotic syndrome Isolated haematuria Acute nephritic syndrome Uraemia	Glomerular	Attach Aggregate Crystallise
Fanconi syndrome Renal acidosis Renal diabetes insipidus Uraemia Oligo-anuria	Tubular	Toxicity Crystal formation Cast formation
Uraemia Oligo-anuria	Global	

physico-chemical characteristics. These have been detailed earlier (p. 3), and their potential for influencing the nephron discussed. Precisely why a given lesion develops is not clear yet, but the identification ex-vivo of the characteristics of a secreted light chain promises rapidly to resolve some of the problems, as is already becoming evident in AL amyloid.

It is clear that in any overt B-cell dyscrasia, virtually any evidence of renal disease might point to a light chain nephropathy and should be investigated (Table 3). The biopsy findings may be startling and may suggest a much longer standing lesion than has been apparent clinically. Frequently, there is evidence of involvement in several parts of the nephron, so that with a predominantly tubulo-interstitial lesion there may be glomerular damage, and vice-versa.

So from a clinical standpoint much can be learnt from analysis of the nephropathies arising in B cell dyscrasias not least that there should be close and repeated search for free urinary light chains by immunoelectrophoresis and for markers of renal damage (albuminuria, microscopic haematuria, declining renal function, low molecular weight proteinuria, NAG). There should be constant awareness that such intercurrent factors as infection and contrast dyes may aggravate renal impairment in any of these dyscrasias and not just in frank myeloma.

However, a light chain nephropathy may arise with no overt evidence of a B cell dyscrasia and with as wide variety of presentation and of renal

Table 3. Suggested investigations for renal involvement in overt B cell dyscrasia. The tests in brackets may be required in selective cases. Both glomerular and tubular damage should be considered, since these may be present simultaneously.

Urine	Immunoelectrophoresis of concentrated urine
	Low molecular weight proteins
	N.A.G.
	(Acid load)
	(Concentrating ability)
	Red cell morphology and excretion rate
Blood	Immunoelectrophoresis
	Anti-nuclear factors
	Complement
	Cryoglobulins
	(Immune complexes)
	Bone marrow with selective staining
	Renal biopsy

damage as described in Table 2. It is commonplace that even florid myeloma may first be diagnosed in a patient presenting with renal failure but less well recognised that careful, repeated analysis may show free monoclonal light chains in the serum or urine of a patient presenting with a less advanced nephropathy, apparently in good health otherwise.

The importance of the sporadic, but now plentiful reports [1—30] confirming this is that with effective chemotherapy, progressive renal damage can be prevented. I wish to underline this point by considering particularly the light chain — associated glomerular nephropathies.

I shall exclude frank amyloid deposition and cases with documented or probable cryoglobulinaemia. All glomerular syndromes have been reported. The cases can be considered in three groups (Table 4).

In the first group, the diagnosis necessarily has been by renal biopsy, but only a few cases have been described in which the search for free urinary light chains has been sufficiently exacting by modern standards. The presentation has been with asymptomatic proteinuria, nephrotic syndrome or impaired renal function, lesions have been predominantly mesangial but with subendothelial basement membrane deposits; the outlook has been poor with terminal renal failure developing usually within a year of biopsy diagnosis, but there are hardly any reports of cases in which vigorous chemotherapy has been offered early in the disease.

Most commonly, the glomerulopathy has occurred in association with free urinary light chains, though these may have been present in small amounts only [29]. Tubular light chain deposition, within and on the anti-luminal [27] side of both proximal and distal tubular cells, tubular atrophy and interstitial fibrosis are found in association with the glomerular pathology and there may be interstitial infiltration of monoclone bearing cells [27]. Typical presentations and glomerular pathology are outlined in Table 5. It is noteworthy that while lesions occur more commonly with free kappa light chains and with kappa light chains in the glomeruli most histopathologies have also been attributed to lambda light chains.

In a few documented cases of B-cell dyscrasia, a glomerulopathy has occurred with immunochemical characteristics distinct from those of the secreted monoclone (Table 6), probably these represent immune complex deposition in patients whose natural immunity is impaired by the underlying disorder has provided speculation. There is evidence that the pI may be

Table 4. Glomerular lesions and B-cell dyscrasias.

Glomerular but not urinary light chain.
Same light chain in glomerulus and urine.
Urinary but not glomerular light chain.

Table 5. Light chain nephropathy; free light chain identified.

Presentation	
Albuminuria	
Nephrotic syndrome	
Macroscopic haematuria	
Microscopic haematuria	
Acute nephritic syndrome	
Impaired renal function	
Glomerular pathology	
No light microscope change	λ
Mesangial proliferation	κ or λ
Nodular mesangial sclerosis	κ
Diffuse proliferative	κ or λ
Mesangiocapillary I	κ
Mesangiocapillary II	κ or λ
Crescentic	κ or λ

Table 6. Light chains present but with a glomerulopathy with immunological characteristics which are not due to light chain deposition.

	Deposit	Monoclone
Membranous	IgG	IgG (k)
Diffuse proliferative	IgG	
Mesangial proliferative	IgG	IgA (k)

important in determining glomerular localisation [26] and that glomerular basement membrane proteins may be produced by the presence of light chain deposits [23].

This wide spectrum of glomerular injury would be only of academic interest if it were not for the potential benefit of therapy. Consider these two personal cases.

In the first, with diffuse, crescentic, mesangial proliferative glomerular disease and no plasma cell increase, repeated episodes of acute renal failure occurred, sometimes with purpura. There was an IgA-k paraprotein, free urinary kappa chains but no cryoglobulin. After repeated courses of quadruple therapy (Cyclophosphamide, Melphalan, BCNU and steroids), the episodes ceased. Kappa light chains were not detected, the monoclone was less evident, and the patient survives with stable, impaired renal function (serum creatinine c 300 mmol/l) 12 years later. There is at least one similar case in the literature [18].

In this second case, nephrotic syndrome was diagnosed and persisted. Two renal biopsies showed mesangial expansion. At the time of the second biopsy, free kappa light chain was found in the urine. There was no skeletal or bone marrow evidence of myeloma and no circulating paraprotein. Quadruple therapy was instituted with prompt, complete remission of proteinuria. There was no recurrence in the twelve years to his death, aged 72, from heart failure.

These are two of the six cases in whom we have discovered light chain nephropathy without myeloma, during the investigation of proteinuria and in whom sustained remission has been achieved by cytotoxic therapy. It is difficult to estimate the incidence of such cases in otherwise idiopathic glomerular disease, but a cautious estimate from our own experience suggests that perhaps 5—8% of patients presenting over 50 years old show eventually evidence of a B cell dyscrasia, and may respond to cytotoxic therapy.

Repeated and exacting search is necessary, however. Concentrated urine should be examined by immunoelectrophoresis at presentation and at 12—18 month intervals, as part of a detailed (re-) assessment. In a patient with albuminuria or haematuria otherwise unexplained evidence of proximal or distal tubular damage may point to light chain nephropathy and should stimulate appropriate analysis.

Nephrologists and haematologists alike have something to learn from our collective experience. Renal involvement in the paraproteinaemias is more common and pleomorphic than is recognised generally. It should be kept in mind, sought for and treated. The effort is worthwhile.

Conclusions

- Evaluate B-cell dyscrasia repeatedly for nephropathy.
- Evaluate glomerular disease repeatedly for B cell dyscrasia.
- Include tests for tubular damage in studying glomerular disease.
- Treatment may cure.

References

1. Kaplan NG, Kaplan KC. Monoclonal gammopathy, glomerulonephritis, and the nephrotic syndrome. Archs intern Med 1970; 125: 696—700.
2. Verroust P, Mery JP, Morel-Maroger L, et al. Glomerular lesions in monoclonal

gammopathies and mixed essential cryoglobulinaemias IgG-IgM. Adv Nephrol 1971; 1: 161—94.

3. Jensen H, Wiik A. Monoclonal immunoglobulinaemia associated with glomerulopathy. Acta med scand 1975; 197: 265—9.
4. Rifle G, Genin R, Chalopin JM. Glomerulonephrite membrano-proliferative hypocomplementaire au cours d'un myelome. Nouv Presse med 1976; 5: 437—8.
5. Sobel AT, Antonucci M, Intrator L, et al. Association d'une gammapathie monoclonale d'une glomerulopathie chronique et d'une hyperlipidemie auto-immune. Nouv Presse med 1976; 5: 2375—8.
6. Avasthi PS, Erickson DG, et al. Benign monoclonal gammaglobulinaemia and glomerulonephritis. Am J Med 1977; 62: 324—9.
7. Case records of the MGH. Case 31—1977. New Engl J Med 1977; 297: 266—74.
8. Dhar SK, Smith EC, Fresco R. Proliferative glomerulonephritis in monoclonal gammopathy. Nephron 1977; 19: 288—94.
9. Mallick NP, Dosa S, Acheson EJ, et al. Detection, significance and treatment of paraprotein presenting with 'idiopathic' proteinuria without myeloma. Q J Med 1978; 196: 145—75.
10. Rao TKS, Nicastri AD, et al. Membranoproliferative glomerulonephritis (MPGN), an unusual manifestation of multiple myeloma (MM) (Abstract). Kidney int 1978; 14: 659.
11. Silva FG, Meyrier A, et al. Proliferative glomerulonephropathy in multiple myeloma. J Path 1980; 130: 229—36.
12. Tubbs DO, Gephardt GN, McMahon JT, et al. Light chain nephropathy. Amer J Med 1981; 71:263—9.
13. Lapenas DJ, Drewry SJ, et al. Crescentic light-chain glomerulopathy. Archs Pathol Lab Med 1983; 107: 319—23.
14. Knobler H, Kopolovic J, et al. Multiple myeloma presenting as dense deposit disease. Light chain nephropathy. Nephron 1983; 34: 58—63.
15. Auletta M, Usberti M, et al. Membranoproliferative glomerulonephritis as an unusual initial manifestation in a case of plasmacytoma. Minerva Med 1984; 75: 479—82.
16. Alpers CE, Hopper J Jr, Biava CG. Light-chain glomerulopathy with amyloid-like deposits. Hum Pathol 1984; 15: 444—8.
17. Rahman A, Mossey RT, et al. Kappa-chain nephropathy associated with plasma cell leukaemia. Arch Int Med 1984; 144: 1689—91.
18. Meyrier A, Simon P, et al. Rapidly progressive ('crescentic') glomerulonephritis and monoclonal gammapathies. Nephron 1984; 38: 156—62.
19. Kebler R, Kithier K, et al. Rapidly progressive glomerulonephritis and monoclonal gammopathy. Am J Med 1985; 78: 133—8.
20. Nakamoto Y, Imai H, et al. IgM monoclonal gammopathy accompanied by nodular glomerulosclerosis, urine-concentrating defect, and hyporeninaemic hypoaldosteronism. Am J Nephrol 1985; 5: 53—8.
21. Sinnah R, Cohen AH. Glomerular capillary aneurysms in light-chain nephropathy. An ultrastructural proposal of pathogenesis. Am J Pathol 1985; 118: 298—305.
22. Alpers CE, Tu WH, et al. Single light chain subclass (kappa chain) immunoglobulin deposition in glomerulonephritis. Hum Pathol 1985; 16: 294—304.
23. Bruneval P, Foidart JM, et al. Glomerular matrix proteins in nodular glomerulosclerosis in association with light chain deposition disease and diabetes mellitus. Hum Pathol 1985; 16: 477—84.
24. McLeish KR, Gohara AF, Gillespie C. Mesangial proliferative glomerulonephritis associated with multiple myeloma. Am J Med Sci 1985; 290: 114— 117.
25. Sano M, Terasaki T, et al. Glomerular lesions associated with the Crow-Fukase syndrome. Virchows Arch 1986A; 409: 3—9.

26. Palant CE, Bonitati J, et al. Nodular glomerulosclerosis associated with multiple myeloma. Role of light chain isoelectric point. Am J Med 1986; 80: 98–102.
27. Silver MM, Hearn SA, et al. Renal and systemic kappa light chain deposits and their plasma cell origin identified by immunoelectron microscopy. Am J Pathol 1986; 122: 17–27.
28. Bradley JR, Thiru S, Evans DB. Light chains and the kidney. J Clin Pathol 1987; 40: 53–60.
29. Bangerter AR, Murphy WM. Kappa light chain nephropathy. A pathologic study. Virchows Arch 1987; 410: 531–9.
30. Alpers CE, Rennke HG, et al. Fibrillary glomerulonephritis: an entity with unusual immunofluorescence features. Kidney Int 1987; 31: 781–9.

2. Effect of light chains on proximal tubule function

E. H. COOPER & I. C. M. MACLENNAN

Introduction

The aetiology of renal failure in myelomatosis is multifactorial. The excretion of light chains in the urine is a common factor, as is extensively discussed in this book. However, many patients excrete large amounts of light chains without any impairment of glomerular filtration rate (GFR). Whilst it is the GFR and indicators of glomerular function such as serum creatinine (scr) that are of major clinical importance in the management of myelomatosis, there are other measurements that can provide sensitive information about renal function.

In health a wide variety of low molecular weight proteins (LMWPs) including plasma proteins, hormones and enzymes are removed from the circulation by glomerular filtration followed by reabsorption and catabolism by the proximal tubular cells [2]. This process is highly efficient, β_2-microglobulin (β_2-m 11.3 kDa) for example is removed from the glomerular filtrate with a >95% efficiency [6]. Free light chains are catabolised by the renal tubular cells [12], it is estimated the kidney has a capacity for catabolising up to 30 g/day, in some myeloma patients [10] but this is considerably reduced in renal failure [12]. Several urinary proteins and enzymes have been demonstrated to be indicators of tubular function and have enabled disorders of the renal tubules previously recognised by SDS polyacrylamide gradient gel electrophoresis [1], to be measured quantitatively and small changes of function revealed.

Several investigators had observed that light chain proteinuria could be accompanied by an increase of excretion of other LMWPs in the urine [16, 18, 19]. We made a more detailed study of this phenomenon in myelomatosis by investigating over 500 patients participating in a multicentre clinical trial [4]. It became apparent that individual monoclonal light chains differ not only in their nephrotoxic effects but also on the reabsorption of LMWPs by the proximal tubular cells. Meanwhile evidence that cationic light chains were more nephrotoxic had been reported [3, 5]. Clyne et al.

Minetti et al. (eds.), The kidney in plasma cell dyscrasias. ISBN 978-94-010-7085-0

[3] isolated light chains from 11 patients and then tested for their nephrotoxicity in the aciduria hydropenic rat, only rats injected with light chains with a pI > 6.2 showed renal failure and intratubular casts. Coward et al. [5] reported that light chain pI and creatinine clearance in 23 patients with multiple myeloma, were positively correlated. This led us to examine the light chain pI spectrotype to see what part this aspect of the physicochemistry of the light chain molecules could influence their behaviour in the kidney [7]. In this paper we review the key features of these studies in the context of kidney disease in myelomatosis and extend our investigation of light chain pIs.

Materials and methods

Patients: Nine hundred and eighty six patients were entered consecutively into the IVth and Vth M.R.C. myelomatosis trials between March 1979 and February 1982 were studied. The patients were examined at admission to the trial, following a 48 h period of hydration, before treatment with chemotherapy.

Specific protein measurements: The determination of α_1-microglobulin (α_1-m), α_1-acid glycoprotein (AGP), β_2-m, retinol binding protein (RBP), urinary free light chains was by radial immunodiffusion [4] and the presence of light chain checked visually using 12% polyacrylamide gel electrophoresis of unconcentrated urine. The light chain concentrations were expressed in units (1 unit is equivalent to 1 g of kappa or lambda standard).

Urinary N-acetyl-β-D-glucosaminidase activity was measured according to Price [15], and expressed as units/l, the upper limit of normal was 13 U/l.

Light chain pI

Two methods were used to measure the pI. In the first study the urinary light chains were isolated by chromatography and their pI subsequently estimated by isoelectric focusing, using 3—9 pH IEF gels [7]. Later we devised a sensitive immunoblotting technique from IEF gels to be used with a Pharmacia PhastSystem which enabled us to study patients excreting low concentrations of free light chains [8].

Results and discussion

The association between urinary light chain excretion, serum creatinine

Table 1. Relationship of light chain excretion and paraprotein type to the incidence of renal failure patients with myelomatosis.

Urinary light chain u/g creatinine*	Serum creatinine μmol/l	Secreted paraprotein of neoplastic clone																Non-secretors
		Gκ		Aκ		Dκ		κ		Gλ		Aλ		Dλ		λ		
		n	(%)	n	(%)	n	(%)	n	(%)	n	(%)	n	(%)	n	(%)	n	(%)	n
< 0.04	< 130	90	(29)	39	(28)	0		0		55	(28)	32	(26)	1	(6)	0		13
< 0.04	> 130 < 300	25	(8)	9	(6)	0		0		15	(8)	12	(10)	0		0		1
< 0.04	> 300	0		1	(1)	0		0		1	(0)	0		0		0		1
> 0.04 < 1	< 130	82	(26)	28	(20)	1	(13)	4	(5)	20	(10)	19	(15)	1	(6)	3	(5)	0
> 0.04 < 1	> 130 < 300	31	(10)	16	(11)	0		4	(5)	8	(4)	6	(5)	0		0		0
> 0.04 < 1	> 300	1	(0)	0		0		1	(1)	2	(1)	1	(1)	0		0		0
> 1	< 130	54	(17)	19	(13)	5	(62)	25	(32)	36	(18)	26	(21)	6	(35)	14	(25)	0
> 1	> 130 < 300	45	(14)	18	(13)	0		25	(32)	43	(22)	13	(10)	3	(18)	19	(33)	0
> 1	> 300	23	(7)	11	(8)	2	(25)	19	(24)	16	(8)	15	(12)	6	(35)	20	(36)	0
Total with paraprotein class		351		141		8		78		196		124		17		56		15

* One unit of urinary free light chain is equivalent to 1 gram of polyclonal free κ or free λ standard. These data are derived from 986 consecutive patients entered into the 4th and 5th MRC myelomatosis trials. Values being obtained before the administration of cytotoxic chemotherapy but after a 48 hour period of hydration.

and paraprotein type for the 986 patients considered in this study are shown in Table 1. Of these patients 120 had serum creatinine levels of 300 μmol/l or above. Only 8 of this renal failure subgroup had a free light chain output in the normal range. Modest rises in serum creatinine 130—300 μmol/l were not infrequently encountered in patients with light chain output in the normal range (62 of 295 patients in this range). These cannot easily be attributed to dehydration as all patients on diagnosis had a 48 hour period of hydration before the serum and urine were taken for analysis.

A survey of tubular protein reabsorption was made using α_1-m as an indicator, the stability of this protein at low pH and its suitability for estimation by simple techniques such as radial immunodiffusion made it the LMWP of choice. From 522 patients studied 357 (68.4%) had a raised urinary α_1-m (> 15 mg/g cr). Considering the 247 patients with a normal scr (< 130 μmol/l) then the Spearman rank coefficient for the urinary α_1-m and free light chain excretion was $r = 0.64$. The relationships of light chain excretion and the other indices of tubular function in this group of patients without impairment of GFR is shown in Table 2. The effect of renal failure produced a significant χ^2 for trend of rise of urinary output of α_1-m and RBP ($p = 0.0002$, and 0.0017 respectively) with increase of scr, but not for AGP or NAG which appeared to have reached their upper limits of excretion as the result of a high concentration of the light chains in glomerular filtrate alone. This is demonstrated in greater detail in Cooper et al. [4]. It appears that light chains have a greater effect on the inhibition of resorption of the glycosylated proteins α_1-m and AGP than the non-glycosylated LMWPs β_2-m and RBP.

The direct effect of the light chain on the glomerular size charge barrier appeared to be relatively slight as 117/118 (99.5%) patients chosen at

Table 2. Correlation between urinary light chain output and the concentrations of other urinary proteins in patients with serum creatinine < 130 μmol/l.

	Light chain v α_1m	AGP	RBP	NAG
Spearman correlation coefficient(r)	0.64	0.64	0.16	0.39
n	247	248	96	245
Significance(p)	< 0.0001	< 0.0001	> 0.1*	< 0.0001

α_1m = α_1-microglobulin, AGP = α_1-acid glycoprotein, NAG = β-N-acetyl-D-glucosaminidase, RBP = retinol binding protein.
* $r = 0.167$.

random had a urinary albumin of <1 g/g cr. During follow up tubular proteinuria usually disappears in patients whose light chain excretion returns to normal in response to chemotherapy. Conversely the reappearance of light chain proteinuria in relapse is accompanied by evidence of tubular dysfunction.

Light chain pI

The light chains exhibited a wide variation of pI ranging from approximately pH 3—9, and within a given light chain there could be evidence of considerable microheterogeneity of charge producing several bands on IEF. This heterogeneity of light chains in urine has been confirmed by other studies [14], especially since IEF and immunoblotting have been advocated as a sensitive method for identifying urinary light chains [14, 17] and has been observed in serum [9].

In our first study of 43 light chain pI spectrotypes, it became apparent there was no correlation between the nephrotoxicity of the light chains pI spectrotype as revealed by comparing the mid-point pI with scr concentration, or clinical course of renal function [7]. In a second study we concentrated on patients without evidence of glomerular impairment (scr <130 μmol/L). The distribution of the light chain mid-point pIs is shown in Fig. 1. Once the conflicting factors arising from renal failure had been eliminated it then appeared that light chains with a high pI tended to have a greater effect on the inhibition of the reabsorption of α_1-m than those with a more acidic pI (Fig. 2). It is known that substances with a terminal positively charged amino or guanidine group inhibit tubular protein reabsorption, lysine can produce an almost complete inhibition [13]. It is uncertain whether a similar mechanism is involved in the way light chains produce their inhibitory action on the tubular cell protein uptake.

Although this data show an association between cationic pI and defective reabsorption of some LMW proteins, we have not seen a correlation between renal failure and light chain pI. Therefore these studies of pI at best only partially support the concept that light chains with a cationic pI are more nephrotoxic as suggested by Clyne et al. [3] and supported by Coward et al. [5]. However, our data agree with that of Melcion et al. [11] who could find no simple relation between isoelectric point and light chain nephrotoxicity. Other characteristics such as the light chain type (kappa or lambda) or the formation of dimers was unrelated to their nephrotoxic action or effect on proximal tubular function.

In summary it appears there is evidence that in the absence of glomerular impairment an increased urinary light excretion will produce progressive impairment of the proximal tubular reabsorption of LMWPs. Some dis-

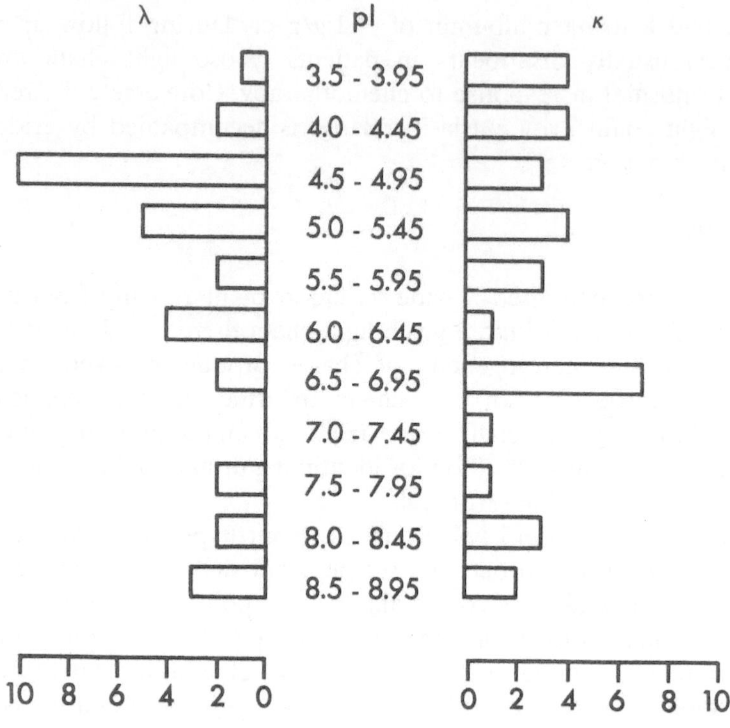

Fig. 1. Distribution of free light chain pIs.

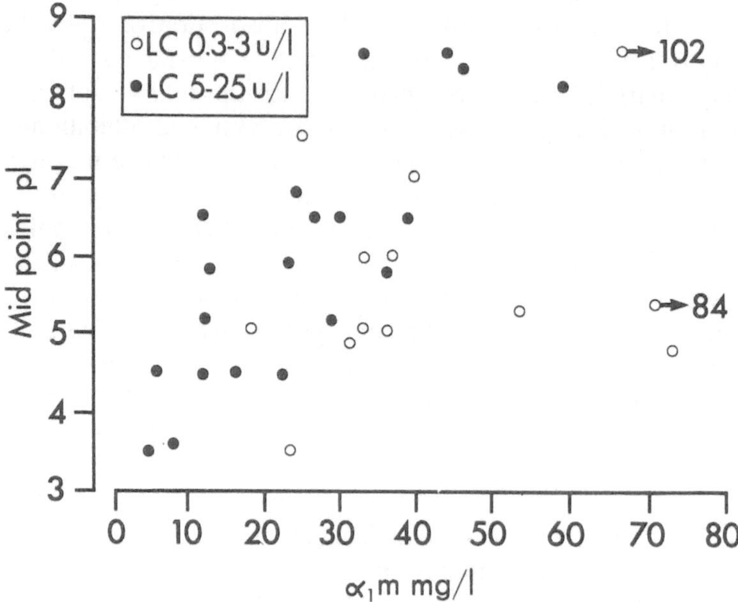

Fig. 2. Relation of light chain mid point pI and α1-microglobulin excretion in patients with serum creatinine $< 130\ \mu$mol/l.

turbance of reabsorption of LMWP and increased NAG excretion can be detected in patients with a light chain excretion within normal limits. This suggests that the tubules may be responding to a toxic effect associated with the neoplasm. The finding of some elevation of serum creatinines in 22 percent of patients with light chain output in the normal range (Table 1) provides further support for additional nephrotoxic factors. A marked increase of urinary NAG excretion occurs in acute myeloid leukaemia [20] and we have observed LMWP-uria in leukaemia. This impairment of protein reabsorption in myelomatosis is accompanied by an increased NAG excretion indicative of some form of lysosomal disorder, possibly reflecting the saturation of the catabolic functions by pinocytosed light chains. There is some evidence of recruitment of the defective reabsorption, α_1-m being more readily affected than RBP and β_2-m and cationic light chains appear to compete with α_1-m more effectively than their anionic counterparts. This reversible phenomenon tends not to leave residual renal damage.

However, once the glomerular filtration rate shows a significant fall, as indicated by a raised scr the proximal tubular dysfunction is the combined result of the increased levels of LMWPs in the glomerular filtrate exceeding their reabsorption threshold, the direct of light chain in the filtrate, and the intrinsic damage to the nephrons produced by casts, micro-obstruction and interstitial nephritis. Under these conditions it is not possible to estimate the extent of tubular alterations alone [6]. In some patients this complex condition can revert back to normal renal function, in others the lesion is irreversible and enters the final common pathway of end stage renal failure.

Acknowledgement

Supported by a grant from the Medical Research Council, UK.

References

1. Boesken W. Die tubulare Proteinurie. Klin Wschr 1975; 53: 473—9.
2. Carone FA, Peterson DR, Oparil S, Pullman TN. Renal tubular transport and catabolism of proteins and peptides. Kidney Int 1979; 16: 271—8.
3. Clyne DH, Pera AJ, Thompson RE. Nephrotoxicity of Bence-Jones proteins: the importance of isoelectric point. Kidney Int 1979; 16: 345—52.
4. Cooper EH, Forbes MA, Crockson RA, MacLennan ICM. Proximal renal tubular function in myelomatosis: observations in the fourth Medical Research Council trial. J Clin Pathol 1984; 37: 852—8.
5. Coward RA, Delamore IW, Mallick NP, Robinson EL. The importance of urinary

immunoglobulin light chain isoelectric point (pI) in multiple myeloma. Clin Sci 1984; 66: 229—32.

6. Gauthier C, Nguyea-Simmonet H, Vincent C, Revillard JP, Pellet MV. Renal tubular absorption of β_2-microglobulin. Kidney Int 1984; 26: 170—5.
7. Johns EA, Turner R, Cooper EH, MacLennan ICM. Isoelectric points of urinary light chains in myelomatosis: analysis in relation to nephrotoxicity. J Clin Pathol 1986; 36: 833—7.
8. Jackson PJ, Sampson CJ, Cooper EH, Heney D, Brocklebank JT. A new method for rapid analysis of proteinuria using PhastSystem. Submitted to Ann Clin Chemistry 1987.
9. McLeod BC, Viernes A, Kyle RA, Sassetti RJ. Analysis of serum light chains by crossed immunoelectrophoresis: comparison with urinary light chains in light chain disease. J Clin Oncol 1984; 2: 1110—4.
10. McLaughlin P, Alexanian R. Myeloma protein kinetics following chemotherapy. Blood 1982; 60: 851—5.
11. Melcion C, Mougenot B, Baudouin B, Ronco P, Moulonguet-Doleris L, Vanhille Ph, Beaufils M, Morel-Maroger L, Venoust P, Richet G. Renal failure in myeloma: relationship with isoelectric point of immunoglobulin light chains. Clin Nephrol 1984; 22: 138—43.
12. Mietten TA, Kekki M. Effect of impaired hepatic and renal function on $[^{131}I]$ Bence Jones protein catabolism in human subjects. Clin Chim Acta 1967; 18: 395—407.
13. Morgensen CE, Sølling K. Studies on renal tubular protein reabsorption partial or near complete inhibition by certain amino acids. Scand J Clin Lab Invest 1977; 37: 477—86.
14. Norden AGW, Fulcher LM, Flynn FV. Immunoglobulin light chain immunoblots of urine proteins from patients with tubular and Bence-Jones proteinuria. Clin Chim Acta 1987; 166: 307—15.
15. Price RG, Dance N, Richards B, Cattell WR. The excretion of N-acetyl-β-glucosaminidase and β-galactosidase following surgery to the kidney. Clin Chim Acta 1970; 27: 65—72.
16. Scarpioni L, Ballochi S, Bergonzi G, et al. Glomerular and tubular proteinuria in myeloma. Relationship with Bence-Jones proteinuria. Contrib Nephrol 1981; 26: 89—102.
17. Sinclair D, Parrott DMV, Stott DI. Quantitation of monoclonal immunoglobulins by immuno-isoelectric focusing and its application to B cell neoplasia. J Immunol Methods 1986; 90: 247—55.
18. Smithline N, Kassier JP, Cohen JJ. Light chain nephropathy tubular dysfunction and light chain proteinuria. N Engl J Med 1976; 294: 71—74.
19. Virella G, Pires MT, Coehlo IM. Analytical characterization of urinary proteins from sixty patients with monoclonal gammopathies. Clin Chim Acta 1974; 50: 63—75.
20. Whiting PH, King DJ, Ireland A, Ratcliffe J, Dawson AA. N-acetyl-β-D-glucosaminidase enzymuria in leukaemia and myelomatosis: effect of treatment in acute myeloblastic leukaemia and myelomatosis in adults. Ann Clin Biochem 1986; 23: 676—80.

3. Pathophysiological aspects of myeloma cast nephropathy

P. RONCO, B. MOUGENOT, P. DOSQUET, Ph. VANHILLE, V. LEMAITRE, M. DE MEYER-BRASSEUR, F. MIGNON & P. VERROUST

Introduction

Myeloma cast nephropathy (MCN) is a frequent complication occurring in more than 50% of patients with multiple myeloma [1, 2, 3, 4]. It may be responsible for severe renal failure (RF) often judged irreversible and generally considered as an ominous prognostic sign [1, 5, 6]. The most typical lesion found on renal biopsies consists of large tubular casts characterized by a macrophagic reaction, almost always associated with tubular damage [7, 8, 9]. By immunofluorescence, these casts are brightly stained by fluorescein conjugated antisera specific for the light chain (LC) constitutive of the monoclonal component (MC) and for Tamm-Horsfall protein (THP), a protein synthesized by cells of the thick ascending limb of Henle's loop and normally restricted to this segment and the early distal convoluted tubule [10]. In addition, they often contain albumin as well as other immunologobulin (Ig) antigenic determinants. Although altered renal function, cast formation and tubular damage are almost exclusively observed in patients excreting LC in urine, there is no direct relation between the excreted amounts of LC and the development and severity of the renal lesions [2]. In particular, it is remarkable that a number of patients produce large amounts of LC without presenting any sign of renal involvement throughout the course of the disease. This may be related to the presence or absence of enhancing factors such as high urinary solute concentration, low pH, hyperuricemia and intravenous pyelogram (IVP), but also suggests that some LC may have a peculiar propensity to induce renal lesions, especially cast formation.

The first aim of the present study was, therefore, to examine some properties of the LC which could be responsible for nephrotoxicity. This analysis was focused on LC isoelectric point (pI) since it had been suggested [11, 12] that at a low urinary pH, LC with a high pI (> 5.6) — then positively charged — could undergo interaction and precipitation with

Minetti et al. (eds.), The kidney in plasma cell dyscrasias. ISBN 978-94-010-7085-0

THP which, with a pI of 3.2, is always negatively charged in the urine pH range.

The second issue investigated in this work relates to the respective role of individual lesions in the impairment of renal function. In particular, although myeloma casts are unusually large and abundant, the mechanical part that they play through tubular obstruction in the development of RF is debated. Studies dealing with nephropathies related to urinary tract obstruction have shown that the presence of THP in the glomerular urinary space (GUS) is a good marker of retrograde flux of tubular urine [13, 14]. Consequently, we took advantage of the availability of monoclonal antibodies. (Mab) previously produced in our laboratory [15] to search for THP in glomeruli of kidney biopsies from myeloma patients. This was complemented by an experimental study performed in mice bearing a K light chain excreting plasmacytoma which developed lesions closely resembling human MCN.

Patients and methods

Light-chain immunochemical study

Patients. 34 patients were studied (Table 1). All had multiple myeloma defined by the simultaneous presence of medullary plasma cell proliferation and a MC detectable by immunoelectrophoresis of serum or urine. Tumor mass, estimated by the Durie and Salmon's staging system excluding hemoglobin values [16], was high in 24 patients, intermediary in 5 and low in 4. Chemotherapy was administered according to tumor mass and age. In general, patients with low tumor mass or over 70 years old received melphalan and prednisone, whereas the combination of vincristine-melphalan-cyclophosphamide-prednisone was given in case of intermediary or high tumor mass. Doses were reduced according to serum creatinine values.

All patients exhibited severe RF as defined by peak serum creatinine concentration higher than 300 μmoles/l (Table 1). They were classified into three groups according to RF outcome: 1. Completely reversible RF was defined as return to normal of serum creatinine concentration (group I). 2. Partially reversible RF was defined as reduction by more than half of serum creatinine level, provided that the recovery concentration was less than 500 μmol/l (group II). 3. Patients with non-reversible RF were themselves categorized into two distinct subgroups according to the fact that they had to be taken on a chronic dialysis program (group IIIb) or not (group IIIa). All patients were given similar symptomatic treatment; in particular, dialysis was performed as long as necessary.

A percutaneous renal biopsy was performed in 28/34 patients. Kidney

Table 1. Characteristics of patients included in the light-chain immunochemical study.

Patient N	Sex/age	MC	Tumor mass	Serum Creatinine Peak (μM/l)	Recovery (μM/l)	Time from peak to recovery	Ca++ (mM/l)*	ECDH	Infect.
Group I									
1	F/77	$\gamma\lambda$	High	1189	115	210 D.	2.70	+	+Ur.
2	M/62	λ	Inter	2000	100	120 D.	2.40	+	+
3	M/33	$(\gamma)\lambda$	High	1575	130	50 D.	3.70	+	—
4	M/60	$\gamma\lambda$	Low	950	130	50 D.	2.50	+	+Ur.
5	M/67	$\gamma\kappa$	High	320	90	23 D.	3.50	+	+Resp.
6	M/73	$\gamma\kappa$	High	445	85	9 D.	2.60	+	+Sep.
7	F/56	$\alpha\kappa$	High	770	125	< 90 D.	3.10	+	—
Group II									
8	F/73	$\alpha\lambda$	High	1525	440	10 M.	2.50	+	+Ur.
9	M/63	λ	High	1500	470	60 D.	3.00	+	—
10	M/46	$\gamma\lambda$	High	830	270	28 D.	4.10	+	—
11	F/51	λ	High	700	220	60 D.	2.90	+	+Ur.
12	M/71	$\gamma\lambda$	High	945	160	11 M.	2.50	—	+Resp.
13	M/75	$\alpha\kappa$	Inter	630	250	115 D.	2.60	—	—
14	F/90	$\gamma\lambda$	High	1480	210	38 D.	2.00	+	+Ur.
15	M/79	$\alpha\lambda$	Inter	520	230	150 D.	2.35	—	—
16	M/68	κ	High	930	340	7.5 M.	2.40	+	—
				First value (μM/l)	Last** value (μM/l)	Time from first to last value			
Group IIIa									
17	F/83	λ	Low	320	1020	55 D.	2.40	+	—
18	F/76	$\gamma\lambda$	High	410	750	8 D.	3.30	+	+Ur.
19	F/71	$(\gamma)\kappa$	Inter	334	600	25 D.	2.03	+	+Sep.
20	F/66	$\gamma\kappa$	High	592	429	9 D.	3.07	+	—
21	F/67	$(\gamma)\lambda$	High	220	500	17 M.	2.85	—	—
22	M/69	$\alpha\lambda$	High	164	440	13 M.	2.37	—	—
23	F/74	$\gamma\lambda$	Low	450	650	15 M.	2.15	—	+Ur.
24	M/58	$\gamma\lambda$	High	620	730	50 D.	3.50	+	—
25	M/47	λ	Inter	740	570	11 M.		—	—
Group IIIb									
26	F/83	$\alpha\kappa$	High	300	980	7 D.	3.05	+	—
27	F/59	λ	High	648	1200	12 D.	2.47	+	—
28	F/72	κ	Low	584	1000	30 D.	2.50	—	+Ur.
29	F/34	$\gamma\kappa$	High	330	670	65 D.	2.10	—	—
30	M/74	$\gamma\lambda$	High	768	1940	7 D.	2.70	+	—
31	F/68	κ	High	1900	1630	3 D.	2.55	—	+UrResp.
32	F/74	$\gamma\kappa$	—	925	1100	3 D.	2.53	+	—
33	F/71	λ	High	—	750	—	2.43	—	—
34	M/57	λ	High	500	910	5 M.	2.40	—	+Ur.

* Value measured at admission or at RF onset.
** Last value before hemodialysis or peritoneal dialysis for patients in group IIIb.
MC: Monoclonal component (Brackets indicate trace amounts of HC monoclonal component), ECDH: Extra-cellular dehydration, Infect: Infection, Inter: Intermediary, Ur: Urinary, Resp: Respiratory, Sep: Septicemia, D: Days, M: Months.

Table 2. Renal histology and isoelectric point (pI) of LC.

Patient	Tubules			Interstitium			
	Casts	Epith. lesions	Tubul. atrophy	Fibro edema	Fibrosis	Cells	LC pI
Group I							
1	No biopsy						5.5—5.7
2	++	+++	0	+F	0	+F	NA
3	++	++	0	+F	0	+F	5.5—5.8
4	0	+++	0	++D	0	+F	7.0—7.5
5	+	+	0	+F	0	+F	6.8—7.4
6	0	+	0	+F	0	0	7.7—7.8
7	No biopsy						8.3—8.8
Group II							
8	+++	+++	+	++D	0	+++F	6.0—6.7
9	++	+++	0	++D	0	+F	5.4—5.8
10	++	+++	+	0	+D	+F	5.5—6.0
11	0	+	+++	0	+++D	+F	6.0—7.0
12	++	+++	+	0	++F	++F	6.1—6.7
13	+++	+++	0	++D	0	++D	5.2—5.5
14	No biopsy						NA
15	0	++	++	0	++D	+F	6.0—7.0
16	++	++	+	0	++F	+D	6.5—7.0
Group IIIa							
17	++	++	+++	0	++D	++F	5.4—6.2
18	No biopsy						5.2—5.7
19	++	+++	+	++D	0	+F	8.8—8.9
20	+	+	+	0	+D	+F	6.6—6.8
21	++	+++	0	++D	0	++F	6.0—6.5
22	++	++	++	0	+D	+D	5.7—6.6
23	++	++	+++	0	+++F	+F	6.5—7.4
24	+++	+++	0	++D	0	++F	5.5—6.0
25	++	++	++	0	++F	+F	5.2—5.6
Group IIIb							
26	++	++	+++	0	++D	+D	5.9—6.1
27	++	++	+	0	++D	+D	7.1—77
28	++	+++	0	+F	0	+F	5.5—6.6
29	++	+++	+	0	++D	+D	8.0—8.2
30	++	++	0	0	++D	+F	5.2—5.5
31	++	+++	0	++D	0	+D	7.1—7.7
32	++	+++	0	0	++F	++F	7.5—7.8
33	++	++	0	+++D	0	+++F	5.3—5.9
34	++	++	+++	0	+++D	+++F	6.0—7.5

Epith. lesions = Epithelial lesions, Tubul. atrophy = tubular atrophy, F = Focal, D = Diffuse, NA = not available.

samples were taken at post-mortem examination in two additional patients. Two-micron sections of tissue fixed in Dubosq-Brazil solution and embedded in paraffin were processed and stained according to methods currently used in our laboratory [17]. Tubular and interstitial lesions were graded from 0 to 3+ depending on the number of tubules involved, the intensity of cell injury and the degree of interstitial damage (Table 2).

Determination of LC isoelectric point. It was achieved without prior purification of the LC through the three following steps:1. Isoelectrofocusing (IEF) of the sample in a polyacrylamide gel 2. Transfer of the focused proteins to a nitrocellulose sheet and 3. Identification of the LC on the nitrocellulose replica by immunoenzymatic techniques. Details of the method have been previously published [18].

Statistical analysis. The chi-square test with Yate's modifications for small samples and the Mann-Whitney-Wilcoxon rank test were used for data analysis.

Distribution of Tamm-Horsfall protein

Patients. 29 patients were studied. 18 had a typical multiple myeloma. The latter include 5 patients (No. 5, 12, 20, 31 and 33) of the LC immunochemical study. Since the frozen kept biopsies from the remaining patients were no longer available, we incorporated 13 other patients more recently referred to us (Table 3). 11 additional patients with a monoclonal gammopathy and renal lesions distinct from MCN (amyloidosis, nodular glomerulosclerosis, proliferative glomerulonephritis, plasmacell infiltration and minimal lesions) were included in the study as controls.

Mice. 13 nine weeks old Balb/c mice were inoculated subcutaneously with 10^6 dispersed cells from either 66.2 (a gift of Dr Preud'homme, Hôpital Saint Louis, Paris) or MOPC41 (Bionetics, Kensington, U.S.A.), two kappa LC excreting plasmacytomas. The mice were killed 4—6 weeks after injection, and their kidneys were processed for light and immunofluorescence microscopy.

Analysis of THP distribution. It was performed by indirect immunofluorescence using 3 previously described Mab (Mab18, 35 and 174) specific for different epitopes expressed on human THP [15]. 2 um cryostat sections were first incubated with a mixture of the 3 Mab at a final concentration of 10 μg/ml in PBS. After thorough washing, fixation of anti-

Table 3. Study of Tamm-Horsfall protein distribution: Characteristics of patients with myeloma cast nephropathy at the time of renal biopsy.

Patient	Sex/age	Monoclonal component	Urinary LC g/24 h (%)	Tumor mass	Creatinine (μM/L)	Ca++ (μM/L)	Triggering events
1	M/67	$\gamma\kappa$	1.4 (85)	High	320	3.50	DH.I.NSAI
2	M/62	$\gamma\kappa$		High	875	3.63	DH
3	F/58	$\gamma\kappa$	1.4 (75)	High	426		
4	M/66	κ	3.5 (78)	High	283		
5	F/73	$\gamma\lambda$	0.6 (73)	High	510	3.93	DH.I
6	M/65	$\alpha\lambda$		High	270	2.30	DH.I.Genta
7	M/71	$\gamma\lambda$	0.4 (60)	High	945	2.50	I
8	F/81	$\gamma\kappa$	5.7 (86)	Inter	309	2.35	I
9	F/77	$\gamma\kappa$	5.4 (90)	High	380	2.90	DH
10	F/66	$\gamma\kappa$	2.2 (88)	High	592	3.07	DH
11	F/68	κ	1.1 (70)	High	1900	2.55	I
12	F/71	λ	0.7 (70)	High	750	2.43	NSAI
13	M/65	λ	2.6 (85)		220		IVP
14	F/77	κ	1.5 (83)	High	840	3.35	DH
15	M/57	λ		High	1500		IVP.NSAI
16	M/57	$\gamma\lambda$	15.2 (95)	High	420	2.50	
17	F/82	κ	5.2 (91)	High	380	2.43	DH.I
18	M/76	κ			815	2.70	

Inter: Intermediary, DH: Dehydration, I: Infection, NSAI: Nonsteroidal antiinflammatory drugs, IVP: Intravenous pyelogram, Genta: Gentamicin.

THP Mab was revealed by FITC species-specific anti-mouse Ig antibodies (Amersham, Les Ulis, France). In the mouse, THP was searched for using specific rabbit polyclonal antibodies followed by FITC species-specific anti-rabbit Ig antibodies (Amersham).

Results

Light-chain immunochemical study

Renal damage. 16 patients experienced reversible RF (Table 1): 7 fulfilled the criteria required for entering group I, the remaining 9 could be included in group II. 18 patients had irreversible RF (group III): 9 of them did not need dialysis (group IIIa) whereas the others did (group IIIb). Peak serum creatinine values were close to 1000 μmol/l in the 3 groups (Table 1): 1035 ± 558 μmol/l in group I, 1017 ± 372 in group II and 927 ± 373 in group III.

Histological lesions are listed in Table 2. Myelomatous casts exhibited characteristic features in most cases. Tubules frequently showed variable degrees of epithelial degeneration or necrosis. These epithelial lesions, which were noted in the three groups of patients, must be clearly distinguished from global tubular atrophy with thickening of tubular basement membrane well correlated with interstitial fibrosis and glomerular sclerosis. Tubular atrophy was only found in groups II and III. In patient 33, striking glomerular lesions were observed, characterized by the presence of huge casts in Bowman's spaces with complete retraction of the floculus and disruption of Bowman's capsule. Glomerular abnormalities were otherwise infrequent and moderate, consisting of a mild increase of mesangial matrix in more than half cases and of mesangial cells in patients 21 and 31.

Immunochemical properties of light chains. λLC were identified in 22/34 patiens (65%), and κLC in the twelve remaining ones. 14 patients had a light chain multiple myeloma (LCMM), most often of the λ type (10/14). The frequency of λLC in the three groups of patients was not significantly different.

Table 2 indicates that LC pI available in 32 patients were scattered from 5.2 to 8.9. 10 patients produced LC with pI lower than 6. LC pI was significantly higher in group I (7.0 ± 1.1) than in group II (6.2 ± 0.5) (p value = 0.04) but no significant difference could be found between group I and group III (6.5 ± 1.0). In addition, there was no correlation between the estimated intensity of casts and the pI value of LC.

Distribution of Tamm-Horsfall protein

Patients. THP deposits were identified in the GUS of 16/18 patients with MCN (Table 4). They were generally very abundant, lining the inner aspect of the Bowman's capsule and penetrating between lobules of the capillary tuft (Fig. 1). In other cases, they were segmental and localized between capillary loops. 55 out of the 119 glomeruli available for study (46%) were

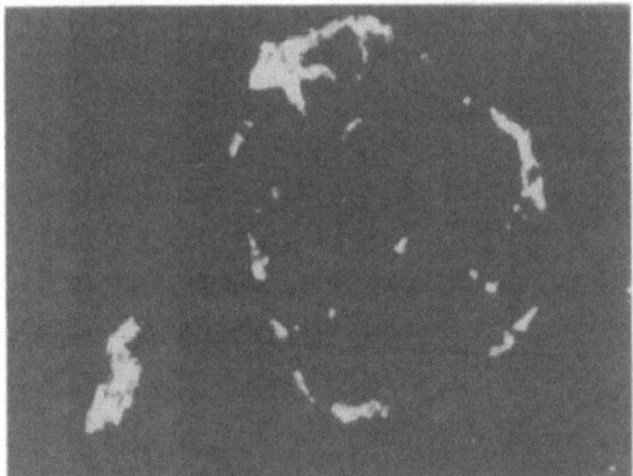

Fig. 1. Indirect immunofluorescence of a frozen kidney section from a patient with MCN, incubated with monoclonal antibodies to THP. Note intense THP deposits in the glomerular urinary space.

Table 4. Analysis of Tamm-Horsfall protein deposits in patients with myeloma cast nephropathy.

Patient	Glomeruli Total number	THP+	Interstitial Deposits
1	6	4	—
2	6	5	—
3	2	1	+
4	5	2	+
5	25	14	+
6	4	2	—
7	4	2	—
8	4	2	—
9	7	3	+
10	6	4	—
11	10	6	+
12	4	2	+
13	2	0	—
14	6	1	—
15	1	0	—
16	5	2	+
17	10	4	—
18	6	1	+
	113	55 (48.7%)	8/18

THP positive. By contrast, in the 11 patients with monoclonal gammopathy and renal lesions distinct from MCN, minimal deposits of THP were detected in only 3 out of the 55 glomeruli examined (5%). Futhermore, THP interstitial deposits were noted in 8 patients with MCN and 3 patients in the control group.

Mice. Plasmacytoma injected mice developed within 4—6 weeks severe renal lesions characterized by numerous lamellar casts associated with cellular reaction and extensive tubular damage. These lesions are similar to those observed in human MCN. THP glomerular deposits were observed in 4/7 and 6/6 mice inoculated with MOPC 41 and 66.2 respectively.

Discussion

The pathogenetic mechanisms leading to renal damage in myeloma as well as the respective contribution to renal failure of elementary histological lesions (including casts, tubular lesions and interstitial damage) are poorly understood. In the present study, we have considered two potentially important issues: the pathogenetic role of some LC immunochemical properties with emphasis on the isoelectric point, and the part played by cast induced tubular obstruction in the development of RF.

LC immunochemical properties were analyzed in 34 patients with multiple myeloma and severe RF. Our study shows a large preponderance of λLC which were detected in 2/3 patients, whereas they account only for 30 % of normal or monoclonal Ig [4]. This finding, at variance with most prior published data, was also noted by Bernstein [19] who suggested an association between λLC and RF. However, LC type does not correlate with the outcome of RF. In addition, we measured the pI of urinary LC since it had been postulated that LC with a pI greater than 5.6 could be more nephrotoxic [11, 12]. When urinary pH falls to 5, those LC which then bear positive charges, are suspected of undergoing electric interaction and precipitation with THP. The role of LC charges was also put forward by Hill et al. [20] who demonstrated a good correlation between decreasing LC electrophoretic mobility and increasing severity of RF, and by Coward et al. [21] who showed a significant negative correlation between pI and creatinine clearance. However, preliminary results from our laboratory on a limited series of 15 patients indicated that there was no simple relationship between pI and nephrotoxicity [18]. This is confirmed by the present study on 32 patients, which leads to three comments. First, severe RF can occur over a wide range of LC pI from 5.2 to 8.9. Second, one-third of LC have a pI lower than 6, so that even at highly acid urinary pH, they are only weakly charged. Potential nephrotoxicity of low pI LC was also demonstrated by Smolens et al. [22] in a rat plasmacytoma model. Under conditions designed to produce acid and maximally concentrated urine, LC with the lowest pI were found to be the most nephrotoxic. Along this line, we observed severe tubular lesions in mice bearing MOPC 41 and 66.2 plasmacytomas which produce acidic kappa LC with pI of 5.0—5.2 and 5.7—5.9 respectively (values assessed in serum). These human and experimental data suggest that pI of LC per se does not play a crucial role in the formation of casts, which are more probably induced by other physico-chemical properties yet unidentified. Third, the prognostic value of LC pI seems to be weak. Although group I differed statiscally from group II, no significant difference could be found between group I and group III.

In addition, we felt it important to analyze the role of cast induced tubular obstruction since this phenomenon could have significant implications for the management of myeloma patients with severe RF. The observation that THP could be detected in the urinary space of glomeruli in obstructive nephropathies [13, 14] prompted us to use monoclonal antibodies to THP to analyze its distribution in our patients. This protein could be localized in the glomerular urinary space in 16/18 biopsies studied, thus suggesting reflux of tubular urine to the glomerulus. These results which extend previous findings by Border [23] and Cohen [24] in two patients, indicate that tubular obstruction by casts may play a substantial part in RF observed in myeloma. Although the number of biopsies studied was too small to conclude, the degree of tubular obstruction estimated according to the percentage of THP containing glomeruli does not seem to correlate with either the peak creatinine value or the RF outcome. In contrast, the latter is well correlated with global tubular atrophy and severe interstitial damage which have pejorative significance. These findings were confirmed by an experimental study performed in the mouse. Mice injected with a K light chain excreting plasmacytoma developed lesions typical of MCN. Numerous large casts associated with severe tubular damage were identified in biopsy specimens taken from 4—6 weeks after inoculation. Analysis of THP distribution confirmed the role of cast induced tubular obstruction as THP could be localized in the GUS in 10/13 mice. The significance of THP interstitial deposits is more controversial. They may be caused by disruptions of tubular basement membranes induced by tubular obstruction. On the other hand, they may result from severe tubular damage due to the LC itself or the cast associated cellular reaction, with release of THP from its normal intracellular and intraluminal locations into the renal interstitium [14]. From a clinical point of view, the role played by obstruction in myeloma RF may explain the slow recovery of renal function noted in many patients, as illustrated by a mean recovery time of 77 days in group I and 145 days in group II [25]. We believe that the mechanical component of myeloma RF is potentially totally reversible, provided that the patients are submitted to prolonged forced diuresis started as soon as possible. The dispersion of LC isoelectric points observed in this study does not provided definite arguments for or against alkaline prescription which remains however logical because of decreased THP solubility at acid urinary pH [10].

References

1. Defronzo RA, Humphrey RL, Wright Jr, Cooke CR. Acute renal failure in multiple myeloma. Medicine 1975; 54: 209—23.
2. Defronzo RA, Cooke CR, Wright Jr, Humphrey RL. Renal function in patients with multiple myeloma. Medicine 1987; 57: 151—66.
3. Ganeval D, Jungers P, Noel LH, Droz D. La néphropathie du myélome. Actual Nephrol Hop Necker 1977; 1: 309—47.
4. Kyle RA. Multiple myeloma: review of 869 cases. Mayo Clin Proc 1975; 50: 29—40.

5. Durie BGM, Salmon SE. The current status and future prospects of treatment for multiple myeloma. Clin Haematol 1982; 11: 181—210.
6. Kyle RA, Elveback LR. Management and prognosis of multiple myeloma. Mayo Clin Proc 1976; 51: 751—60.
7. Heptinstall RH. Amyloidosis, multiple myeloma and Waldenström's macroglobulinemia. London: Little Brown Publ, Pathology of the Kidney 571, 1966.
8. Morel Maroger L, Beaufils M. Richet G. The kidney in dysproteinemias. In: Hamburger, Crosnier, Grünfeld, eds. Nephrology. Second ed. New York, Paris: Wiley-Flammazion, 1980: 711.
9. Pirani CL, Silva FG, Appel GB. Tubulo-interstitial disease in multiple myeloma and other nonrenal neoplasias. In: Cotran RS, Brenner BM, Stein JH, eds. Tubulo-interstitial Nephropathies. New York: Churchill Livingstone, 1983: 287—334.
10. Ronco P, Brunisholz M, Geniteau-Legendre M. Chatelet F, Verroust P, Richet G. Physiopathologic aspects of Tamm-Horsfall protein: a phylogenetically conserved marker of the thick ascending limb of Henle's loop. Grünfeld, Maxwell, eds. In: Advances in Nephrology (Vol. 16) from the Necker Hospital. Chicago, London: Year Book Medical Publisher, 1987: 231—44.
11. Clyne DH, Kant KS, Pesce AJ, Pollak VE. Nephrotoxicity of low molecular weight serum proteins: physicochemical interactions between myoglobin, hemoglobin, Bence-Jones proteins and Tamm-Horsfall mucoprotein. Curr Probl Clin Biochem 1979; 1: 299—308.
12. Clyne DH, Pesce AJ, Thompson RE. Nephrotoxicity of Bence-Jones proteins in the rat: importance of protein isoelectric point. Kidney Int 1979; 16: 345—52.
13. Dziukas LJ, Sterzel RB, Hodson CJ, Hoyer JR. Renal localization of Tamm-Horsfall protein in unilateral obstructive uropathy in rats. Lab Invest 1982; 47: 185—93.
14. Resnick JS, Sisson S, Vernier R. Tamm-Horsfall protein. Abnormal localization in renal diseases. Lab Invest 1978; 38: 550—5.
15. Brunisholz M, Geniteau-Legendre M, Ronco P, Moullier P, Pontillon F, Richet G, Verroust P. Production and characterization of monoclonal antibodies specific for human Tamm-Horsfall protein. Kidney Int 1986; 29: 971—6.
16. Durie BGM, Salmon SE. A clinical staging system for multiple myeloma. Correlation of measured myeloma cell mass with presenting clinical features, response to treatment, and survival. Cancer 1975; 36: 842—54.
17. Morel Maroger L, Leathem A, Richet G. Glomerular abnormalities in nonsystemic diseases. Relationship between findings by light microscopy and immunofluorescence in 433 renal biopsy specimens. Am J Med 1972; 53: 170—84.
18. Melcion C, Mougenot B, Baudouin B, Ronco P, Moulonguet-Doleris L, Vanhille PH, Beaufils M, Morel-Maroger L, Verroust P, Richet G. Renal failure in myeloma: relationship with isoelectric point of immunoglobulin light chains. Clin Nephrol. 1984, 22: 138—43.
19. Bernstein SP, Humes HD. Reversible renal insufficiency in multiple myeloma. Arch Intern Med 1982; 142: 2083—6.
20. Hill GS, Morel Maroger L, Mery J PH, Brouet J Cl., Mignon F. Renal lesions in multiple myeloma: their relationship to associated protein abnormalities. Am J Kidney Dis 1983; 2: 423—38.
21. Coward RA, Delamore IW, Mallick NP, Robinson EL. The importance of urinary immunoglobulin light chain isoelectric point (pI) in nephrotoxicity in multiple myeloma. Clin Science 1984; 66: 229—32.
22. Smolens P, Venkatachalam M, Stein JH. Myeloma kidney cast nephropathy in a rat model of multiple myeloma. Kidney Int 1983; 24: 192—204.
23. Border WA, Cohen AH, Renal biopsy diagnosis of clinically silent multiple myeloma. Ann Intern Med 1980; 93: 43—6.

24. Cohen AH, Border WA. Myeloma kidney. An immunomorphogenetic study of renal biopsies. Lab Invest 1980; 42: 248–56.
25. Rota S, Mougenot B, Baudouin B, De Meyer-Brasseur M. Lemaitre V, Michel C, Mignon F, Rondeau E, Vanhille PH, Verroust P, Ronco P. A clinico-pathological study of 34 patients with multiple myeloma and severe renal failure: reappraisal of outcome and prognostic factors. Medicine 1987; 66: 127–39.

4. Light chain nephrotoxicity: Insights from a rat model of myeloma

PETER SMOLENS & JAY H. STEIN

Renal dysfunction is frequently observed in patients with multiple myeloma and a wide spectrum of renal alterations may be seen. These include isolated tubular defects, glomerulopathies, acute renal failure, and chronic renal failure. Up to two thirds of the patients are found to have a serum creatinine of greater than 1.5 mg% and 10—20% develop end-stage renal disease [1]. A variety of renal pathological lesions are also found in these patients. For example, some patients with myeloma and renal failure may have the typical cast nephropathy of 'myeloma kidney' while others may have a paucity of casts but show severe tubular atrophy and tubular dropout [2]. Others may have glomerular or tubular cell deposits of the Bence Jones proteins (BJP).

Much evidence suggests that the BJP may be an important factor in the genesis of the renal dysfunction in these patients. Most myeloma patients with renal failure have Bence Jones proteinuria and in some studies a rough correlation has been found between the degree of renal impairment and the amount of Bence Jones proteinuria [3]. Patients with plasma cell dyscrasias where Bence Jones proteinuria does not occur (such as heavy chain disease) do not develop renal failure. Typically, morphologic studies of the kidneys show a cast nephropathy and immunofluoresent study of these casts has shown them to be composed (at least in part) of the BJP [4]. In addition, patients with Bence Jones proteinuria and tubular dysfunction have often been found to have droplets and/or crystals of the BJP in their renal tubular cells [5].

In view of the wide spectrum of renal alterations that may be seen in myeloma patients with Bence Jones proteinuria, it would appear that the renal response to exposure to BJP is not uniform. Indeed, some patients may excrete large amounts of certain BJPs for years and yet maintain normal renal function [6].

If in fact, the renal manifestations of multiple myeloma are due primarily to the effects of the BJP, how can one explain the diversity of renal

Minetti et al. (eds.), The kidney in plasma cell dyscrasias. ISBN 978-94-010-7085-0

functional and pathologic alterations that occur in these patients? Several possibilities may be considered. First it may be due to differences in the physicochemical nature of individual BJPs such as net electric charge [7], degree of glycosylation [8] or polymerization [9] or light chain type (κ or λ) [10]. A second possibility is that certain factors other than the BJP may be present in these patients which can modulate or trigger the nephrotoxicity of BJPs. It is conceivable, as well that both of these possibilities may obtain. That is, the ability of other factors to modulate the nephrotoxicity of a BJP may be dependent on certain physicochemical features of the BJP. Alternatively, the diversity in the renal manifestations of myeloma may suggest that the BJP is not as important as is currently thought and that factors independent of the BJP are what actually determine the renal outcome in these patients.

Investigating these possibilities is often difficult in patients with myeloma. It is particularly hard to obtain a clear picture of the role of the BJP when multiple other factors such as dehydration, hypercalcemia, and nephrotoxin exposure are present, as is common, in these patients. A number of investigators have utilized animal models to study the pathophysiology of BJP nephrotoxicity in a more easily controlled fashion [7, 11, 12]. In most of these studies, human BJPs were given to mice or rats. While these studies have proved useful, conclusions from them need to be somewhat guarded since heterologous BJPs were employed and renal handling of these foreign proteins might differ from that of native proteins. In addition, because of the possibility of an immune response to these heterologous proteins, only acute exposure to these BJPs could be evaluated.

To circumvent these problems, we have utilized a rat model of myeloma which was developed by Bazin and co-workers [13]. These investigators discovered a unique strain of rats, known as LOU/c, which spontaneously developed immunoglobulin synthesizing tumors located in the ileocecal region of the abdomen, It was found that when the tumors were removed and transplanted into other histocompatible rats, the immunoglobulin synthetic capability of the tumor remained intact. These other histocompatible rats, known as LOU/m do not develop spontaneously growing tumors. With this model, the effects of chronic exposure of the kidney to homologous BJP under controlled conditions can be evaluated. We elected to examine this rat model of myeloma to see if alterations in renal function and morphology occurred and if so to use it to further investigate the role of the BJPs in the genesis of the renal failure. For all of our studies, four kappa light chain synthesizing tumors were utilized. Isoelectric focusing of these kappa light chains showed them to have isoelectric points (pI's) of 4.3, 5.2, 6.7, and 7.6. The molecular weight was determined with sodium dodecyl sulphate polyacrylamide gel electropheresis (SDS-PAGE). Most of the BJPs were found to be excreted as 24,000 dalton monomers. Only small amounts appeared to be excreted as dimers or trimers.

In our first study [14], rats were implanted with these different kappa light chain synthesizing tumors and the effects on renal function and morphology were examined. To enhance the likelihood of demonstrating a nephrotoxic effect, animals were kept hydropenic and aciduric by placing them on a high acid ash, water restricted diet. Renal function was monitored by serum creatinine measurement and renal histology was evaluated at the time the animals succumbed to the effects of the tumor. The findings of this study are summarized in Fig. 1. The tumor bearing rats excreted 30—200 mg of protein per day in the urine and greater than 90% of this protein was the kappa light chain (BJP). Duration of survival after implantation of the tumor ranged from 15—40 days and was a reflection of the aggressiveness of the tumor. Rats excreting a BJP with a pI of 5.2 were found to have an elevated serum creatinine and a distal nephron light chain containing cast nephropathy. Rats excreting the pI 4.3 BJP also had an elevated serum creatinine, but the renal histologic changes were primarily those of acute tubular necrosis. In contrast to these two groups, rats excreting the pI 6.7 BJP maintained a normal serum creatinine and renal histology in these rats was virtually normal despite the fact that they had prolonged exposure to large amounts of the BJP. Rats excreting the pI 7.6 BJP also had normal serum creatinine.

Thus, as in human myeloma, a spectrum of renal lesions was demonstrable in this animal model. With this study it was not possible to ascertain whether the different renal outcomes were actually a function of the different BJPs to which the kidneys were exposed. It is conceiveable that tumor related factors other than the BJP (degree of tumor infiltration into the body, metabolic effects of the tumor, release of other tumor derived

Group	n	Serum Creat. Mean $\pm$ SEM	P Value	Histology	Duration Survival	24 Hour Urinary Protein
Control	9	0.96		Normal	30 days	6 mg.
pI 4.3	12	1.61	0.01	ATN w/myeloma cast	40 days	100-200 mg.
pI 5.2	12	1.91	0.001	Myeloma cast nephropathy	15 days	30-60 mg.
pI 6.7	18	1.07	(NS)	Normal	40 days	100-150 mg.
pI 7.6	15	1.23	(NS)	Variable	20 days	100-150 mg.

Fig. 1. Effect on renal function and histology of implantation of different BJP synthesizing tumors. Group refers to the pI of the BJP synthesized by the tumor. N refers to the number of rats studied in each group. P values were determined by comparing serum creatinine values in tumor groups to that seen in sham operated controls.

factors etc), differed among the different tumor groups and may have contributed to the renal outcomes. In addition, since the survival of the animals was variable as was the BJP excretion, the amount of BJP to which the kidney was exposed was not the same in all groups.

The next study was designed, therefore, to circumvent these factors, and to control both the amount of BJP to which the kidney was exposed and the interval of time during which this exposure occurred. For this study [15], the different BJPs were collected from the tumor bearing animals. Non tumor bearing LOU/m rats were placed on a water restricted high acid ash diet which resulted in a urine pH of about 5.5 and urine osmolality of >2000. These rats were then given 100 mg/d for 5 days of either the pI 4.3, 5.2, or 6.7 BJP. Inulin clearance was measured prior to the administration of the BJPs and again after the 5 days of BJP administration had been completed.

Shown in Fig. 2 are the changes in GFR which occurred with administration of these different proteins. As may be seen, the most severe fall in GFR was observed in the rats receiving the pI 5.2 BJP. A significant decrement in GFR was also observed in the rats receiving the pI 4.3 BJP. No significant change in GFR, however, was noted in the rats receiving the pI 6.7 BJP.

The pI 5.2 group of rats was found to have a severe distal nephron cast nephropathy. In addition, a proximal tubule injury was also noted in this group. As shown in the left panel of Fig. 3, there was intense vacuolization in the proximal tubule cells. When the vacuoles were examined with electron microscopy, they appeared to represent accelerated autophago-

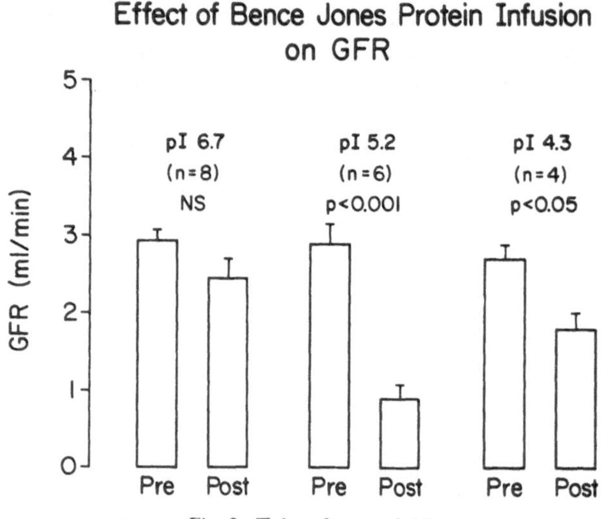

Fig. 2. Taken from ref. 15.

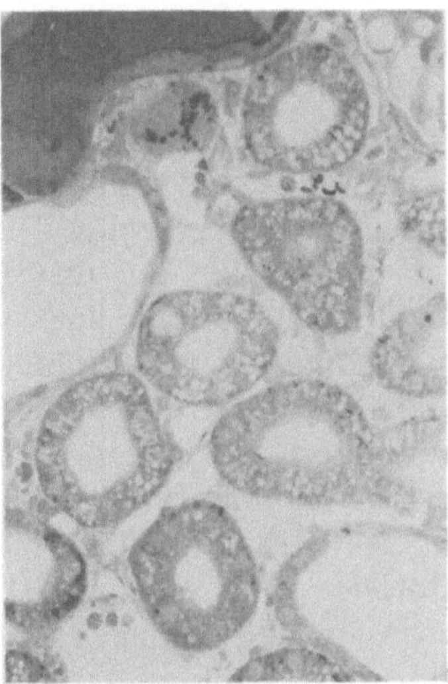
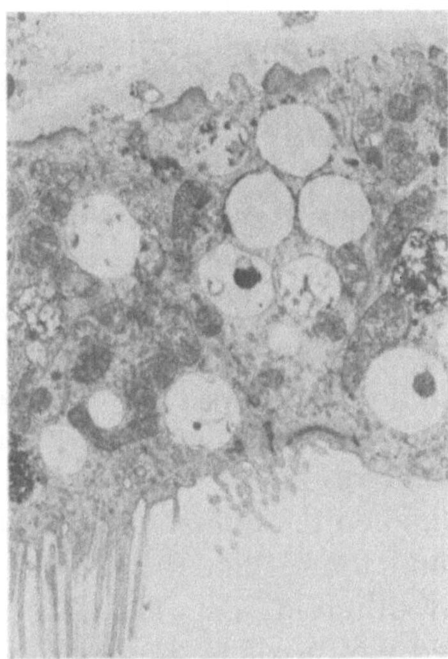

Fig. 3. Effect of infusion of pI 5.2 BJP on renal histology: in the left panel is a toluidine blue stained plastic section showing severe vacuolar change in proximal tubular cells. On the right is the ultrastructural appearance of these injured cells (adapted from ref. 15).

cytosis. Many of the vacuoles contained mitochondrial remnants and many mitochondria not enveloped in vacuoles were abnormal appearing due to swelling and disruption of their cristae. Because of these findings, we re-evaluated the renal histology from the tumor bearing animals from the first study and, in fact, similar vacuolar changes were present in the tumor bearing pI 5.2 animals. Similar but less severe changes were seen in the rats receiving the pI 4.3 BJP infusion. In contrast, renal histology remained largely unaltered in the pI 6.7 group. Thus the findings in the tumor bearing rats were, in large part, reproduced by the chronic administration of the different BJPs to non tumor bearing rats.

Several conclusions seemed to be supported by the results of these studies. First, they confirmed the idea that BJPs have a unique inherent nephrotoxic potential. Second, a given BJP was demonstrated to be able to induce both a distal cast nephropathy and a proximal tubular injury. While it is not clear whether the two were related, the sublethal proximal tubular injury which we noted after 5 days exposure to certain BJPs may be a forerunner of the tubular atrophy and dropout that may be seen in the absence of casts in a sizable number of myeloma patients. Lastly, since nephrotoxicity was observed only in the animals with the negatively charged BJPs, these studies provided further evidence that the nephrotoxic potential of BJPs does not seem to be a function of it carrying a positive net electric charge as some authors have suggested [7, 16].

We next turned to investigate factors which could cause this variability in BJP nephrotoxicity. Whether or not tubular cell injury occurs may be a function of how much of the BJP accumulates in the cell. An overload of BJP in the tubular cell could lead to cellular injury by a number of mechanisms. Since proteins of this type are compartmentalized after absorption into phagolysosomes [17], an overload could result in release of toxic lysosomal enzymes into the cell interior. Alternatively, if the cells' activities become devoted to the degradation of BJPs, this may interrupt other necessary functions of the cell and/or result in accumulation of toxic metabolites. The amount of BJP which accumulates in the tubular cell is determined both by the rate of absorption and the rate of degradation. It is conceivable that the rate of absorption of different BJPs may vary or that susceptibility to proteolytic digestion may not be uniform. Falconer-Smith et al. examined the uptake of different human BJPs in isolated perfused rat kidney and found that the tubular absorption rates of these BJPs were markedly different [18]. The difference in absorptive rates could not be correlated with toxicity, however, because none of the proteins appeared to be nephrotoxic.

Studies with proteins other than the BJPs have suggested that electric charge interactions between the protein and the brush border anionic glycocalyx are the major determinants of the rate of tubular uptake [19]. These studies indicate that proteins which carry a positive net electric charge would be reabsorbed to a greater degree than are those carrying a negative net electric charge. Whether or not this is true for BJPs is not known. If the absorption rates are different, it is possible that this is an important determinant of the nephrotoxic potential of a given BJP.

To examine this issue, we have begun to evaluate the rate of proximal tubule uptake of the different BJPs whose putative nephrotoxicities have been characterized as reviewed above [20]. For these studies, the BJPs were obtained from the urine of the tumor bearing rats. They were then purified with ion exchange and gel filtration chromatography. They were then labelled with ^{125}I. Our first experiments were designed to examine the role of net electric charge in the uptake of BJPs. The BJPs selected for study were the pI 5.2 and the pI 7.6 BJPs. They were placed in a tubular perfusate solution which had a pH of 7.0. At this pH, the pI 5.2 BJP is negatively charged and the pI 7.6 is positively charged. The absorption of these BJPs was then measured with in-vivo microperfusion techniques in the superfical proximal convoluted tubule of the rat. The concentration of the BJP in the perfusate was approximately 5 μg/ml. This relatively low concentration was chosen because it was felt that at this level the effect of factors such as net electric charge would be enhanced. Preliminary results of this study are shown in Table 1. The average length of the proximal tubule segment which was studied ($\pm$SD) was 2.55 $\pm$ 0.66 mm. The rate of absorption ($\pm$SD) of the pI 5.2 BJP was 12.8 $\pm$ 9.1 pg/mm/min (N =

Table 1. Proximal tubular uptake of Bence Jones proteins

BJP (pI)	n # tubule	BJP conc μg/ml	Tubule length (mm) ± SD	Reab %/mm/min ± SD	Jprot pg/mm/min ± SD	Jv nl/mm/min ± SD
5.2	9	5	2.70 ± 0.66	8.21 ± 5.4	12.8 ± 9.1	2.12 ± 0.94
7.6	7	5	2.35 ± 0.80	12.2 ± 9.4	18.3 ± 14.1	2.54 ± 1.12
7.6	9	50	2.22 ± 0.40	3.75 ± 1.82	56.3 ± 27.3	2.94 ± 0.87
Control	7	0	2.77 ± 0.81	—	—	2.37 ± 0.88

9 tubules) while that of the pI 7.6 BJP was 18.3 ± 14.1 pg/mm/min (N = 7 tubules). The difference in these values was not statistically significant. Although the uptake for the pI 7.6 BJP appeared to be greater, we believe this difference is probably not of physiologic significance either. It may be noted that the fractional uptake of these 2 proteins was only 8.2 and 12.2 %/mm/min for the pI 5.2 and 7.6 BJPs respectively. At the low concentration of BJP which was used, one would think that if preferential absorption of the cationic pI 7.6 BJP were really occurring, the fractional uptake of this protein would be substantially greater. Thus in contrast to what would be predicted from studies of other proteins, the cationic pI 7.6 BJP was not more avidly absorbed than was the anionic pI 5.2 light chain. It is to be noted that these preliminary results do not preclude the possibility that at higher delivery rates of the BJPs, differences in uptake of these two BJPs could occur. After the uptake of the pI 5.2 and 7.6 BJPs have been completed, the uptake of the non-toxic pI 6.7 BJPs will be examined to see if the lack of toxicity is related to diminished tubular uptake.

In another study, this rat model of myeloma was used to evaluate whether the nephrotoxic potential of a BJP could be modified by hypercalcemia [21]. Hypercalcemia is frequently seen in patients with myeloma and may be found in up to 2/3 of those with renal failure [22]. Hypercalcemia, by itself, can lower GFR via several mechanisms, including renal vasoconstriction [23] and alterations in the glomerular permeability coefficient (Kf) [24]. In addition, in vitro studies have demonstrated that the aggregability of Tamm-Horsfall protein is markedly enhanced in the presence of calcium ions [25]. BJPs have also been postulated to increase the aggregability of Tamm-Horsfall proteins.

We wondered if hypercalcemia might also directly potentiate the nephrotoxicity of BJPs in the setting of myeloma. To evaluate this possibility, we examined the effect of hypercalcemia superimposed on the infusion of one of our previously characterized BJPs into rats. The BJP chosen was the pI 6.7 BJP. This was the BJP which was found to have little, if any, nephrotoxicity in the previous studies. Three groups of rats were studied. All were anesthetized and underwent a baseline measurement of inulin clearance. Following this, group 1 (N = 13) rats were given 2 ml of vehicle (phosphate buffered saline) and were then made hypercalcemic with an infusion containing 0.048M $CaCl_2$. At the end of 2 hours a second inulin clearance was measured. Group 2 rats (N = 8) were given 100 mg of the pI 6.7 BJP in 2 ml of the vehicle and were kept on a non calcium containing infusate. Group 3 rats (N = 11) were given 100 mg of the BJP in 2 ml of the vehicle and were then started on the calcium containing infusate used in group 1. Rats in groups 2 and 3 also had a second inulin clearance measured at the end of 2 hours. At the completion of the second clearance, kidneys were processed for renal histology.

The serum calcium level measured during the second inulin clearance period was 13.5 mg% for group 1, 7.9 mg% for group 2 and 13.7 mg% for group 3. The effects of these maneuvers on GFR are shown in Fig. 4. Hypercalcemia alone (group 1) and administration of BJP alone (group 2) had no significant effect on GFR. In contrast, the combination resulted in a dramatic 46% fall in GFR. To evaluate the mechanism by which the GFR was suppressed, we examined the effects of these maneuvers on renal blood flow (electromagnetic flow probe) and renal histology. We found that RBF in the group 3 animals did not fall and thus vasoconstriction cannot be invoked to explain and the decrememt in GFR. Morphologic alterations which could have explained the suppression of GFR include the formation of casts with intratubular obstruction, severe tubular necrosis

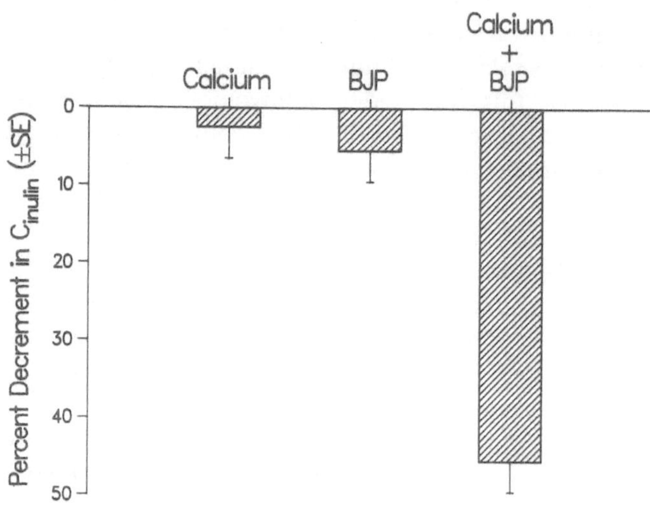

Fig. 4. Effect of infusion of calcium, BJP or both on inulin clearance (taken from ref. 21).

with rents in the tubular wall, and alterations in the glomerular capillaries such as necrosis or thrombosis. None of these alterations, however, were found in any of the rat groups. Thus the mechanism of the fall in GFR that occured was unclear. In view of the absence of tubular findings or alterations in renal blood flow, one might speculate that the mechanism of this nephrotoxic synergism could involve an alteration of glomerular dynamics such as a fall in glomerular permeability (Kf) or filtration pressure. (ΔP)

The results of this study highlight an additional point which is of potential clinical significance. In recent years, a number of studies have been undertaken to evaluate the physicochemical characteristics of different BJPs to see if one could predict those patients most at risk for renal injury to occur [8, 16, 7, 26]. Implicit in these types of studies is the idea that each BJP has an inherent nephrotoxic potential. The findings of the present study suggest that prediction of nephrotoxicity or non-toxicity of BJPs may be somewhat complex and that utilization of physicochemical markers of the BJPs to predict toxicity may be complicated by the fact that other factors such as hypercalcemia (and probably other factors as well) may markedly alter the intrinsic nephrotoxic properties of a given BJP.

In summary, we have utilized a unique rat model of multiple myeloma to examine how BJPs mights injure the kidney and why there is such a diversity of renal effects upon exposure to BJP. We have found that a spectrum of renal lesions similar to that seen in man occur in animals bearing these kappa LC synthesizing tumors. In addition, we have shown that chronic administration of these proteins for 5 days can reproduce, in large part, the findings in the tumor bearing rats — thus confirming the importance of the BJP in these processes. To determine why these different nephrotoxicities obtain, we have begun to examine if differences in tubular uptake of the different BJPs can account for this. Lastly we have utilized this model to show that hypercalcemia can markedly potentiate the nephrotoxicity of a BJP which by itself is normally non-nephrotoxic. These observations offer a new mechanism by which renal failure can occur in myeloma. In addition they highlight the need to realize that the nephrotoxic potential of a BJP is, in part, a function of other factors which may be present in the setting of multiple myeloma.

Acknowledgements

Studies done in this laboratory were supported by National Institutes of Health grants PO1 DDK17387 and R23 DDK34858.

References

1. Bernstein SP, Humes HD, Reversible renal insufficiency in multiple myeloma. Arch Int Med 1982; 142: 1083—2086.
2. Silva GF, Pirani CL, Mesa-Tejeda R, Williams G. The kidney in plasma cell dyscrasias: A review and a clinopathologic study of 50 patients. In: Fenoglio CE, Wolff M, eds. Progress in surgical pathology. New York: Masson, 1982: 131—76.
3. DeFronzo RA, Cooke CR, Wright JR, Humphrey RL. Renal function in patients with multiple myeloma. Medicine 1978; 57: 151—66.
4. Cohen AH, Border WA. Myeloma kidney, an immunomorphogenetic study of renal biopsies. Lab Invest 1980; 42: 248—56.
5. Maldonado JE, Velosa JA, Kyle RA, Wagoner RD, Holley KE, Salassa RM. Fanconi syndrome in adults. Am J Med 1975; 58: 354—64.
6. Woodruff R. Sweet B. Multiple myeloma with massive Bence Jones proteinuria and preservation of renal function. Aust NZ Med 1977; 7: 60—2.
7. Clyne DH, Pesce AJ, Thompson RE. Nephrotoxicity of Bence Jones protein in the rat. Importance of protein isoelectric point. Kid Int 1979; 16: 345—52.
8. Johns EA, Turner R, Cooper EH, Maclennan ICM. Isoelectric points of urinary light chains in myelomatosis: analysis in relation to nephrotoxicity. J Clin Pathol 1986; 39: 833—7.
9. Solling K, Solling J, Lanng Nielsen J. Polymeric Bence Jones proteins in serum in myeloma patients with renal insufficiency. Acta Med Scand 1984; 216: 495—502.
10. Alexanian R, Haut A, Khan AU, Lane M, McKelvey EM, Migliore PJ, Stuckey WJ, Wilson HE. Treatment for mutiple myeloma: Combination chemotherapy with different melphalan dose regimes. JAMA 1969; 208: 1680—5.
11. Koss MN, Pirani CL, Osserman EF. Experimental Bence Jones cast nephropathy. Lab Invest 1976; 34: 579—91.
12. Weis JH, Williams RH, Galla JH, Gottschall J, Rees ED, Bhathena D, Luke RH. Pathophysiology of acute Bence Jones protein nephrotoxicity in the rat. Kid Int 1981; 20: 198—210.
13. Bazin HC, Beckers A, Heremans JF. Transplantable immunoglobulin secreting tumours in rats. 1. General features of Lou/Wsl strain rat immunocytomas and their monoclonal proteins. Int J Cancer 1972; 10: 568—80.
14. Smolens P, Venkatachalam M, Stein JH. Myeloma kidney cast nephropathy in a rat model of multiple myeloma. Kid Int 1983; 24: 192—204.
15. Smolens P, Barnes JL, Stein JH. Effect of chronic infusion of Bence Jones proteins on rat renal function and histology. Kid Int 1986; 30: 874—82.
16. Coward RA, Delamore IW, Mallick NP, Robinson EL. The importance of urinary immunoglobulin light chain isoelectric point (pI) in nephrotoxicity in multiple myeloma. Clin Sci 1984; 65: 229—32.
17. Christensen EI, Maunsback AB. Intralysosomal digestion of lysozyme in renal proximal tubular cells. Kidney Int 1974; 6: 296—407.
18. Falconer Smith JF, Van Hegan RI, Esnouf MP, Ross BD. Characteristics of renal handling of human immunoglobulin light chain by the perfused rat kidney. Clin Sci 1979; 57: 113—20.
19. Sumpio BE, Maack T. Kinetics, competition, and selectivity of tubular absorption of proteins. Am J Physiol 1982; 243: F379—92.
20. Smolens P, Miller V. Renal tubular uptake of light chains of different isoelectric points (pI). Tenth Int Cong Neph (Abst) 1987; 591.

21. Smolens P, Barnes JL, Kreisberg R. Hypercalcemia can potentiate the nephrotoxicity of Bence Jones proteins. J Lab Clin Med (in press Oct 1987).
22. Cohen DJ, Sherman WH, Osserman EF, Appel GB. Acute renal failure in patients with multiple myeloma. Am J Med 1984; 76: 247—56.
23. Chomdeg B. Bell PD, Navar LG. Renal hemodynamic and autoregulatory responses to acute hypercalcemia. Am J Physio 1977; 232: 490—6.
24. Humes HD, Ichikawa I, Troy JL Brenner BM. Evidence for a parathyroid hormone dependent influence of calcium on the glomerular ultrafiltration coefficient. J Clin Invest 1978; 61: 32—40.
25. Stevenson FK, Cleave AJ, Kent PW. The effect of ions on viscometric ultracentrifugal behaviour of Tamm-Horsfall glycoprotein. Biochem Biophys Acta 1971; 236: 59—66.
26. Melcion C, Mougenot B, Baudouin B, Ronco P, Moulonguet-Doleris L, Vanhille PH, Beaufils M, Morel-Maroger L, Verroust P, Richet G. Renal failure in myeloma: relationship with isoelectric point of immunoglobulin light chains. Clin Nephrol 1984; 22: 138—43.

5. Light chain-related tubulointerstitial nephropathy

PAUL W. SANDERS, GUILLERMO A. HERRERA & JOHN H. GALLA

Renal failure remains a major complication of multiple myeloma, occurring in about half of the patients with this disease; its presence is associated with a markedly shortened patient survival [1, 2, 3]. Although several different renal lesions may develop, the one most commonly recognized is a tubulointerstitial nephropathy often referred to as 'myeloma kidney' [1]. The characteristic features of this lesion include proximal tubule damage with atrophy and distal nephron cast formation. Bence Jones proteins (BJP), which are immunoglobulin LC's in monomeric, dimeric, and aggregated forms, have been shown to be the most important association with renal failure [4, 5]. Also parenteral administration of LC's has reproduced this tubulointerstitial lesion in mouse and rat models.

The current proposed pathogenetic mechanisms of tubule injury by BJP's include direct toxicity to the epithelial cells of the proximal tubule and intratubular obstruction. Both of these mechanisms have been demonstrated in our laboratory [6, 7]. They are not mutually exclusive and may produce renal damage in concert.

In the first series of experiments, we examined the propensity of BJP's to produce proximal tubule injury in humans. Renal biopsy specimens of patients (BJP group) who had LC proteinuria, no recent exposure to nephrotoxic agents, and no evidence of distal nephron cast formation were examined using light, transmission electron and immunoelectron microscopy. The morphology of the proximal tubules was compared to a control group of patients who had glomerular lesions and nephrotic-range proteinuria. The two groups were comparable with respect to mean ages, serum creatinine concentrations, creatinine clearances, and urine protein excretion (Table 1).

Using light microscopy, semi-quantitiative evaluation of the morphology of the proximal tubules was performed. In the control group, the only significant finding was vacuolation of three of the 12 controls; desquamation and necrosis were not seen. In contrast, the proximal tubules of all 11

Minetti et al. (eds.), The kidney in plasma cell dyscrasias. ISBN 978-94-010-7085-0

Table 1. Comparisons of the two groups of patients.

	Controls	BJP	P
Age, years	49.0 ± 4	59.0 ± 3	NS
Serum creatinine, mg/dl	2.4 ± 0.5	3.2 ± 1.5	NS
Creatinine clearance, ml/min	65.0 ± 13	63.0 ± 12	NS
Urine protein, gm/24 h	9.9 ± 1.7	5.8 ± 1.7	NS
Number	12	11	

specimens exposed to monotypical LC's demonstrated significant vacuolation, desquamation and necrosis. Electron microscopy also demonstrated the relatively-normal appearance of the control tubules that were exposed to high intraluminal concentration of protein. However, the proximal tubules of the BJP group were abnormal, showing focal loss of the microvillus border, cell fragmentation and desquamation, and atypical lysosomes which were enlarged and distorted in appearance. These atypical lysosomes were peculiar to those proximal tubules exposed to monotypical LC's. Immunoelectron microscopy using an indirect immunogold-labeling technique demonstrated localization of monotypical LC's to the endolysosomal system of the experimental tubules.

These results suggested that:

1. Patients with monotypical LC proteinuria developed accumulation of the LC in the endolysosomal system of the proximal tubule cells. Associated with this lysosomal overload was necrosis and damage of the cells. These changes occurred in the absence of distal nephron cast formation.
2. Activation of the lysosomal system and atypical lysosomes were ubiquitous findings in those tubules exposed to LC's.
3. In contrast, with the exception of vacuolation of three of the specimens, none of these changes were demonstrated in the 12 control tubules that were exposed to protein other than LC.

Male Sprague-Dawley rats were anesthetized and prepared for microperfusion in standard fashion [7]. After identifying a suitable nephron that had multiple surface proximal convoluted tubule (PCT) segments, a bone wax cast was injected into the earliest accessible surface convolution. A pipet attached to a microperfusion pump was then inserted into the next available segment just distal to the wax block and the remaining nephron perfused for 20 minutes at 20nl/min. Trace amounts of [^{3}H]-inulin and [^{14}C]-glucose were also added to the ATF to calculate perfusion rate and unidirectional glucose flux, respectively.

Three different human BJP's, 2 kappa and 1 lambda, were used. These were purified from the urine of patients who had multiple myeloma and renal failure with the use of a combination of ammonium sulfate precipitation, ion exchange chromatography, and extensive dialysis. The proteins were added to the ATF in a concentration of 5 g/dl.

After perfusion for 20 minutes, a collection pipet was inserted into the latest accessible surface proximal convolution, an oil block was injected and a complete timed collection of tubule fluid made. The perfused segment was then injected with Microfil® and the tubules subsequently dissected and their lengths measured directly with a micrometer.

Results of each protein perfusion were compared to control perfusions that were obtained contemporaneously using artificial tubule fluid (ATF) alone. All values are expressed as mean ± standard error. Comparisons were made using an unpaired t-test with significance set at the 5% level.

In all of the following series of perfusions, the mean calculated perfusion rate and the length of the perfused segment of proximal convoluted tubule were not different from the appropriate controls.

In separate experiments, after perfusion of the nephron for 20 minutes, the nephron was reperfused with Carson Millonig fixative, dissected, and processed for routine transmission electron microscopy using standard techniques.

Perfusion of the PCT's with the first kappa BJP resulted in significant decreases in water, chloride and glucose absorptions, compared to the control perfusions (Table 2). Morphologic changes of the proximal tubule were found and included activation of the lysosomal system with appearance of atypical lysosomes, cell desquamation, and focal loss of the microvillus border. Thus, these changes were very similar to those described in

Table 2. Absorption characteristics of the in vivo microperfusion groups.

Group	Volume Absorption nl/min/mm	Chloride Absorption pEq/min/mm	Glucose Absorption pmol/min/mm
BJP1	1.37 ± 0.11	138 ± 16	32 ± 3
ATF1	2.30 ± 0.27	198 ± 23	44 ± 4
P	<0.05	<0.05	<0.05
BJP2	1.76 ± 0.22	195 ± 37	37 ± 3
ATF2	2.00 ± 0.23	179 ± 20	39 ± 3
P	NS	NS	NS
BJP3	1.62 ± 0.32	175 ± 24	38 ± 4
ATF3	1.40 ± 0.16	145 ± 16	42 ± 3
P	NS	NS	NS

those human proximal tubules exposed to monotypical LC's In addition, in the lumen of the distal tubule was a cellular cast.

The second protein was also a kappa LC. Water absorption, chloride absorption, and glucose absorption were not different from perfusions with ATF alone (Table 2). Unlike the first kappa LC, this protein did not alter proximal tubule morphology. In the distal nephron, however, there was a dense, homogeneous, acellular cast.

The last protein was a lambda LC. Volume absorption, chloride absorption, and glucose absorption were also not affected by the presence of the lambda protein (Table 2). This protein did not alter tubule morphology and precipitated in the distal nephron, forming an acellular cast.

We have also examined the perfused tubules for the presence of the LC with standard ultrastructural immunogold-labeling techniques similar to those used in the preceeding series of experiments with the human specimens. All three BJP's which labeled with the antibodies that were attached to 40 nm gold particles, were localized to the endolysosomal system of the perfused proximal tubules.

In summary, one of three human BJP's produced acute toxicity to rat proximal convoluted tubules, while the other two were nontoxic but appeared to produce distal nephron casts.

From these studies, we conclude that:

1. Some, but not all human BJP's are toxic to the epithelium of the proximal convoluted tubule of the rat and man.
2. Isotype does not appear to be a factor associated with toxicity.
3. More than one mechanism appears to be responsible for acute tubule damage that occurs with nephrotoxic BJP exposure. Intratubular obstruction from intraluminal precipitation of the BJP may occur independently of proximal tubule damage. Proximal tubule injury may decrease glomerular filtration rate by leaking or by causing intratubular obstruction from cellular casts resulting from desquamation of cell fragments. Finally, some patients with Bence Jones proteinuria may present without any renal damage. The reason for these phenomena is uncertain, but may relate to distinctive physicochemical properties of the BJP's.

Acknowledgement

This research is supported by Veterans Administration Merit Review and Career Development Awards.

References

1. Martinez-Maldonado M, Yium J, Suki WN, Eknoyan G. Renal complications in multiple myeloma: pathophysiology and some aspects of clinical management. J Chron Dis 1971; 24: 221—37.
2. Alexanian R, Balcerzak S, Bonnet JD, Gehan EA, Haut A, Hewlett JS, Monto RW. Prognostic factors in multiple myeloma. Cancer 1975; 36: 1192—1201.
3. Kyle RA: Multiple Myeloma. Review of 869 cases. Mayo Clin Proc 1975; 50: 29—40.
4. Defronzo RA, Humphrey RL, Wright JR, Cooke CR: Acute renal failure in multiple myeloma. Medicine (Baltimore) 1975; 54: 209—23.
5. Defronzo RA, Cooke CR, Wright JR, Humphrey RL. Renal function in patients with multiple myeloma. Medicine (Baltimore) 1978; 57: 151—66.
6. Weis JH, Williams RH, Galla JH, Gottschall JL, Rees ED, Bhathena D, Luke RG. Pathophysiology of acute Bence Jones protein nephrotoxicity in the rat. Kidney Int 1981; 20: 198—210.
7. Sanders PW, Herrera GA, Galla JH. Human Bence Jones protein toxicity in rat proximal tubule ephithelium in vivo. Kidney Int 1987; 32 (in press).

References

6. The pathogenesis of cast nephropathy

ARTHUR H. COHEN

Introduction

The initial description of the disease we now know as multiple myeloma occurred in 1848 when Bence Jones [1] described a novel protein in the urine of MacIntyre's patient with bone pain, edema, and constitutional symptoms. However, it was not until 1920 that Thannhauser and Krauss [2] reported unusual renal tubular structural abnormalities in a myeloma patient with proteinuria who succumbed from the illness. They described and illustrated a peculiar type of tubular cast; following contributions by other investigators, this renal lesion eventually became known as myeloma kidney, or more recently since the elucidation of the composition of the cast [3], Bence Jones cast nephropathy [4]. It is somewhat surprising that almost 75 years elapsed before the recognition of the distinctive pathological change in the kidneys, for it is well known that in excess of 50% of patients with multiple myeloma develop renal failure [5—11] and that the cast lesion is the most common structural feature [10, 12]. It is also surprising that virtually all patients with multiple myeloma do not develop renal impairment and cast formation, for it has been shown that abnormal free light chains are directly responsible for renal damage [7, 8, 13]. Finally, although the morphological features of the casts are well characterized [11], the events leading to their formation and the tissue reaction to their presence are controversial [6, 10, 15—21].

Definition

Myeloma kidney or Bence Jones cast nephropathy is that renal lesion evolving from precipitation of abnormal light chains in renal tubules, the formation of a unique cast, and the accumulation of cells around it [6, 10, 11, 18, 22, 23]. By light microscopy, the casts are typically large, refractile,

Minetti et al. (eds.), The kidney in plasma cell dyscrasias. ISBN 978-94-010-7085-0

contain numerous 'fracture' lines, may incorporate crystals, and/or may be layered or lamellated. They are frequently in tubules with discontinuities in basement membranes [23], are among the largest casts known [24], and have been found in the proximal nephron, including glomerular urinary spaces [6]. They have distinctive tinctorial features with the commonly employed stains. The casts are usually surrounded by various cells including desquamated tubular epithelium, polymorphonuclear leukocytes, lymphocytes, monocytes, and large multinucleated giant cells [6, 11, 23]. Knowledge of these characteristic morphologies may allow for precise diagnosis in the absence of a clinical history [25].

The composition of the casts has been studied in tissue sections, primarily with immunofluorescence microscopy [3, 10, 23, 26]. In most instances, at least the abnormal light chain is present, although it is invariably accompanied by the other light chain, immunoglobulins, albumin, and, when sought, Tamm-Horsfall protein [10, 23]. The casts may have a central less intense staining zone and a more heavily staining 'rim' with all antisera [3, 23].

The ultrastructural appearance of the casts is extremely variable; they may be of medium or deep electron density and may be coarsely or finely granular and/or crystalline [23]. The pale fibrillar matrix of Tamm-Horsfall protein may often be observed. The casts incorporate crystals, entire cells, or cytoplasmic debris [6, 23].

Pathogenetic considerations

The initial sophisticated studies of animal models of light chain renal damage by Clyne and coworkers [27] and Koss and colleagues [4], both groups ably supported by the keen morphological observations of Pirani, advanced our knowledge of the pathogenesis of renal tubular damage in multiple myeloma. Following injection of kappa light chains, purified from the urine of a myeloma patient, into the peritoneum of rats, Clyne et al. [27] demonstrated the formation of many kappa light chain-containing cytoplasmic droplets in proximal tubular cells. They also noted various "empty" and dense body-containing single membrane bound vacuoles and vesicles in these cells. Furthermore, dense crystals representing light chains were also in both intra- and extracellular sites. While ultrastructural and functional evidence of extensive tubular damage was produced, casts were not a feature of this model, perhaps because of the relatively short-term nature of the experiment. On the other hand, Koss, Pirani, and Osserman [4], using lambda light chain purified from another patient with myeloma, induced a nephropathy characterized by tubular cell protein crystals,

Bence Jones protein (lambda light chain) containing casts, and tubular cell degeneration. Large multinucleated cells were an infrequent feature of the damage, although polymorphonuclear leukocytes more commonly surrounded the casts. The ultrastructural and tinctorial properties of the casts were similar to the human lesion. These investigators also showed that the casts were composed initially of the injected light chain, and that after one day, Tamm-Horsfall protein was also present. These two models served as an impetus for further experimental work and represented important data clearly applicable to the human lesion.

In normal individuals, the small quantity of circulating free light chains is freely filtered by glomeruli and approximately 90% is reabsorbed and catabolized by proximal tubular cells [28—30]. In these cells, the light chains are taken up by a saturable, high-capacity low-affinity process of endocytosis. At the luminal surface of the cells, ingested light chains are incorporated in vesicles which fuse with lysosomes where proteases degrade the proteins [30,31]. Indeed, infusion of light chains in experimental animals causes a profound increase in phagolysosomes in proximal tubular cells [4, 21, 27]. Although lysosomal degradation is not usually a rate-limiting step for their disposition, it may not be adequate to handle large quantities of filtered light chain, as in multiple myeloma [31].

A variety of changes have been shown to affect the proximal tubular cells exposed to increased light chains. Functionally, there is diminished organic ion transport and gluconeogenesis [32] and inhibition of sodium-dependent uptake of amino acids and glucose by brush border preparations [33]. There is also low molecular weight proteinuria, even in patients with normal renal function [17, 34]. Structurally, in addition to phagolysosomes, there are swollen mitochondria which have partial loss of cristae in both experimental animals and human myeloma [21, 35, 36], and there are numerous clear and mitochondrial-remnant containing cytoplasmic vacuoles (autophagic vacuoles) [21]. With ultimate frank necrosis, tubular cells and fragments accumulate in the lumina and are incorporated into casts during their formation; this explains the constant ultrastructural finding of cytoplasmic debris in the pleomorphic myeloma casts, as described above [23].

Thus, in the face of deranged proximal tubular function and structure, the increased load of abnormal light chains in myeloma is not completely handled by the proximal tubules, thereby allowing light chains to advance to the distal nephron. In this location, they can co-precipitate with Tamm-Horsfall protein which is produced by cells of the thick ascending limb of the loop of Henle [37—39]. In vitro studies have demonstrated that Tamm-Horsfall and Bence Jones proteins coprecipitate [40, 41] and, therefore, lead to cast formation. There are several factors which further promote precipitation of Tamm-Horsfall protein, especially in conjunction with light chains. Radiographic dyes are well known to interact with Tamm-Horsfall protein [37], a fact that perhaps explains the observation that radiocontrast studies may promote the development of acute renal failure and cast nephropathy in some myeloma patients [7]. In addition, hypercalcemia may also cause direct precipitation of light chains [7], or may influence urine flow rate and composition because of dehydration, thereby favoring precipitation of Tamm-Horsfall protein with light chains [37, 39]. Clinically it is known that patients with cast nephropathy are more likely to have hypercalcemia [6, 7], and experimentally, increased serum calcium levels can worsen renal function and enhance nephrotoxicity of Bence Jones proteins [42].

Controversies

As noted above, Bence Jones protein casts are not a universal feature of the kidneys in myeloma, and not all patients with myeloma develop renal failure. These observations have generated considerable interest to attempt to determine what quality or qualities the abnormal light chains possess which are responsible for nephrotoxicity. Although it was once thought that lambda light chains were more toxic, studies by Cooper et al. [34] among others, demonstrated that there is no preferential toxicity based upon light chain class. Other properties, including amino acid composition, degree of polymerization [43], solubility, and quantity excreted do not relate to the development of renal failure or cast formation [7, 8]. Perhaps the most intensely studied characteristic of light chains in relation to renal damage is the net electrical charge. In humans, experimental animals, and in vitro conditions, it has been suggested that light chains with high isoelectric points (pI) are more nephrotoxic than those with low or lower pIs, especially if the urine pH is lower than the light chain pI. Clyne and coworkers [41] were the first to focus attention on this property, and have caused many investigators to examine the role of electrical charge [10, 15, 16, 18, 19, 20, 21, 39, 45]. This concept appears to have certain validity for cast formation, especially since the pI of Tamm-Horsfall proteins is 3.2 [37, 39]; this would allow greater interaction between and precipitation of cationic Bence Jones and anionic Tamm-Horsfall proteins. Indeed, in a study of myeloma patients with renal damage, Hill and associates [18] found that anionic light chains usually were not associated with myeloma casts, whereas more cationic light chains did have casts, their frequency and prominence increasing with higher pIs. These morphological findings correlated with clinical data of Coward et al. [16] who demonstrated a direct relationship between urinary cationic light chains and diminished renal function in myeloma patients.

However, these observations have not been confirmed by others in studies of both human disease and a rat model of cast nephropathy [10, 15, 19, 20, 21, 39]. For functional aspects in humans, Johns et al. [19], Cooper et al. [34], Melcion et al. [15], and Rota et al. [10] found no relationship between the pI of urinary light chains and renal function. The study of Rota [10] also included tissue examination of most patients; there was also no correlation between light chain pI and presence of Bence Jones cast nephropathy. Perhaps the most convincing evidence against a primary nephrotoxic role of light chain pI is from the innovative experimental works of Smolens and coworkers [20, 21]. They used a rat model of myeloma in which four different plasma cell tumors, each producing kappa light chains of different pI, were transplanted into the same strain of animals. In their experiments, they demonstrated the development of cast nephropathy in animals excreting light chains of pI 5.2, tubular necrosis in animals excreting light chains of pI 4.3, and no cast nephropathy in animals excreting light chains with pI 6.7 or 7.6. The discrepancies in results from the different groups of investigators are clearly unexplained; however at the present time, the bulk of evidence suggests that the isoelectric charge of light chains is neither an important nor the only factor in the pathogenesis of Bence Jones cast nephropathy.

The basic description of morphology of the casts is agreed upon by most investigators. It is the nature of the large multinucleated cells which often surround them that has generated considerable controversy throughout the years. Early reports indicated that the cells were multinucleated giant cells similar to those in foreign body reactions or granulomata [2, 46]. However, beginning in the early 1950's and for many years beyond, the prevalent view was that they were a peculiar 'syncytium' of tubular epithelial cells [47, 48, 49]. Since the mid-1970's, however, this view has been challenged; several ultrastructural studies identified the cells to be of histiocytic (monocyte) origin [23, 50, 51, 52]. They were shown to gain access to the tubules through basement membrane discontinuities [23]. Nevertheless, even at the present time there is continued dissent; among others, Sessa and colleagues [14] have described multinucleated tubular epithelium to surround the casts in electron microscopic studies. In the first report of its kind to date, Sedmak and Tubbs [53], using monoclonal antibodies to renal tubular epithelium and to monocytes/macrophages, demonstrated the giant cells surrounding casts to be of macrophage origin in the single patient evaluated. Furthermore, Start and colleagues [54] have very recently found similar results in a larger group of patients studied. It seems reasonable to conclude that monocytes and histiocytes must play a major role in the reaction to the abnormal light chains. This is postulated not only on the above information, but on the basis of observations, both in the kidney and in other organs, of the tissue reaction to crystalline light chains. As is well known, light chains may crystallize in cells and tissues [27]; crystals in non-renal and intra- and extravascular sites may be ingested by histiocytes or may be incorporated within granulomata [6]. While this rare form of tissue damage in plasma cell dyscrasias is usually associated with an abnormal kappa light chain [55, 56], we (Cohen AH, Schoenfeld L, Guziel L, unpublished observations) and others [57] have studied patients with monoclonal lambda light chain, widespread crystals and associated granulomata present throughout both kidneys and other tissues. As light chains in crystalline form can be associated with granuloma and giant cell formation, it is entirely conceivable that non-crystalline light chains can induce a similar cellular reaction when exposed to tissue or blood borne monocytes or histiocytes. This can occur in the kidney as the casts come into contact with interstitial leukocytes through breaks in the tubular basement membranes [23].

The reasons for the development of tubular basement membrane discontinuities are unknown. It is possible that they result from lesions of tubular necrosis, as has been demonstrated previously [58, 59, 60]. Alternatively, it is possible that the breaks are a consequence of the piercing action of light chain crystals within tubular cells or casts; this is highly unlikely, in that crystals of any size were an inconstant feature of our cases [23] and were not specifically identified in the study of Rota et al. [10] which also noted tubular basement membrane ruptures. It is possible that breaks result from collagenase and other proteases produced by infiltrating monocytes and other inflammatory cells, similar to lesions in acutely rejecting renal transplants [61].

Regardless of pathogenesis, Bence Jones protein casts and light chain proteinuria may contribute to permanent or temporary renal functional impairment by one or all of several mechanisms. Damage to tubular cells, discussed above, is quite obvious and probably results in tubular dysfunction, including partial or complete Fanconi syndrome, and necrosis. With formation of large casts, there may be nephron obstruction. This is supported by the demonstration of Tamm-Horsfall protein in glomerular urinary spaces both by us [23] and Rota and colleagues [10]. This finding has been shown to be indicative of intratubular urinary back-flow [62], and the increased tubular pressure may cause diminution of glomerular filtration. Finally interstitial edema and inflammation consequent to tubular necrosis, cast formation, and/or tubular basement membrane ruptures may be associated with altered function by well described means [63].

References

1. Bence Jones H. On a new substance occurring in the urine of a patient with 'mollities ossium'. Phil Tr Royal Soc London 1848; 138: 55.
2. Thannhauser SJ, Krauss E. Uber eine degenerative Erkrankung der Harnkanalchen (Nephrose) bei Bence-Jones'scher Albuminurie mit Nierenschwund (kleine, glatte, weisse Niere). Dtsch Arch Klin Med 1920; 133: 183—92.
3. Levi DF, Williams RC, Lindstrom FD. Immunofluorescent studies of the myeloma kidney with special reference to light chain disease. Am J Med 1968; 44: 922—33.
4. Koss MN, Pirani CL, Osserman EF. Experimental Bence Jones cast nephropathy. Lab Invest 1976; 34: 579—91.
5. DeFronzo RA, Cooke CR, Wright JR, Humphrey RL. Renal function in patients with multiple myeloma. Medicine 1978; 57: 151—66.
6. Silva FG, Pirani CL, Mesa-Tejeda R, Williams G. The kidney in plasma cell dyscrasias: a review and clinicopathologic study of 50 patients. In: Fenoglio CE, Wolff M, eds. Progress in Surgical Pathology. New York: Masson, 1982: 131—176.
7. Fang LST. Light-chain nephropathy. Kidney Int 1985; 27: 582—92.
8. Soloman A. Clinical implications of monoclonal light chains. Semin Oncol 1986; 13: 341—9.
9. Hamble TJ. The kidney in myeloma. Br Med J 1986; 292: 2—3.
10. Rota S, Mougenot B, Baudouin B, de Meyer-Brasseur M, Lemaitre V, Michel C, Mignon F, Rondeau E, Vanhille P, Verroust P, Ronco R. Multiple myeloma and severe renal failure: a clinicopathologic study of outcome and prognosis in 34 patients. Medicine 1987; 66: 126—37.
11. Cohen AH. Pathology of light chain nephropathies. In:Robinson RR, ed. Nephrology. New York: Springer-Verlag, 1984: 895—904.
12. Pasquali S, Zucchelli P, Cassanova S, Cagnoli L, Confalonieri R, Pozzi C, Banfi G, Lupo A, Bertani T. Renal histological lesions and clinical syndromes in multiple myeloma. Clin Nephrol 1987; 27: 222—8.
13. Bradley JR, Thiru S, Evans DB. Light chains and the kidney. J Clin Pathol 1987; 40: 53—60.
14. Sessa A, Torri Tarelli L, Meroni M, Ferrario G, Giordano F, Volpi A. Multinucleated giant cells in myeloma kidney: an ultrastructural study. Appl Pathol 1984; 2: 185—94.
15. Melcion C, Mougenot B, Baudouin B, Ronco P, Moulonguet-Doleris L, Vanhille Ph, Beaufils M, Morel-Maroger L, Verroust P, Richet G. Renal failure in myeloma: relationship with isoelectric point of immunoglobulin light chains. Clin Nephrol 1984; 22: 138—43.
16. Coward RA, Delamore EW, Mallick NP, Robinson EL. The importance of urinary immunoglobulin light chain isoelectric point (pI) in nephrotoxicity in multiple myeloma. Clin Sci 1984; 66: 229—32.
17. Coward RA, Mallick NP, Delamore IW. Tubular function in multiple myeloma. Clin Nephrol 1985; 24: 180—5.
18. Hill GS, Morel-Maroger L, Mery J-P, Brouet JC, Mignon F. Renal lesions in multiple myeloma: their relationship to associated protein abnormalities. Am J Kid Dis 1983; 2: 423—38.
19. Johns EA, Turner R, Cooper EH, MacLennan ICM. Isoelectric points of urinary light chains in myelomatosis: analysis in relation to nephrotoxicity. J. Clin Pathol 1986; 39: 833—7.

20. Smolens P, Venkatachalam M, Stein JH. Myeloma kidney cast nephropathy in a rat model of multiple myeloma. Kidney Int 1983; 24: 192—204.
21. Smolens P, Barnes JL, Stein JH. Effect of chronic administration of different Bence Jones proteins on rat kidney. Kidney Int 1986; 30: 874—82.
22. Cohen AH, Adler SG. Nephrotoxicity of myeloma proteins. Plasma Ther Transfus Technol 1984; 5: 531—41.
23. Cohen AH, Border WA. Myeloma kidney, an immunomorphogenetic study of renal biopsies, Lab Invest 1980; 42: 248—56.
24. Oliver J. New directions in renal morphology: a method, its results and its future. Harvey Lect 1944—45; 40: 102—55.
25. Border WA, Cohen AH. Renal biopsy diagnosis of clinically silent multiple myeloma. Ann Intern Med 1980; 93: 43—6.
26. Isobe T, Matsumoto J, Fujita T, Maeda S, Sugiyama T. Localization of Bence Jones proteins in the kidney of myeloma patients. Jap J Med 1982; 21: 12—6.
27. Clyne DH, Brendstrup L, First MR, Pesce AT, Finkel PN, Pollak VE, Pirani CL. Renal effect of intraperitoneal kappa chain injection. Lab Invest 1974; 31: 131—42.
28. Strober W, Waldmann TA. The role of the kidney in the metabolism of plasma proteins. Nephron 1974; 13: 35—66.
29. Solling K. Free light chains of immunoglobulins. Scand J Clin Lab Invest 1981; 41: Suppl 157: 1—83.
30. Falconer Smith JF, Van Hegan RI, Esnouf MP, Ross BD. Characteristics of renal handling of human immunoglobulin light chain by the perfused rat kidney. Clin Sci 1979; 57: 113—20.
31. Maack T, Park CH, Camargo MJF. Renal filtration, transport, and metabolism of proteins. In: Seldin DW, Giebisch G, eds. The Kidney: Physiology and pathophysiology. New York: Raven Press 1985: 1773—1803.
32. Preuss HG, Hammack WJ, Murdaugh HV. The effects of Bence Jones protein on the in vitro function of rabbit renal cortex. Nephron 1967; 5: 210—6.
33. Batuman V, Sastrasinh M, Sastrasinh S. Light chain effects on alanine and glucose uptake by renal brush border membranes. Kidney Int 1984; 30: 662—5.
34. Cooper EH, Forbes MA, Crockson RA, MacLennan, ICM. Proximal renal tubular function in myelomatosis: observations in the fourth Medical Research Council trial. J Clin Pathol 1984; 37: 852—8.
35. Costanza DJ, Smoller M. Multiple myeloma with the Fanconi syndrome: a study of a case with electron microscopy of the kidney. Am J Med 1963; 34: 125—33.
36. Fisher ER, Perez-Stable E, Zawadski ZA. Ultrastructural renal changes in multiple myeloma with comments relative to the mechanism of proteinuria, Lab Invest 1964; 13: 1561—74.
37. Hoyer JR, Seiler MW. Pathophysiology of Tamm-Horsfall protein. Kidney Int 1979; 16: 279—89.
38. Cohen AH. Morphology of renal tubular hyaline casts. Lab Invest 1981; 44: 280—7.
39. Ronco P, Brunisholz M, Geniteau-Legendre M, Chatelet F, Verroust P, Richet G. Pathophysiologic aspects of Tamm-Horsfall protein: a phylogenetically conserved marker of the thick ascending limb of Henle's loop. Adv Nephrol 1987; 16: 231—50.
40. Kant KS, Pease AJ, Clyne DH, Pollak VE. Co-precipitation of Tamm-Horsfall protein with myoglobin, hemoglobin, Bence Jones protein and albumin: effect of pH. Clin Res 1977; 25: 594A.
41. Clyne DH, Kant KS, Pesce AJ. Nephrotoxicity of low molecular weight serum proteins: physico chemical interactions between myoglobin, hemoglobin, Bence Jones proteins and Tamm-Horsfall mucoprotein. Curr Probl Clin Biochem 1979; 9: 299—308.
42. Smolens P, Kreisberg JR. Modest hypercalcemia can markedly increase the nephrotoxicity of Bence Jones protein, Kidney Int 1985; 27: 238.

43. Solling K, Solling J, Nielsen JL. Polymeric Bence Jones proteins in serum in myeloma patients with renal insufficiency. Acta Med Scand 1984; 216: 495—502.
44. Clyne DH, Pesce AJ, Thompson, RE. Nephrotoxicity of Bence Jones proteins in the rat: importance of protein isoelectric point. Kidney Int 1979; 16: 345—52.
45. Holland MD, Galla, JH, Sanders PW, Luke RG. Effect of urinary pH and diatrizoate on Bence Jones nephrotoxicity in the rat. Kidney Int 1985; 27: 46—50.
46. Fishberg AM. Hypertension and Nephritis. 5th ed. Philadelphia: Lea and Febiger, 1954: 440.
47. Allen AC. The kidney: medical and surgical diseases. New York: Grune and Stratton, 1951: 280.
48. Heptinstall RH. Pathology of the kidney. 2nd ed. Boston: Little Brown & Co, 1974: 762.
49. Dunnill MS. Pathologic Basis of Renal Disease. Philadelphia: WB Saunders, 1976: 281—284.
50. Jones, DB. Myeloma nephropathy, a light chain storage disease. Am J Pathol 1975; 78: 49a—50a.
51. Factor SM, Winn RM, Biempica L. The histiocytic nature of the multinucleated giant cells in myeloma kidney. Human Pathol 1978; 9: 114—20.
52. Papadimitriou JM, Matz LR. The origin of multinucleate giant cells in myeloma kidney from mononucluear phagocytes: an ultrastructural study. Pathol 1979; 11: 583—93.
53. Sedmak DD, Tubbs RO. The macrophagic origin of multinucleated giant cells in myeloma kidney: an immunohistologic study. Human Pathol 1987; 18: 304—6.
54. Start DA, Silva FG, David LD, D'Agati V, Pirani C. Myeloma cast nephropathy: immunohistochemical and lectin studies. Kidney Int (In press).
55. Terashima K, Takahashi K, Kojima M, Imai Y, Tsuchida S, Migita S, Ebina S, Itoh C. Kappa-type light chain crystal storage histiocytosis. Acta Pathol Jpn 1978; 28: 111—38.
56. Takahashi K, Naito M, Takatsuki K, Kono F, Chitose M, Ooshima S, Mori N, Sakuma H, Uchino F. Multiple myeloma, IgAK type, accompanying crystal-storing histiocytosis and amyloidosis. Acta Pathol Jpn 1987; 37: 141—54.
57. Dornan TL, Blundell JW, Morgan AG, Burden RP, Reeves WG, Cotton RE. Widespread crystallisation of paraprotein in myelomatosis. Quart J Med 1985; 57: 659—67.
58. Bywaters EGL, Dible JH. The renal lesion in traumatic anuria, J Path Bact 1942; 54: 111—20.
59. Solez K, Morel-Maroger L, Sraer J-D. The morphology of 'acute tubular necrosis' in man: analysis of 57 renal biopsies and a comparison with the glycerol model. Medicine 1979; 58: 362—76.
60. Ooi BS, Weiss MA, Kant KS, Hong CD, Pollak VE, Andriole VT. Antibody to Tamm-Horsfall protein after acute tubular necrosis. Am J Nephrol 1981; 1: 48—51.
61. Cohen AH, Border WA, Rajfer J, Dumke A, Glassock RJ. Interestitial Tamm-Horsfall protein in rejecting renal allografts: identification and morphologic pattern of injury, Lab Invest 1984; 50: 519—25.
62. McGiven AR, Hunt JS, Day WA, Bailey RR. Tamm-Horsfall protein in the glomerular capsular space. J Clin Pathol 1978; 31: 620—5.
63. Kourilsky O, Solez K, Morel-Maroger L, Whelton A, Duhoux P, Sraer J-D. The pathology of acute renal failure due to interstitial nephritis in man with comments on the role of interstitial inflammation and sex in gentamicin nephrotoxicity. Medicine 1982; 61: 258—68.

7. Light chain nephrotoxicity: A forum

N. P. MALLICK, E. H. COOPER, R. A. COWARD, P. RONCO, G. WILLIAMS, P. SMOLENS, J. S. CAMERON, G. GALLO, C. L. PIRANI, A. SOLOMON, A. H. COHEN & S. PASQUALI

MALLICK: I wonder whether there is another biochemical marker of light chain nephrotoxicity that might be more valuable than the ones we have been considering. It is really a pity that the pI of light chains has not proved to be a more obvious marker of damage, because that would have really helped out: something between biochemistry and the clinician would have been really valuable.

COOPER: Because of certain advances in chromatography you can now pull basic proteins out of urine very easily. Of course the classic examples are lysozime and postgamma globulin, and any light chains which are of a basic nature. If we could narrow the window of protein spectra we might manage to get some more information. In many patients the light chain load diminishes in response to therapy, so that the tubular disfunction, as measured by the reabsorption of other indicator proteins, will gradually improve. Many of them will go to a stage of having a normal tubular function and still be maintaining their chemotherapy; the chemotherapy agents that seem to particularly upset the tubular function are drugs like methotrexate, which is not widely used at the moment.

COWARD: We found the highest level of NAG in a patient with crystal deposits in tubular cells, and normal renal function. Following chemotherapy the paraprotein responded and the urinary NAG levels fell.

COOPER: In the follow-up patients who had normal serum creatinine at presentation had still a high probability to develop a fall of renal function in the succeeding years.

RONCO: The Tamm-Horsfall protein has become the subject of great interest, since it was recently reported that this protein is homologous or identical with uromodulin, which would have very significant immunoregulatory function. However a definite convincing evidence that the two proteins are identical has not yet been provided.

WILLIAMS: About the potential toxicity of THP on its own, I wonder whether we have to regard THP as a toxicity marker through its attachement to light chains or ascribe to it an intrinsic toxicity.

Minetti et al. (eds.), The kidney in plasma cell dyscrasias. ISBN 978-94-010-7085-0

RONCO: I think the THP deposits either in the interstitium, or in the basal space are only a marker of disease. My guess is that THP does not induce further damage to the kidney. The reason of my guess is that, first, the humoral immunoresponse to THP is often very low and is made of antibodies with very low affinity. In addition, and most important, immunoglobulin deposits, and they were never detected along the thick ascending limb of the Henle's loop, where the protein is synthesized. Regarding the cellular immuneresponse, it is possible that cellular immuneresponse directed to THP plays some role, but I don't think this role is crucial, since in many cases THP interstitial deposits were not associated with any cellular inflammatory reactions.
SMOLENS: We did look for bound light chains by immunoflourescence and we found they were present in the casts. We also found it in some of the tubular cells but we did not find it bound to basement membranes. The light chains we used in our experimental model were all monomers, but a couple of percent that were dimers or trimers.
MALLICK: There are a 50% of patients with myeloma who develop uremia at some stage and 50% do not. I wonder where this damage is coming from? Primarily the tubule, only the cast or a combination of both?
CAMERON: I would focus on the interstitial infiltrate, which has been mentioned, but soon dismissed. We see a number of patients with myeloma and a decrease of renal function, without renal infiltration with plasma cells, in which there is a considerable tubulo-interstitial infiltrate, predominantly or not exclusively composed of T-helper lymphocites, with a minority of macrophages and, interestingly enough, some eosinophils. I don't think we should write off this infiltrate. I think this may well be, if not an initiating factor, a continuing factor in the damage. One possible mechanism we might like to speculate about is the one recently suggested of non-immunologic activation of complement within the interstitium. This mechanism was studied first of all within a rat remnant kidney model, and more recently within hypokalemia-induced interstitial nephropathy. It seems very likely that this mechanism operates in all interstitial nephropathies, and myeloma would therefore be no exception. The mechanism is the non immunologic cleavage of C3 by ammonia at ambient concentrations, which leads to deposition of the C 5—9 membrane attack complex of complement. Thus, I would like to ask Dr Ronco and perhaps Dr Smolens: even though immunoglobulins were not there, was there any complement which you would just dismiss, or did you not look for complement? I think we may be all ignoring the complement just because, if immunoglobulines are not there, its presence may be considered an artefact, as may have occurred in the past in a number of situations of which myeloma may be one.

RONCO: With regard to the experimental model, we have not looked for complement in the interstitium or the glomeruli. As far as the patients are concerned, C3 deposits have been searched in all the biopsies, and fixation of C3 antiserum has been occasionally observed on proximal tubular epithelium and in some casts, but not in interstitium.
SMOLENS: In our experimental model we did not look for complement deposition in the kidney.
GALLO: We have never seen complement in the interstitium in our human cases of light chain nephropathy. Occasionally in tubular basement membranes we see complement as in other different diseases, but there was nothing significant in terms of C3 or Clq in patients with LCDD.
PIRANI: Dr Smolens raised a very good point that in experimental models, when you inject human light chain proteins, you can produce antibodies to these light chains and introduce immunologic phenomena. What is the evidence that light chains, either normal or abnormal, can produce antibodies? Could the abnormal light chain become antigen?
SOLOMON: It is certainly possible to induce anti-human light chain antibodies by immunizing mice or rats with human Bence Jones proteins. In our mouse model, we have not seen such antibodies. Certain human rheumatoid factors with specificity for human light chain determinants have been reported. We have not found such autoantibodies in our patients with myeloma.
CAMERON: We have heard from other people's data that there is not a terribly good correlation between the presence or the absence of casts and the degree of renal function impairment in people with myeloma. By the way, you might take the easy way out and say that the casts were there and that they had been washed away after having done their damage.
COHEN: From a morphological point of view, the development of renal functional impairment in patients with myeloma must be multifactorial. As we have heard, the presence of Tamm-Horsfall protein in the urinary space is a marker of urine obstruction. There is a functional and structural damage to tubular cells, and perhaps interstitial inflammation. It is clear that all of these do play some role. I am just not prepared to take a stand on which is the most important. In our own renal biopsy experience which, by definition, is tilted toward patients who either present with acute renal failure in the absence of diagnosis of multiple myeloma or who have multiple myeloma in whom renal failure apparently appears unexpected, the vast majority of the patients have combined tubular cell damage, vacuoles, mytochondial damage, and casts. In fact, in my experience, the casts are seen more commonly than the tubular cell damage. As far as the washing away of the casts, they are actually quite large and I suspect that, even though in follow-up tissue examination the casts do disappear, some

of them must be so large that they do get stuck and stay for a long time. I might emphasize that there are many anatomically peculiar things about the tubular casts. They are among the only casts that seem to be fractured or broken. I didn't read anything in the literature that would tell me why the casts have these peculiar fractures, nor do I have any reasonable explanation of my own except perhaps for the influence of crystallization of protein.

PIRANI: In a case of cast nephropathy what is the percentage of casts that you would consider typical myeloma casts?

COHEN: All patients with multiple myeloma and casts do not necessarily have casts that are surrounded by giant cells (these are macrophages phenotypically as they bear all the appropriate markers with monoclonal antibodies) and, indeed, just the tinctorial and structural properties of the casts, rather than the cellular reaction to them, are sufficient to be able to recognize them as being predominantly of light chain composition. As for the percent of casts with surrounding giant cells within the average renal biopsy, with myeloma cast nephropathy, I would say in the range of 25 to 33%. A smaller number of tubules have clearcut discontinuities in the walls but not necessarily giant cells, but with either polymorphs or other cells, including desquamated tubular epithelium surrounding them. It is by no means a universal feature.

WILLIAMS: May I return to the tubular rhexis and invite Dr Cohen to outline perhaps the sequence of events which lead up to it. If this is related to, or based on macrophage lytic activity, how do you see this actually evolving? Does lysis proceed from interstitial macrophages outside the lumen attracted possibly by the cast composition or by macrophages entering through 'intact' basement membranes and then causing lytic damage secondary to their reaction with the luminal casts?

COHEN: I think that either explanation is possible. If you consider non myeloma associated acute tubular necrosis, not necessarily of the nephrotoxic type, breaks in tubular basement membranes do occur, and in fact are often associated with spillage of cast matrix, i.e. Tamm-Horsfall protein cast, into the interstitium. This was well described in the initial reports of traumatic anuria by Bywaters and coworkers in the early 40s. In addition, it is entirely possible that either through those breaks, or for some other reason through intact tubular basement membranes, the monocytes may migrate and then may either cause initial or further tubular basement membrane damage through their production of various proteases. So I think therefore, that both mechanisms are entirely possible.

PASQUALI: How do you explain the presence of all immunoglobulin classes — IgG, IgA, IgM — and albumin in addition to light chains in the casts of some myeloma patients?

COHEN: In the absence of demonstrable glomerular damage, which these patients do not have, the only way that I can postulate the presence of other plasma protein, except for the other light chain, is that they are incorporated into the casts through the breaks of the tubular membrane by diffusion out of the peritubular capillaries, across the interstitium, into the tubule. The presence of the other light chain can easily be explained by continued normal glomerular filtration of small quantities of normal light chain, which in face of proximal tubular cell damage, can pass into the distal nephron, where it is incorporated into the cast.

PIRANI: I would like to provide a possible answer to the previous question, about IgG and C3 in the casts. I think that normal urine contains small amounts of IgG and C3. Immunofluorescence notoriously is not a quantitative type of determination, so even a very small amount of these proteins could give a positive reaction even if the glomeruli are perfectly normal. I concur with Dr Cohen that the intensity of the fluorescence in these casts is rather exceptional.

Part III. The kidney involvement in plasma cell dyscrasias

1. Kidney in multiple myeloma and related disorders

ROBERT A. KYLE

Proteinuria was a major feature in the case of multiple myeloma described by Macintyre in 1850 [1]. Despite the excretion of 60 g of protein daily, the kidneys appeared normal on both gross and microscopic examinations. The kidneys had 'proved equal to the novel office assigned them' and had 'discharged the task without sustaining, on their part, the slightest danger.' Little attention was paid to this disease until 1889 when Otto Kahler [2] described a striking case with the same urinary characteristics that had been described by Henry Bence Jones in 1848 [3].

The plasma cell dyscrasias are a group of disorders characterized by the proliferation of plasma cells that produce a homogeneous monoclonal (M) protein.

Analysis of urine for the evaluation of monoclonal proteins

The analysis of urine is essential in all cases of plasma cell dyscrasias. The use of sulfosalicylic acid, or Exton's reagent, is best for the detection of protein. In many laboratories, dipsticks are used to screen for protein. However, dipsticks are often insensitive to Bence Jones protein and should not be used when the possibility of Bence Jones proteinuria exists.

Almost from the time of the discovery of the unique thermal properties of urinary light chains, screening tests for the detection of these light chains have been in use. All such tests have shortcomings, but the heat test of Putnam et al. [4] is the simplest. Most, but not all, monoclonal light chains in the urine precipitate at 40°C to 60°C, dissolve at 100°C, and reprecipitate on cooling to between 40°C and 60°C. Occasionally, the result of the heat test is positive even though there is no sharp peak or localized globulin band on urine electrophoresis and no evidence of a single monoclonal light chain on urine immunoelectrophoresis. Such urine usually produces a broad-based gamma band and normal-appearing κ and λ arcs. Presumably, the positive result of the test is due to an excess of polyclonal

Minetti et al. (eds.), The kidney in plasma cell dyscrasias. ISBN 978-94-010-7085-0

light chains. These false-positive results occur often in renal insufficiency. However, the results of the Bence Jones heat test have been negative in some instances in which large amounts of a monoclonal light chain are present. In addition, the heat test is not sensitive and will not recognize small amounts of Bence Jones protein. The heat test for Bence Jones protein has many shortcomings and should not be used except as a rough screening procedure. The recognition of Bence Jones proteinuria depends on the demonstration of a monoclonal light chain by immunoelectrophoresis or immunofixation of an adequately concentrated urine specimen.

Electrophoresis, as well as immunoelectrophoresis or immunofixation, should be done in all instances of plasma cell dyscrasia. Immunoelectrophoresis or immunofixation of urine also should be done in evaluation of older patients who have an apparently idiopathic nephrotic syndrome.

First, a 24-hour collection of urine must be made for determination of the total amount of protein excreted each day. This determination is important when following the course of a patient, because the amount of monoclonal light chain correlates directly with the size of the plasma cell burden. A urinary monoclonal protein is seen as a dense, localized band on the cellulose strip or as a tall, narrow, homogeneous peak on the densitometer tracing (Fig. 1). Immunoelectrophoresis establishes the pre-

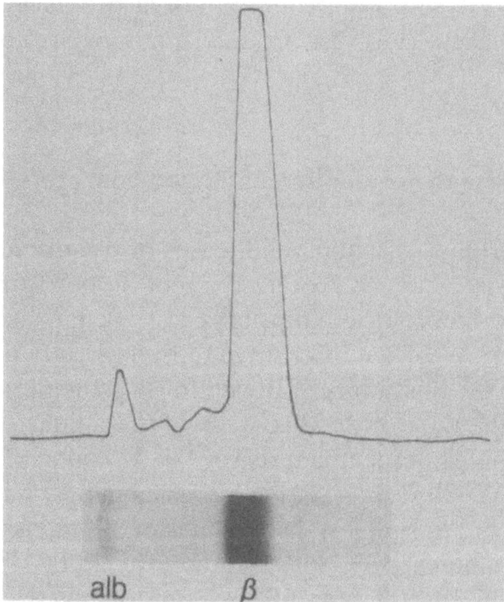

Fig. 1. Monoclonal urine protein. Top, Densitometer tracing showing a tall, narrow-based peak of β mobility; bottom, cellulose acetate electrophoretic pattern showing a dense band of β mobility. This is consistent with a monoclonal urine protein (Bence Jones protein). (From Kyle RA, Garton JP. Laboratory monitoring of myeloma proteins. Semin Oncol 1986; 13: 310—7. By permission of Grune & Stratton.)

sence or absence of light chains and determines whether they are monoclonal or polyclonal. It is not unusual for the protein reaction to be negative and for immunoelectrophoresis of concentrated urine to reveal a monoclonal light chain. Immunofixation is helpful in detecting a monoclonal protein and is more sensitive than immunoelectrophoresis [5]. Immunofixation is most helpful when a monoclonal light chain occurs in the presence of a polyclonal increase in light chains and is also useful in the detection of monoclonal heavy chains or fragments in the urine (Fig. 2).

The presence of a monoclonal light chain in the urine of a patient with a large amount of albumin and insignificant amounts of globulin (nephrotic syndrome) most often indicates the presence of a primary systemic amyloidosis (AL) or light-chain deposition disease.

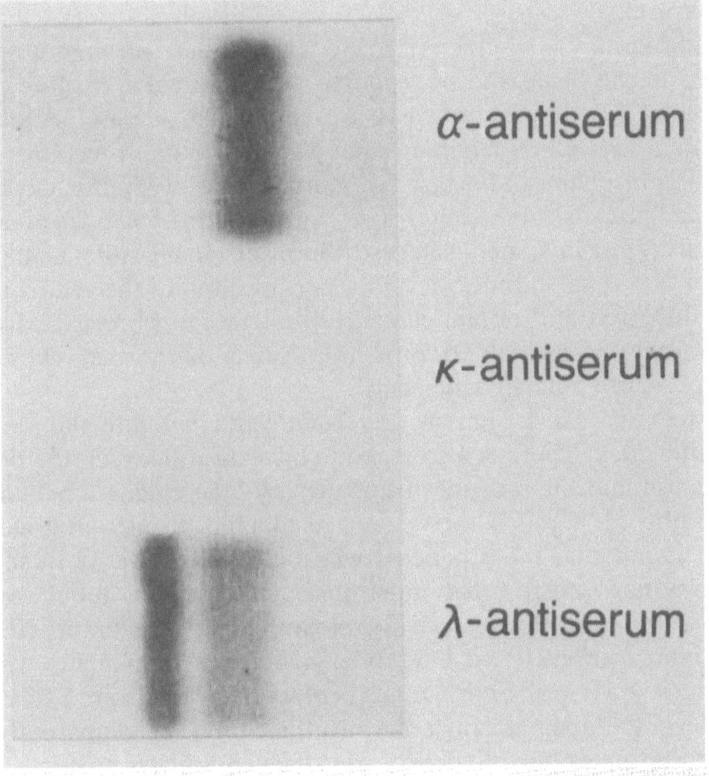

Fig. 2. Immunofixation of urine. Top, Narrow localized band with IgA (α) antiserum; middle, no reaction with κ antiserum; bottom, two discrete bands with λ antiserum. This patient has a monoclonal λ protein plus an IgA λ fragment. (From Kyle RA, Garton JP. Laboratory monitoring of myeloma proteins. Semin Oncol 1986; 13: 310–7. By permission of Grune & Stratton.)

Multiple myeloma

Proteinuria, detected on routine urinalysis, was present in 65% of 456 patients with multiple myeloma who were seen at the Mayo Clinic from 1981 to 1986. At the time of diagnosis, the serum creatinine level was above normal (> 1.2 mg/dl) in 55% and ⩾ 2 mg/dl in 28%. A monoclonal light chain, detected by immunoelectrophoresis or immunofixation, was present in the urine in 79% of the patients at the time that they were first seen at the Mayo Clinic.

The two major causes of renal insufficiency are 'myeloma kidney' and hypercalcemia [6]. Dehydration, infection, nonsteroidal anti-inflammatory agents, antibiotics, roentgenographic contrast media, hyperuricemia, infiltration of the kidney by plasma cells, and increased blood viscosity may all contribute to renal insufficiency. In most patients, the cause of renal failure is multifactorial.

Myeloma kidney is characterized by the presence of large waxy, laminated casts in the distal and occasionally the proximal convoluted tubules and collecting tubules. These casts are composed of precipitated Bence Jones protein as well as albumin, IgG, Tamm-Horsfall mucoprotein, and polyclonal light chains. The casts are surrounded by multinucleated syncytial epithelial cells (giant cells). The giant cells originate from epithelial tubular cells [7] or in some instances from macrophages [8]. Dilatation and atrophy of the renal tubules develop, and eventually the entire nephron becomes distorted and nonfunctional [9]. Interstitial fibrosis and nephrocalcinosis may occur. Blood pressure usually is normal even in the presence of severe renal insufficiency.

The extent of cast formation correlates positively with the severity of renal insufficiency. There is also a good correlation between the degree of cast formation and the amount of free urinary light chains. The amount of interstitial fibrosis parallels the amount of tubular atrophy [10]. DeFronzo et al. [11] found that most patients who excreted > 1 g of Bence Jones protein daily had severe renal impairment and extensive tubular atrophy, while those without Bence Jones proteinuria had creatinine clearances > 50 ml/min. However, we have seen a number of patients who have excreted 1 to > 10 g of Bence Jones protein daily for from 5 to 21 years without developing significant renal insufficiency [12]. Apparently, some Bence Jones proteins have a nephrotoxic effect and others do not.

The mechanism of nephrotoxicity of Bence Jones proteinuria is unknown. Clyne and co-workers [13] suggest that Bence Jones proteins with an isoelectric point above 5.5 become positively charged when the urine pH is below 5.5 and co-precipitate with negatively charged Tamm-Horsfall mucoprotein that normally coats the tubule, thus forming tubular casts.

However, the role of the isoelectric point (pI) of Bence Jones protein is controversial. In a study of 23 patients with multiple myeloma, Coward and associates [14] found no correlation between urinary light chain excretion and the level of creatinine clearance. They reported a significant negative correlation between the pI of the light chain and the clearance of creatinine, implying a deleterious effect of Bence Jones proteins when pI values were higher. Other investigators suggested that pI values above 6.0 were associated with moderate renal failure [15]. However, Smolens et al. [16] suggested that the nephrotoxic effects of a Bence Jones protein resulted from factors other than its electrical charge, while Rota et al. [17] reported that pI did not have a crucial role in renal failure.

The immunologic type of Bence Jones protein probably has no significant role in nephrotoxicity. In a series of 119 patients with multiple myeloma seen at the Mayo Clinic from 1960—1971, no significant differences were found in the serum creatinine levels or in the amount of urinary light chain excretion [18]. Our recent experience with 263 patients seen from 1982—1986 showed that the median creatinine level was 1.2 mg/dl for patients with κ light chains and 1.3 mg/dl for patients with λ light chains. Also, 26% of patients with κ light chains had levels $\geqslant 2.0$ mg/dl whereas 34% of patients with λ light chains had levels $\geqslant 2.0$ mg/dl. Cooper et al. [19] reported that, in a series of 522 patients with myeloma, the serum creatinine level was elevated as frequently in patients with κ light-chain proteinuria as in those with λ light-chain proteinuria.

Nonsteroidal anti-inflammatory agents may have a role in the renal failure of myeloma. Rota et al. [17] reported that oliguria occurred in six of eight patients with severe renal failure who had been treated with nonsteroidal anti-inflammatory agents or analgesics. Another patient was treated with indomethacin and was found to have renal failure and myeloma kidney [20]. Craig and Powell [21] reported two patients with acute oliguric renal failure and two others with permanent worsening of renal function temporally related to the institution of nonsteroidal anti-inflammatory drugs.

Amyloid deposition also may produce the nephrotic syndrome or renal insufficiency or both. In one study [22], histologic documentation of amyloidosis was found in 7% of patients with multiple myeloma. The actual incidence of amyloidosis in myeloma is higher because biopsy for amyloid is not generally done unless the patient has symptoms or findings of amyloidosis. In addition, histologic proof is not sought in patients with myeloma in whom amyloidosis is suspected on the basis of such conditions as nephrotic syndrome, congestive heart failure, or carpal tunnel syndrome because finding such proof will not alter the therapy.

Acute renal failure has occurred after intravenous urography [23], although the risk probably is slight if dehydration from water deprivation and laxatives is minimized and if abdominal compression and hypotension are avoided during the procedure [24]. Cohen et al. [25] stated that infection, hypercalcemia, and dehydration in the presence of Bence Jones proteinuria were the major causes of acute renal failure.

Of 34 patients with multiple myeloma who presented with severe renal failure (creatinine >300 μM/liter), 16 recovered renal function [17]. Recovery of renal function was unexpectedly slow, ranging from 9 to 210 days (mean, 77 days) in patients whose creatinine level returned to normal and from 28 to 334 days (mean, 145 days) in patients whose renal failure was partially reversed. Kidney biopsy, performed in 30 cases, revealed myeloma cast nephropathy in 26. Rota et al. [17] found that dehydration, infection, or the use of nonsteroidal anti-inflammatory agents had a significant role in the development of renal failure. The most reliable prognostic indicator of recovery from renal failure was the absence of tubular atrophy and interstitial damage. The presence of cast-induced tubular obstruction did not seem to influence the outcome of renal failure.

Cavo et al. [26] reported that 56% of 26 patients with renal insufficiency (creatinine >2 mg/dl) had renal failure reversed by the administration of fluids, sodium bicarbonate, methyl prednisolone, and chemotherapy. All but one patient with complete recovery of normal renal function experienced the recovery within 1 month from the beginning of treatment. In another series, 6 of 10 patients with multiple myeloma who presented with acute renal failure had recovery. Three of the six who had recovery of renal function had been oliguric [25]. Lazarus et al. [27] reported that none of eight patients presenting simultaneously with multiple myeloma and acute renal failure regained renal function. All eight required hemodialysis.

Multiple myeloma may be associated with the acquired Fanconi syndrome. This syndrome is characterized by dysfunction of the proximal renal tubules, resulting in glycosuria, phosphaturia, and aminoaciduria [28]. In these patients, Bence Jones proteinuria is almost always of the κ type [29]. The Fanconi syndrome may be present for years before overt multiple myeloma develops [28]. Crystalline cytoplasmic inclusions are commonly seen in the plasma cells of the bone marrow and in the renal tubular cells. These crystalline deposits are probably lysosomal inclusions composed of altered κ light chains [30, 31]. Some manifestations of Fanconi's syndrome have improved when Bence Jones proteinuria was reduced by chemotherapy given because of the underlying multiple myeloma [32]. Rarely, hyporeninemic hypoaldosteronism, hyperkalemia, and hyperchloremic metabolic acidosis may be seen in multiple myeloma [33].

Distal renal tubular dysfunction measured by the inability to produce a urine pH <5.3 and the inability to produce a urine of >600 mosm is usually seen as part of global renal impairment and is rarely seen as an isolated defect [34]. However, the prevalence of functional impairment of the distal tubules is probably high [35].

Myeloma cells have been found in the urine of patients with myeloma. The source of the plasma cells is usually not found, although Neal et al. [36] reported that the plasma cells in the urine in a well-documented case of IgA κ myeloma came from an extramedullary plasmacytoma involving the trigone of the urinary bladder. Pringle et al. [37] found no correlation among the presence of plasma cells in the urine, the type of light chain, and the presence of renal insufficiency.

Rapidly progressive glomerulonephritis characterized by the formation of epithelial crescents in the glomeruli and rapidly progressive renal insufficiency has been recognized [38]. Six additional patients with rapidly progressive glomerulonephritis and monoclonal gammopathies have been reported. Only two of four patients studied had glomerular deposition of the same monoclonal protein, while some patients have had no detectable deposits on immunofluorescence. A direct association between monoclonal gammopathies and rapidly progressive glomerulonephritis is uncertain [39].

Light-chain deposition disease

Monoclonal light chains are deposited in the renal glomerulus and produce renal insufficiency or the nephrotic syndrome. The clinical spectrum ranges from patients with overt multiple myeloma or Waldenström's macroglobulinemia to patients without evidence of a malignant lymphoplasmacytic disorder [40, 41]. Typically, nodular glomerulosclerosis is present. Electron microscopy shows finely granular, electron-dense deposits on the outer aspect of the tubular basement membrane [42]. The deposits consist of κ or λ light chains [43], but experience has shown that almost all light chains are κ. Gallo et al. [44] reported that both normal-sized light chains and shorter polypeptides were synthesized in patients with light-chain deposition disease. The monoclonal light chains may be deposited in the liver, heart, and spleen [45].

Waldenström's macroglobulinemia

The basic abnormality of this disorder is the uncontrolled proliferation of cells, with lymphocyte and plasma cell characteristics producing a large monoclonal IgM protein. Weakness, fatigue, oronasal bleeding, and blurred vision are common symptoms. Pallor, hepatosplenomegaly, and peripheral lymphadenopathy are the most common physical findings. Anemia is almost always present. The bone marrow contains increased numbers of abnormal lymphocytes and plasma cells. Renal insufficiency is uncommon in macroglobulinemia. In our series [46] only 6 of 71 patients had a creatinine level >1.5 mg/dl; and 2 had levels >2.0 mg/dl. One of these had a nephrotic syndrome which responded to prednisone, and the other had a serum creatinine level of 2.2 mg/dl at diagnosis but was stable until his death 7 years later.

We have found that 80% of patients have a monoclonal light chain in the urine. Deposits of IgM on the endothelial aspect of the basement membrane may become large enough to occlude the capillary lumen and resemble thrombi. Presumably, these deposits result from the passive deposition of circulating IgM [47]. Nephrotic syndrome is rare in Waldenström's macroglobulinemia and when present is usually due to amyloidosis. However, Hory et al. [48] described a patient with Waldenström's macroglobulinemia who had the nephrotic syndrome from minimal change lesions. They reviewed three additional cases in the literature. Acute renal failure may be precipitated by dehydration. Hyponatremia due to inappropriate antidiuresis has been reported in macroglobulinemia [49].

Primary systemic amyloidosis (AL)

At the time of diagnosis, approximately 80% of patients with primary systemic amyloidosis (AL) have proteinuria, more than half have renal insufficiency, approximately one-fourth have a serum creatinine level >2 mg/dl, and about one-third have the nephrotic syndrome. Involvement of the kidneys is very common in amyloidosis and is one of the major clinical problems. Amyloid is often first deposited in the mesangium of the glomerulus and later extends along the basement membrane. In some patients, amyloid deposits are seen both in the mesangium and in the capillary walls distal from it [50]. Renal findings are essentially the same in primary (AL) and secondary (AA) amyloidosis. The degree of proteinuria in the nephrotic syndrome does not correlate well with the extent of amyloid deposition in the kidneys [51]. Dikman et al. [52] have noted that the severity of proteinuria correlated better with the presence of spicules and podocyte destruction. The greatest loss of protein probably occurs in areas where the basement membrane is penetrated by amyloid and is denuded of its epithelial covering [53]. Although the kidneys are believed to be enlarged in amyloidosis, normal-size or even small and contracted kidneys have been seen. Gross hematuria is rare in primary amyloidosis.

Also reported have been the occurrence of the adult Fanconi syndrome [54], renal vein thrombosis, retroperitoneal fibrosis [55], and priapism.

Acknowledgement

Supported in part by research grants CA-16835 and CA-15083 from the National Institutes of Health, Public Health Service.

References

1. Macintyre W. Case of mollities and fragilitas ossium, accompanied with urine strongly charged with animal matter. Med Chir Trans Lond 1849—1850; 33: 211—32.
2. Kahler O. Zur Symptomatologie des multiplen Myeloms: Beobachtung von Albumosurie. Prager Med Wschr 1889; 14: 45.
3. Bence Jones H. On a new substance occurring in the urine of a patient with mollities ossium. Phil Trans R Soc Lond, 1848: 55—62.
4. Putnam FW, Easley CW, Lynn LT, Ritchie AE, Phelps RA. The heat precipitation of Bence Jones proteins. I. Optimum conditions. Arch Biochem Biophys 1959; 83: 115—30.
5. Whicher JT, Hawkins L, Higginson J. Clinical applications of immunofixation: a more sensitive technique for the detection of Bence Jones protein. J Clin Path 1980; 33: 779—80.
6. Seney FD Jr, Silva FG. Plasma-cell dyscrasias and the kidney. Am J Med Sci 1987; 293: 407—18.
7. Sessa A, Torri Tarelli L, Meroni M, Ferrario G, Giordano F, Volpi A. Multinucleated giant cells in myeloma kidney: an ultrastructural study. Appl Path 1984; 2: 185—94.
8. Sedmak DD, Tubbs RR. The macrophagic origin of multinucleated giant cells in myeloma kidney: an immunohistologic study. Hum Path 1987; 18: 304—6.
9. Levi DF, Williams RC Jr, Lindstrom FD. Immunofluorescent studies of the myeloma kidney with special reference to light chain disease. Am J Med 1968; 44: 922—33.
10. Hill GS, Morel-Maroger L, Mery JP, Brouet JC, Mignon F. Renal lesions in multiple myeloma: their relationship to associated protein abnormalities. Am J Kidney Dis 1983; 2: 423—38.
11. DeFronzo RA, Cooke CR, Wright JR, Humphrey RL. Renal function in patients with multiple myeloma. Medicine, Balt 1978; 57: 151—66.
12. Kyle RA, Greipp PR. 'Idiopathic' Bence Jones proteinuria: long-term follow-up in seven patients. New Engl J Med 1982; 306: 564—7.
13. Clyne DH, Pesce AJ, Thompson RE. Nephrotoxicity of Bence Jones proteins in the rat: importance of protein isoelectric point. Kidney Int 1979; 16: 345—52.
14. Coward RA, Delamore IW, Mallick NP, Robinson EL. The importance of urinary immunoglobulin light chain isoelectric point (pI) in nephrotoxicity in multiple myeloma. Clin Sci 1984; 66: 229—32.
15. Melcion C, Mougenot B, Baudouin B, Ronco P, Moulonguet-Doleris L, Vanhille P, Beaufils M, Morel-Maroger L, Verroust P, Richet G. Renal failure in myeloma: relation-

ship with isoelectric point of immunoglobulin light chains. Clin Nephr 1984; 22: 138—43.
16. Smolens P, Barnes JL, Stein JH. Effect of chronic administration of different Bence Jones proteins on rat kidney. Kidney Int 1986; 30: 874—82.
17. Rota S, Mougenot B, Baudouin B, De Meyer-Brasseur M, Lemaitre V, Michel C, Mignon F, Rondeau E, Vanhille P, Verroust P, Ronco P. Multiple myeloma and severe renal failure: a clinicopathologic study of outcome and prognosis in 34 patients. Medicine, Balt 1987; 66: 126—37.
18. Kyle RA, Elveback LR. Management and prognosis of multiple myeloma. Mayo Clin Proc 1976; 51: 751—60.
19. Cooper EH, Forbes MA, Crockson RA, MacLennan IC. Proximal renal tubular function in myelomatosis: observations in the fourth Medical Research Council trial. J Clin Path 1984; 37: 852—8.
20. Rose PE, McGonigle R, Michael J, Boughton BJ. Renal failure and the histopathological features of myeloma kidney reversed by intensive chemotherapy and peritoneal dialysis. Br Med J 1987; 294: 411—2.
21. Craig JB, Powell BL. Multiple myeloma (letter to the editor). Arch Intern Med 1984; 144: 863, 868.
22. Kyle RA. Multiple myeloma: review of 869 cases. Mayo Clin Proc 1975; 50: 29—40.
23. Brown M, Battle JD Jr. The effect of urography on renal function in patients with multiple myeloma. Can Med Ass J 1964; 91: 786—90.
24. Myers GH Jr, Witten DM. Acute renal failure after excretory urography in multiple myeloma. Am J Roentgenol Radium Ther Nucl Med 1971; 113: 583—88.
25. Cohen DJ, Sherman WH, Osserman EF, Appel GB. Acute renal failure in patients with multiple myeloma. Am J Med 1984; 76: 247—56.
26. Cavo M, Baccarani M, Galieni P, Gobbi M, Tura S. Renal failure in multiple myeloma. A study of the presenting findings, response to treatment and prognosis in 26 patients. Nouv Rev Fr Hematol 1986; 28: 147—52.
27. Lazarus HM, Adelstein DJ, Herzig RH, Smith MC. Long-term survival of patients with multiple myeloma and acute renal failure at presentation. Am J Kidney Dis 1983; 2: 521—5.
28. Sewell RL, Dorreen MS. Adult Fanconi syndrome progressing to multiple myeloma. J Clin Path 1984; 37: 1256—8.
29. Maldonado JE, Velosa JA, Kyle RA, Wagoner RD, Holley KE, Salassa RM. Fanconi syndrome in adults. A manifestation of a latent form of myeloma. Am J Med 1975; 58: 354—64.
30. Raman SB, Van Slyck EJ. Nature of intracytoplasmic crystalline inclusions in myeloma cells (morphologic, cytochemical, ultrastructural, and immunofluorescent studies). Am J Clin Path 1983; 80: 224—8.
31. Chan KW, Ho FC, Chan MK. Adult Fanconi syndrome in kappa light chain myeloma. Arch Path Lab Med 1987; 111: 139—42.
32. Gailani S, Seon BK, Henderson ES. κ-Light chain — myeloma associated with adult Fanconi syndrome — response of nephropathy to treatment of myeloma. Med Pediatr Oncol 1978; 4: 141—7.
33. Mehta BR, Cavallo T, Remmers AR Jr, DuBose TD Jr. Hyporeninemic hypoaldosteronism in a patient with multiple myeloma. Am J Kidney Dis 1984; 4: 175—8.
34. Coward RA, Mallick NP, Delamore IW. Tubular function in multiple myeloma. Clin Nephrol 1985; 24: 180—5.
35. Fang LS. Light-chain nephropathy. Kidney Int 1985; 27: 582—92.
36. Neal MH, Swearingen ML, Gawronski L, Cotelingam JD. Myeloma cells in the urine. Arch Path Lab Med 1985; 109: 870—2.

37. Pringle JP, Graham RC, Bernier GM. Detection of myeloma cells in the urine sediment. Blood 1974; 43: 137—43.
38. Lapenas DJ, Drewry SJ, Luke RL III, Leeber DA. Crescentic light-chain glomerulopathy. Report of a case. Arch Path Lab Med 1983; 107: 319—23.
39. Alpers CE, Cotran RS. Neoplasia and glomerular injury. Kidney Int 1986; 30: 465—73.
40. Noel LH, Droz D, Ganeval D, Grunfeld JP. Renal granular monoclonal light chain deposits: morphological aspects in 11 cases. Clin Nephr 1984; 21: 263—9.
41. Alpers CE, Tu WH, Hopper J Jr, Biava CG. Single light chain subclass (kappa chain) immunoglobulin deposition in glomerulonephritis. Hum Path 1985; 16: 294—304.
42. Verroust P, Morel-Maroger L, Preud'Homme JL. Renal lesions in dysproteinemias. Springer Semin Immunopath 1982; 5: 333—56.
43. Tubbs RR, Gephardt GN, McMahon JT, Hall PM, Valenzuela R, Vidt DG. Light chain nephropathy. Am J Med 1981; 71: 263—9.
44. Gallo GR, Feiner HD, Buxbaum JN. The kidney in lymphoplasmacytic disorders. Path Annu 1982; 17 (Pt 1): 291—317.
45. Ganeval D, Noel LH, Preud'homme JL, Droz D, Grunfeld JP. Light-chain deposition disease: its relation with AL-type amyloidosis. Kidney Int 1984; 26: 1—9.
46. Kyle RA, Garton JP. The spectrum of IgM monoclonal gammopathy in 430 cases. Mayo Clin Proc 1987; 62: 719—31.
47. Morel-Maroger L, Basch A, Danon F, Verroust P, Richet G. Pathology of the kidney in Waldenström's macroglobulinemia. Study of sixteen cases. New Engl J Med 1970; 283: 123—9.
48. Hory B, Saunier F, Wolff R, Saint-Hillier Y, Coulon G, Perol C. Waldenström macroglobulinemia and nephrotic syndrome with minimal change lesion. Nephron 1987; 45: 68—70.
49. Braden GL, Mikolich DJ, White CF, Germain MJ, Fitzgibbons JP. Syndrome of inappropriate antidiuresis in Waldenström's macroglobulinemia. Am J Med 1986; 80: 1242—4.
50. Gise HV, Christ H, Bohle A. Early glomerular lesions in amyloidosis. Electronmicroscopic findings. Virchows Arch [A] 1981; 390: 259—72.
51. Watanabe T, Saniter T. Morphological and clinical features of renal amyloidosis. Virchows Arch [A] 1975; 366: 125—35.
52. Dikman SH, Kahn T, Gribetz D, Churg J. Resolution of renal amyloidosis. Am J Med 1977; 63: 430—3.
53. Gise HV, Mikeler E, Gruber M, Christ H, Bohle A. Investigations on the cause of the nephrotic syndrome in renal amyloidosis. A discussion of electron microscopic findings. Virchows Arch [A] 1978; 379: 131—41.
54. Finkel PN, Kronenberg K, Pesce AJ, Pollak VE, Pirani CL. Adult Fanconi syndrome, amyloidosis and marked kappa-light chain proteinuria. Nephron 1973; 10: 1—24.
55. Littman E. Renal amyloidosis with nephrotic syndrome associated with retroperitoneal fibrosis. Ann Intern Med 1971; 74: 240—1.

2. Histological, histochemical and ultrastructural features of myeloma kidney

CONRAD L. PIRANI

Renal disease is a common and serious complication of plasma cell dyscrasias (PCD). In most clinical nephrology centers, a significant number of patients 50 years old or older presenting with proteinuria and/or renal insufficiency are diagnosed every year by serum and urine protein studies and by bone marrow biopsy as having developed kidney disease related to PCD. However, in some cases these laboratory studies are not revealing or are not done and such a diagnosis is made first by renal biopsy. Further, only by renal biopsy will it be possible to determine with certainty which of the several different patterns of renal involvement associated with PCD is present in an individual patient. There are six major morphologic patterns (Table 1) which have now been clearly characterized and differentiated and rarely occur in combination. These patterns have different pathogenetic mechanisms, different prognosis and different responses to therapy [1–9].

In this brief review only Bence Jones cast nephropathy (myeloma kidney), by far the most common of all these different types of renal involvement, will be considered. The term 'myeloma kidney' is properly used interchangeably with 'Bence Jones cast nephropathy', since this type of renal disease is much more likely to be associated with classic myelomatous changes in the bone marrow than any of the other types listed in Table 1.

Table 1. Morphologic patterns of renal disease in plasma cell dyscrasias.

1. Bence Jones cast nephropathy
2. Light chain deposit disease
3. Amyloidosis
4. Waldenstrom's macroglobulinemic glomerulonephropathy
5. Cryoglobulinemic membranoproliferative glomerulonephropathy
6. Plasma cell infiltration

Minetti et al. (eds.), The kidney in plasma cell dyscrasias. ISBN 978-94-010-7085-0

Pathology of Bence Jones cast nephropathy (myeloma kidney)

This type of renal involvement develops only, but not always, in patients who have Bence Jones proteinuria (BJP) but appears to be independent from the quantity of BJP present in the urine [7—9]. It is relatively more common in light chain disease and IgD than in IgG, IgM, IgA myeloma and when the light chain protein is of the lambda type. Its development is often rapid and may be precipitated by such factors as dehydration, infection, hypercalcemia, radiographic contrast media and antibiotic therapy [6—8].

The characteristic lesions consist of generally numerous, large casts which are present almost exclusively in the distal tubules and often have a 'hard' and/or a 'fractured' appearance. Such casts are frequently surrounded by mononuclear cells, multinucleated giant cells, exfoliated tubular cells and, less commonly, by polymorphonuclear leukocytes. The *light microscopic* (*LM*) features and the tinctorial properties of Bence Jones protein casts are listed in Table 2. Although some of these features are suggestive of PCD, none of them 'per se' are absolutely diagnostic, except for the presence of crystals, not commonly recognizable in sections from paraffin blocks. The angular or crystalline shape of Bence Jones casts is best recognized by LM in one micron thick sections from Epon blocks. However, under polarized light, these large crystals are not or are only weakly birefringent no matter what the stain used. Polychromatism of the casts in trichrome preparations, a feature emphasized by some [3], can also be seen in other renal diseases not related to PCD. Not infrequently the casts have a stratified or laminated appearance especially in their more peripheral portion. These areas tend to be more strongly positive with Congo red, colloidal iron and alcian blue stains suggesting the presence of

Table 2. Light microscopic characteristics of 'myeloma' casts.

Appearance	Tinctorial properties
Large	Eosin +
"Hard"	PAS +
Fractured*	Fuchsin +
Laminated*	Polychromatism +*
Angular*	Congo Red ±
Crystals**	Alcian Blue +
Refractile	Colloidal Iron +

* Suggestive feature.
** Diagnostic feature.

amyloid and of acidic mucopolysaccharides. However, the typical apple-green birefringence of amyloid under polarized light, in my experience, is not seen in these casts. The diagnosis of myeloma kidney by LM can be definitely confirmed if foreign body type multinucleated giant cells are present. These cells are often seen engulfing the casts and at times actually phagocyting fragments of the casts. On the other hand, the presence of other types of inflammatory cells is non-specific and can be seen around the casts of other infectious and non-infectious renal diseases (Figs 1—6).

It should be emphasized that in most myeloma kidneys, there is an extreme variability in the percentage of casts with typical Bence Jones features as well as of multinucleated giant cells around them. In many instances, most casts have non-specific characteristics by LM even if by immunofluorescence the great majority is seen to consist predominantly of either kappa or lambda light chain protein. When the diagnosis of PCD is being considered such a possibility cannot be excluded unless the search for typical casts has been conducted with great diligence on all available sections including those from plastic embedded tissue [10, 11].

A considerable degree of tubular damage is almost alway present in myeloma kidney. The cells of the proximal convoluted tubules often exhibit atrophic and other nonspecific degenerative changes. Frank necrosis is uncommon and may be associated with vacuolar changes in patients

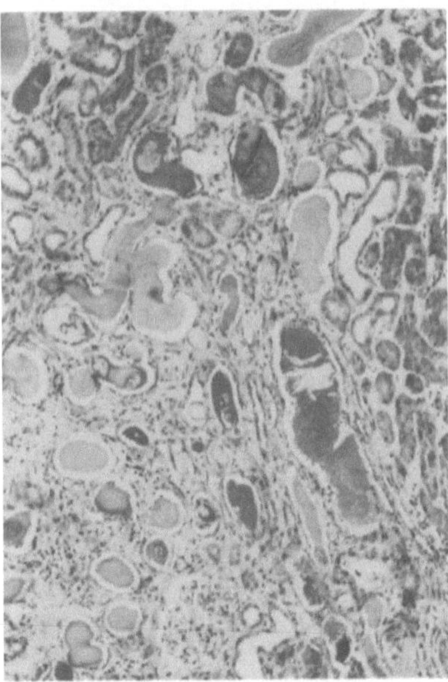

Fig. 1. Bence Jones cast nephropathy. Note the numerous large casts in the distal tubules. The casts vary in size and density and are often polychromatic. There is severe tubular atrophy and moderate interstitial inflammation. Trichrome, X 70.

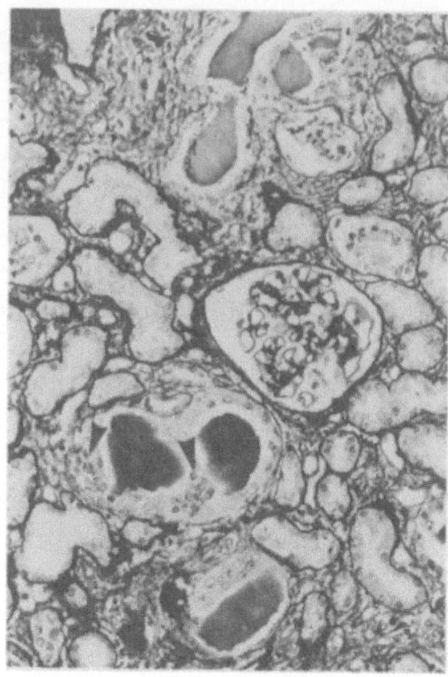

Fig. 2. Several casts in the distal tubules are partially surrounded by multinucleated giant cells (arrows). Silver methenamine, X 140.

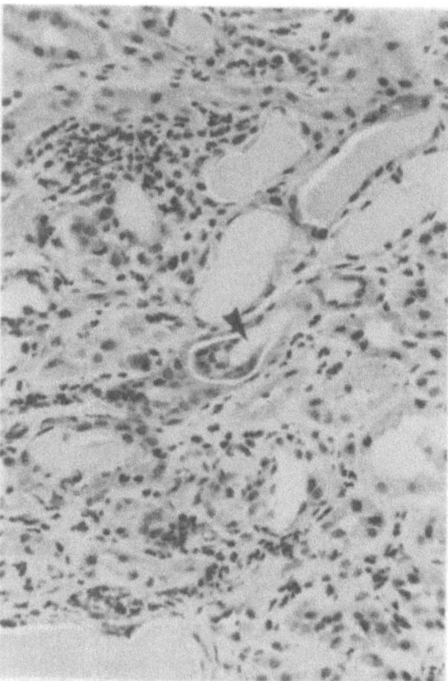

Fig. 3. In the distal tubules, most of the casts are not associated with an inflammatory cell reaction. In one tubule, a small elongated cast is engulfed and partially phagocyted by a multinucleated giant cell (arrow). Hematoxylin-Eosin, X 175.

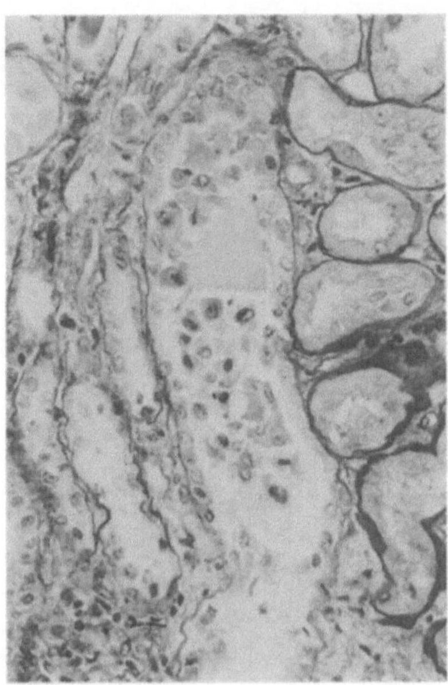

Fig. 4. In a dilated distal tubule a large, angular cast fragment is surrounded by a large number of mononuclear cells, probably macrophages. Hematoxylin-Eosin, X 250.

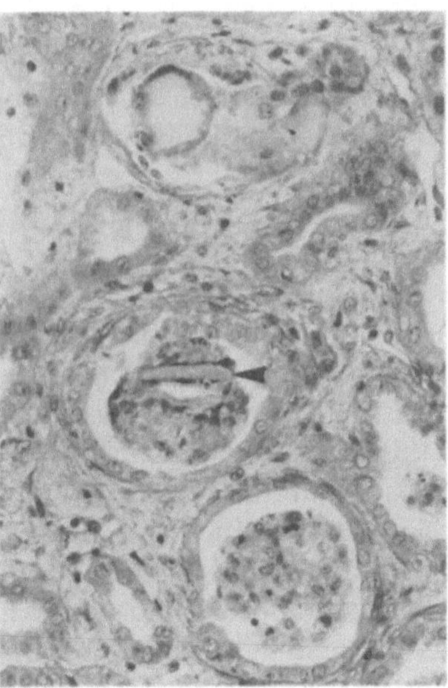

Fig. 5. Two distal tubules contain clumps of mononuclear inflammatory cells probably macrophages. In one of the cellular clumps, elongated fragments of a cast (arrow) can be recognized. Hematoxylin-Eosin, X 250.

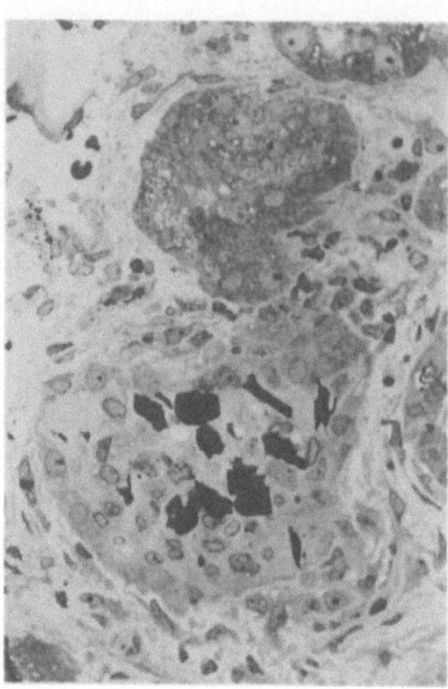

Fig. 6. Crystalline cast fragments in the lumen of a distal convoluted tubule. Toluidine blue, 2 microns, Epon section, X 120.

receiving radiocontrast media. In the distal tubules where the casts are usually located, dilatation of the lumen and flattening of the lining epithelium are common findings. At times the epithelial cells are exfoliated with denudation and occasionally gaps in the continuity of the tubular basement membrane. In these cases inflammatory cells around the tubules and around the casts are more likely to be numerous and at times are arranged in granulomatous-like formations. In general, however, the degree of interstitial inflammation is only mild or moderate consisting primarily of mononuclear cells with only rare plasma cells and polymorphonuclear leukocytes. Interstitial fibrosis varies greatly in severity depending on the chronicity of the cast nephropathy and on the degree of tubular atrophy as well as on that of arterial and arteriolar sclerosis which is invariably present in this older group of patients [6, 10, 11].

The glomeruli are usually normal except for mild mesangial sclerosis and small clusters of globally sclerotic glomeruli, changes which are both related to arteriosclerosis. When mesangial sclerosis is more prominent and glomeruli have a lobulated appearance, the possibility of an associated light chain deposit disease should be considered.

By *electronmicroscopy* (*EM*) (Table 3) casts which by immunofluorescence are found to consist predominantly of either kappa or lambda light chain protein can be divided into four major categories:

1. Finely granular electron dense homogeneous casts.

Table 3. Electronmicroscopic (EM) and immunopathologic (IF or IP) characteristics of 'myeloma' casts.

EM	IF or IP
Electron dense	Kappa + or Lambda +**
Granular or Globular	IgG
Microspherical Particles	IgA
Fibrils (TH)	C_3, C^1
Crystals**	Tamm-Horsfall (TH)
c̄ or s̄ Substructure	Albumin
Cell Debris	Fibrinogen

** Diagnostic feature.

2. Coarsely granular and/or globular casts.
3. Casts consisting predominantly of microspherical particles of undetermined origin frequently associated with small, electron dense needle-shaped crystals.
4. Casts characterized by large elongated crystals, or fragments thereof, with a rectangular shape when cut longitudinally and a pentagonal or hexagonal contour when seen in cross section.

These larger crystals can also be associated with fine, coarse or globular granules and, less commonly, with microspherical particles. At higher magnification, these cyrstals may have a substructure consisting of parallel linear arrays arranged longitudinally.

Cellular debris and fibrillar material consistent with Tamm-Horsfall protein are not infrequently seen in all four types of casts, especially in their peripheral portion. Types 1 and 2 casts are non-specific and can also be commonly seen in renal diseases not associated with PCD. Type 3 casts are definitely more common in Bence Jones cast nephropathy but occasionally are also seen in chronic renal diseases unrelated to PCD but associated with severe renal insufficiency. Type 4 casts with the large crystals, in my experience, have been found only in myeloma kidney. Small and large crystals are also occasionally seen within the cystoplasm of either proximal or distal tubular cells as a rule surrounded by a single smooth membrane suggesting that they are located within lysosomes. Crystals quite similar in size and shape to those of casts type 3 and 4 can also be found within plasma cells associated with either inflammatory processes or myeloma. Electron dense protein resorption droplets, often identifiable by IF to consist of light chain protein, are not infrequently present within the proximal tubular epithelial cells. Other tubular epithelial cell degenerative changes seen by EM are non-specific (Figs 7—14) [6, 7, 8, 10, 11]. The nature of the inflammatory cells, including the multinucleated giant cells

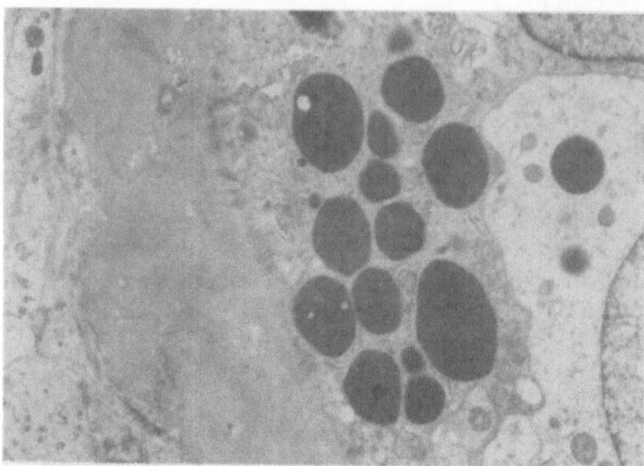

Fig. 7. Segment of atrophic proximal tubule. Within the cytoplasm of a tubular cell are many electron dense droplets (lambda light chain positive by IF). Electronmicrograph, X 9,000.

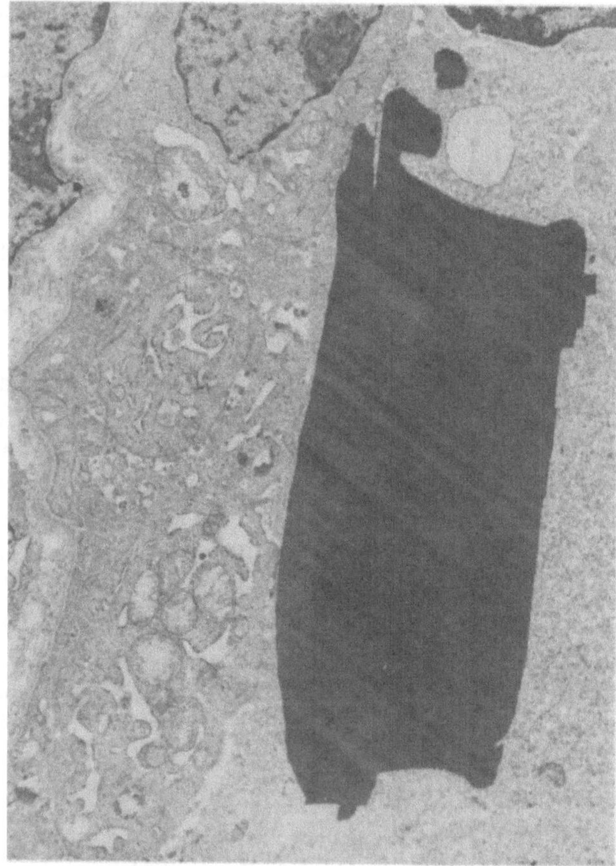

Fig. 8. Large angulated cast in a distal tubule. Electronmicrograph, X 7,200.

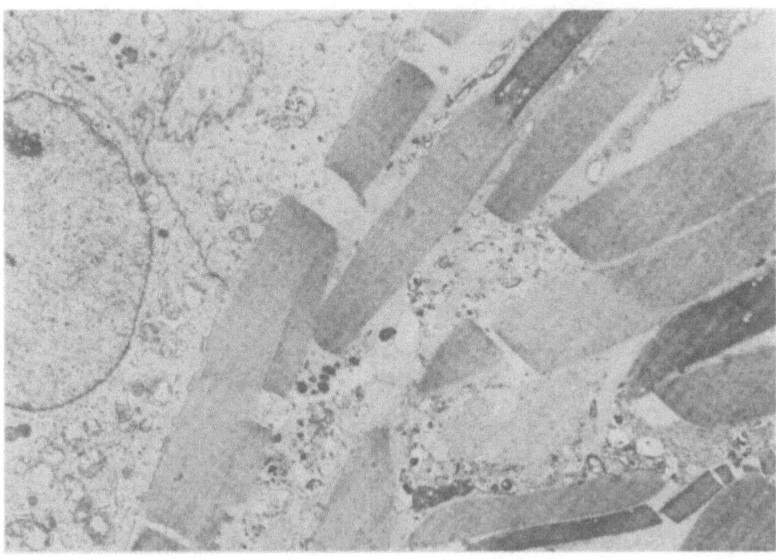

Fig. 9. Multiple crystalline cast fragments are surrounded by cellular debris in the lumen of a distal tubule. Electronmicrograph, X 5,600.

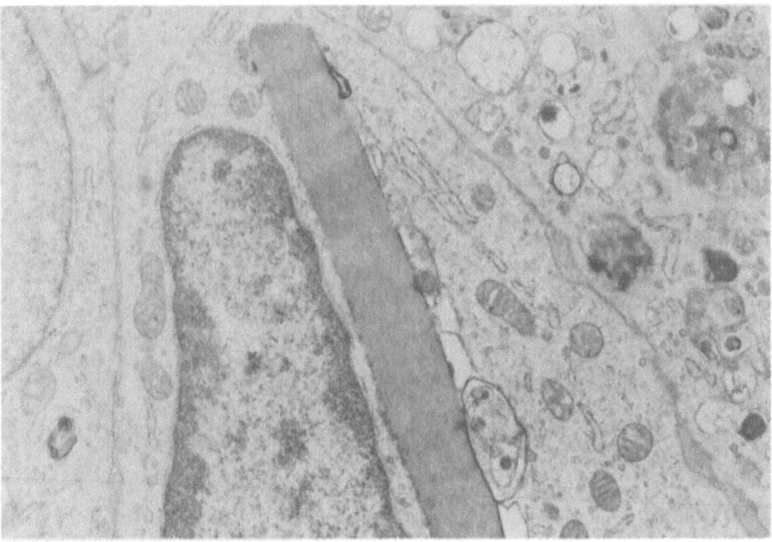

Fig. 10. Intracellular crystal in a tubular cell of a distal tubule. A filamentous substructure can be recognized within the crystal. Electronmicrography, X 12,600.

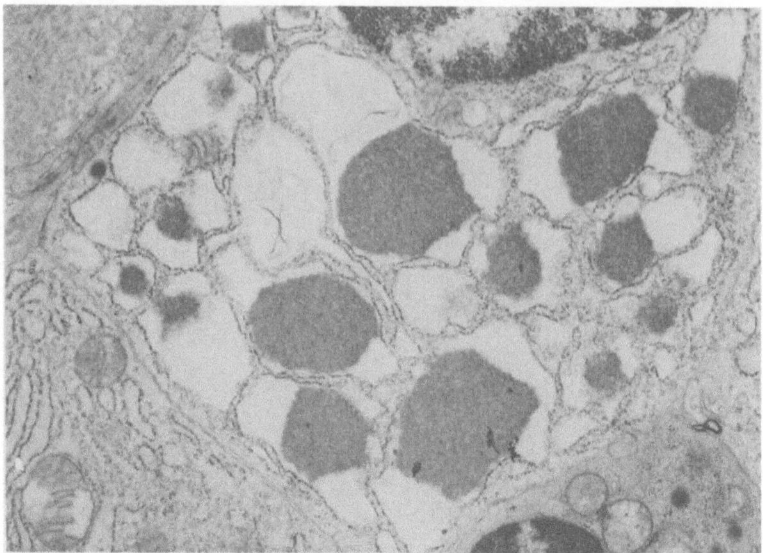

Fig. 11. Segment of a renal interstitial plasma cell from a case of Wegener's granulomatosis and crescentic glomerulonephritis. The patient had no evidence of PCD. The crystalline bodies within the rough endoplasmic reticulum resemble cross sections of the crystals seen in Figs 8,9, and 10. Electronmicrograph, X 10,800.

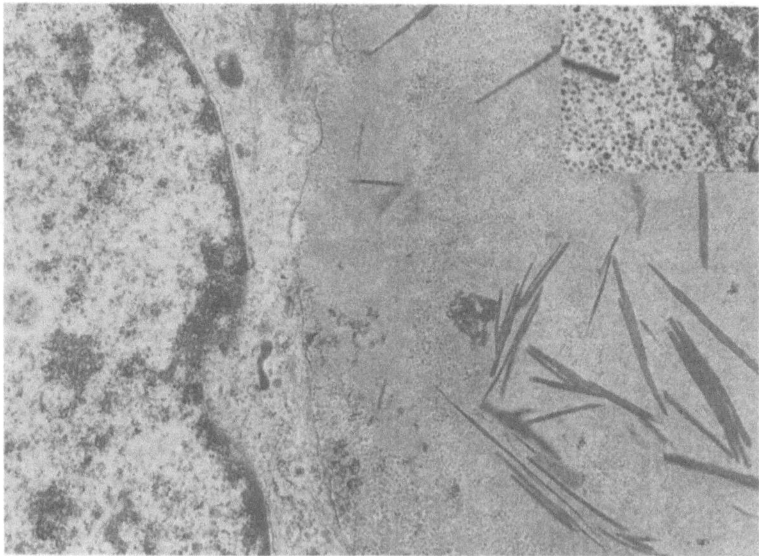

Fig. 12. Distal convoluted tubule filled by a cast consisting of a finely granular matrix in which numerous needle-shaped crystals are embedded. Electronmicrograph, X 9,600. At higher magnification, many granules in the matrix are seen to consist of microspherical particles (Inset, X 16,800).

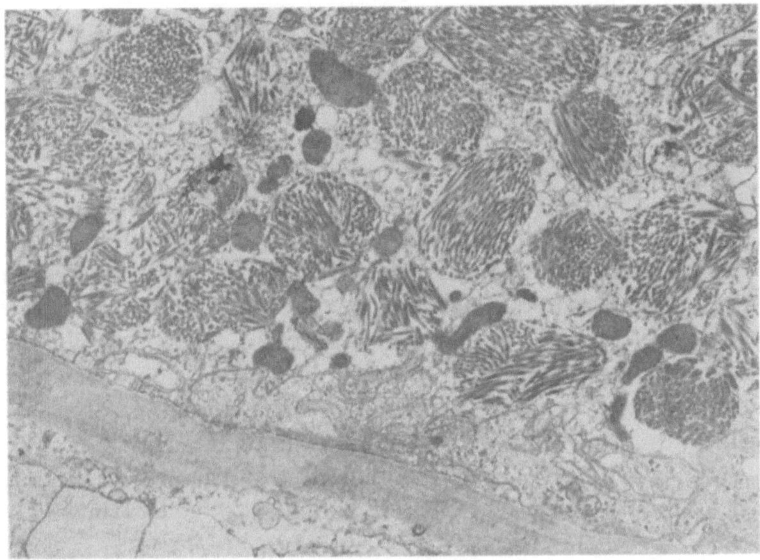

Fig. 13. Segment of proximal tubular cell in which the lysosomes are packed with needle-shaped crystals cut longitudinally or in cross section. Electronmicrograph, X 6,000.

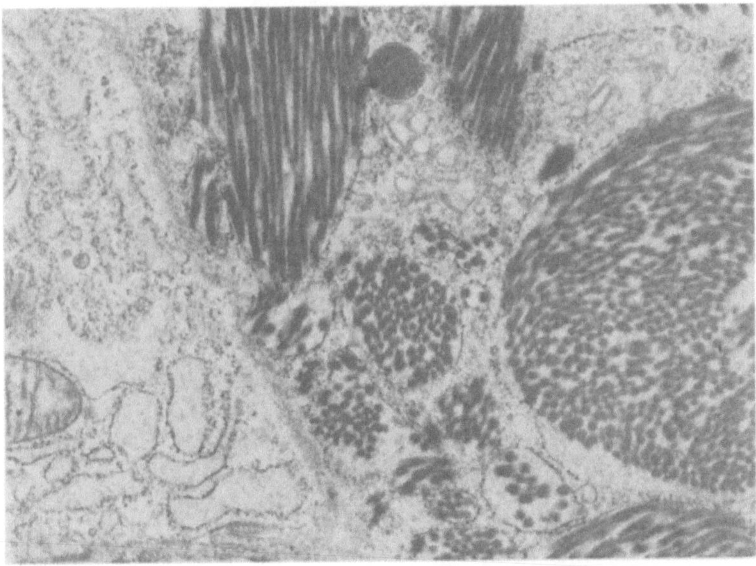

Fig. 14. Segment of a plasma cell in the renal cortex of a case of IgA glomerulonephritis with chronic active interstitial inflammation. The crystals within the sacs of rough endoplasmic reticulum closely resemble those of Fig. 13. Electronmicrograph, X 10,800.

surrounding the casts has not been entirely clarified by EM alone. However, the ultrastructural features of these cells are much more consistent with those of cells of hematopoietic than of epithelial tubular origin [10, 11, 12].

By *immunofluorescence* (*IF*) or *immunoperoxidase* (*IP*), it has been reported that in the great majority of cases the casts are stained exclusively or predominantly with antisera to either kappa or lambda light chain protein. However, in my experience, in about 25% of the cases, immunopathologic studies fail to reveal clear cut difference in the intensity of the stain between kappa or lambda light chain protein. When positive, the stain almost invariably is more intense in the peripheral portion of the casts. On the other hand, the crystals which are located in the more central portion of the casts are either weakly positive or completely negative. The tubular cells, particularly those of the proximal tubules, may contain IF or IP, kappa or lambda positive granules or exhibit a diffuse staining at times more intense than that of the casts [7, 10, 11, 13].

In recent immunohistochemical studies by our group [14], the origin of the multinucleated giant cells around Bence Jones casts has been clarified. Using lectins and antisera, and immunoperoxidase staining methods, epithelial cell markers including epithelial membrane antigen and keratins have been found to be almost always positive for tubular cells but in-

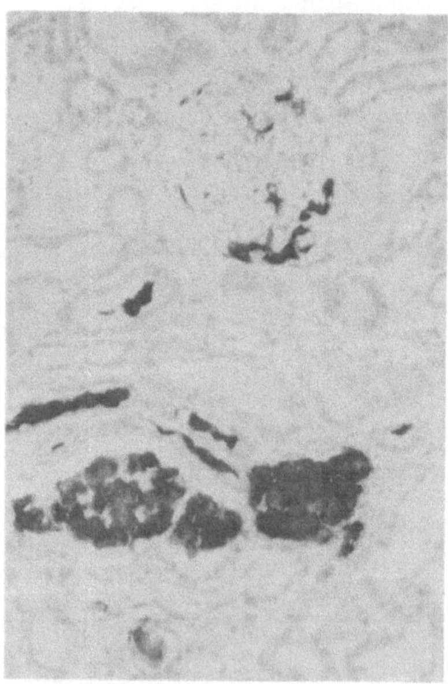

Fig. 15. Myeloma casts in distal tubules positively stained with antiserum to Tamm Horsfall protein. smaller amounts of TH protein are also present in Bowman's space probably owing to reflux. Immunoperoxidase, X 280.

variably negative for giant cells. Conversely antisera to markers for cells of hematopoietic origin such as alpha-1-trypsin or chymotrypsin, lysozyme and vimentin were found to stain positively the majority of multinucleated giant cells. Thus, the longstanding controversy about the origin of these cells appears to have been settled as had originally been suggested [15], i.e., giant cells around myeloma casts originate from fusion of histiocytes or macrophages just as those present in granulomas not related to light chain proteins (Figs 14—18) [7, 10, 11, 16].

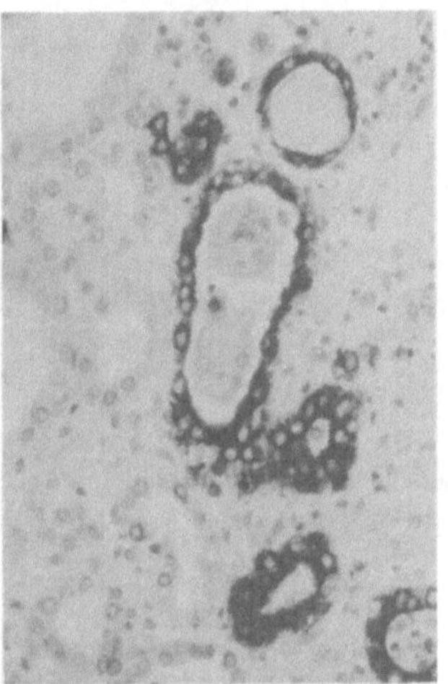

Fig. 16. Myeloma casts in distal tubules with a multinucleated giant cell. Antiserum to low molecular keratin stain the cell of some tubules but the giant cell is negative. Immunoperoxidase, X 390.

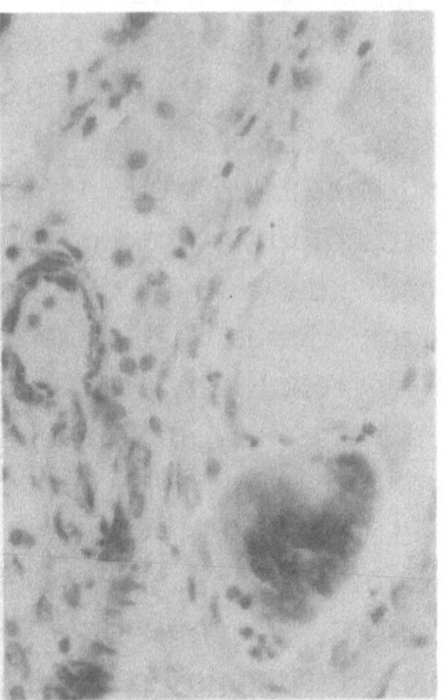

Fig. 17. Antiserum to Vimentin. A multinucleated giant cell in a distal tubule is positively stained. Note the fractured cast. Immunoperoxidase, X 430.

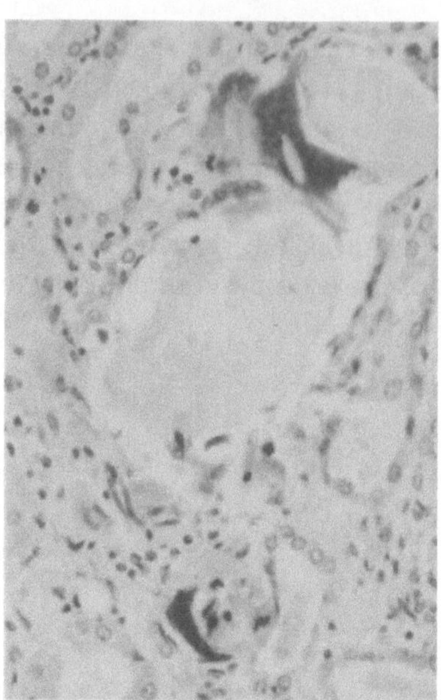

Fig. 18. Antiserum to lysozyme. The multinucleated giant cells around the casts in distal tubules are positively stained. Immunoperoxidase, X 390.

Discussion

As a rule, Bence Jones cast nephropathy is not associated with light chain deposits in the mesangial areas and along the glomerular and tubular basement membranes. This suggests that differences in the properties of the light chain proteins may be responsible for these two different morphologic patterns of renal disease. Indeed, light chain deposit disease in the great majority of cases is caused by kappa and Bence Jones cast nephropathy by either kappa or lambda light chain protein. Although the concomitant presence of the two patterns of renal disease has been reported in a small proportion of cases, when it occurs typical Bence Jones casts tend to be much less prominent. Bence Jones casts are even more rarely present, if at all, in cases of renal amyloidosis secondary to PCD (predominantly lambda) and in Waldenstrom's macroglobulinemia, even when light chain proteins are present in the urine [7]. It should be pointed out that in these two diseases, as well as in light chain deposit disease, excretion of light chain proteins is usually mild or absent [9].

Further, in all three conditions, glomerular lesions due to light chain protein, amyloid or IgM deposits usually cause significant and not uncommonly, severe and non-selective proteinuria. Although not proven, the possibility also exists that the presence of albumin and other serum proteins in the glomerular filtrate and within the distal tubules might modify the local conditions, thereby reducing or preventing the formation of Bence Jones casts [8, 17].

The 'hard', 'fractured' and 'angular' appearance of the casts seems to relate to the presence of crystals. The excellent correlation between the presence of crystals and that of multinucleated giant cells indicate that the crystals acting as foreign bodies are responsible for their formation [11]. Immunohistochemical studies have now demonstrated convincingly that these cells are hematopoietic and not epithelial in origin [10, 14]. In some instances of myeloma kidney, there is weak or absent positive staining of the casts with antisera to either kappa or lambda light chain protein. This is not surprising since it may be caused by a number of factors acting alone or in combination. The commonly used polyclonal antisera are directed against normal light chain proteins and rarely will react with light chain fragments [9]. In addition, there might be loss of antigenicity as a result of degradation by enzymes from tubular lysosomes or from macrophages present in the lumen of the tubules. Further the complex and differing composition of the casts, which include the presence of albumin, immunoglobulins and Tamm-Horsfall protein may mask the reactive sites of the light chain proteins.

With regard to the crystals within the casts, these appear to be much more common than originally thought [2, 18]. With rare exceptions, these cyrstals are not stained by immunohistochemical methods. Degradation and/or polymerization of the light chain proteins are probably responsible for their poor immunological reactivity. However, there is overwhelming indirect evidence that these crystals derive from light chain proteins including: [1] Their unique (at least for large crystals) occurrence in Bence Jones cast nephropathy; [2] the presence of crystals of similar size and shape in normal and abnormal plasma cells; and [3] the formation of quite similar crystals within the tubules of experimental animals after intraperitoneal injection of human light chain proteins [11, 19, 20].

The pathogenesis of Bence Jones cast nephropathy is unquestionably related to the excessive synthesis and great variability in the properties of light chain proteins produced by clones of plasma cells in myeloma. Such variability include abnormalities of the aminoacid sequence in the variable portion, isoelectric point, glycosylation, polymerization and other physico chemical and possibly immunological properties of light chain proteins [9, 21, 22]. However, development of renal disease, at least in part, is dependent on local functional factors involving particularly the ability of the kidney to eliminate and catabolize light chain proteins. Normally the kidneys eliminate light chain proteins by glomerular filtration and then by the more specific resorption and lysosomal enzymatic degradation in the proximal convoluted tubules [23—27]. Previously existing chronic glomerular and/or tubular disease with reduction in the number of functioning nephrons may greatly reduce the catabolic capacity of the kidneys and make them less capable of handling an increased load of light chain proteins. Similarly, an acutely developing tubular malfunction due to a variety of factors may also reduce catabolism and/or create an intraluminal environment in the distal tubules which will facilitate the formation of casts. In general while it is accepted that some light chain proteins are more likely than others to cause cast nephropathy, the role of qualitatively or quantitatively abnormal renal catabolism of these proteins remains to be determined.

References

1. Verroust P, Mery JP, Morel-Maroger L, Clauvel RP, Richet G. Glomerular lesions in monoclonal gammopathies and mixed essential cryoglobulinemias IgG-IgM. In: Hamburger J, Crosnier J, Maxwell MH, eds. Advances in Nephrology. Vol. 1, Chicago: Year Book Publishers 1971: 161—94.
2. Schubert GE, Veigel J, Lennert K. Structure and function of the kidney in multiple myeloma. Virchows Arch A — Pathologic Anatomy 1972; 355: 135—57.
3. Ganeval D, Junger P, Noel LH, Droz D. La nephropathie du myelome. Actual Nephrol Hop Necker 1977; 7: 309—47.
4. Ganeval D, Mignon F, Preud'Homme JL, Noel LH, Morel-Maroger L, Droz D, Brouet JC, Mery J Ph, Grunfeld JP. Depots de chaines légères et d'immunoglobulines monoclonales: Aspects nephrologiques et hypotheses physiopathologiques. Actual Nephrol Hop Necker 1981; 11: 179—214.
5. Gallo GR, Feiner HD, Buxbaum J. The kidney in lymphoplasmacytic disorders. In: Sommers SC, Rosen PP, eds. Pathology Annual 1982, Part I. Norwalk, Connecticut: Appleton-Century-Crofts 1982: 291—317.
6. Hill GS. Multiple myeloma, amyloidosis, Waldenstrom's macroglobulinemia, cryoglobulinemias and benign monoclonal gammopathies. In: Heptinstall RH, ed. Pathology of the Kidney, 3rd ed. Boston: Little, Brown and Company 1983: 993—1068.
7. Pirani CL, Silva FG, Appel. Tubulo-interstitial disease in multiple myeloma and other non-renal neoplasias. In: Cotran R, ed., Brenner BM, Stein JR, series eds. Contemporary Issues in Nephrology, Vol. 10. New York: Churchill, Livingstone, 1983: 287—384.
8. Silva FG, Pirani CL, Mesa-Tejada R, Williams GS. The kidney in plasma cell dyscrasias: A review and a clinicopathologic study of 50 patients. In: Fenoglio C, Wolff M, eds. Progress in Surgical Pathology. New York: Masson Publishers, 1984: 131—76.
9. Solomon A. Clinical implications of monoclonal light chains. Seminars in Oncology 1986; 13: 341—9.
10. Cohen AH, Border WA. Myeloma kidney. An Immunomorphognetic study of renal biopsies. Lab Invest 1980; 42: 248—56.
11. Pirani CL, Silva F, D'Agati V, Chander P, Striker LMM. Renal lesions in plasma cell dyscrasias: Ultrastructural observations. Am J Kid Dis 1987; 10: 208—21.

12. Sessa A, Torri Tarelli L, Meroni M, Ferrario G, Giordano F, Volpi A. Multinucleated giant cells in myeloma kidney: An ultrastructural study. Applied Path 1984; 2: 185—94.
13. Levi DF, Williams RC Jr, Lindstron FD. Immunofluorescent studies of the myeloma kidney with special reference to light chain disease. Amer J Med 1968; 44: 922—33.
14. Start DA, Silva FG, Davis LD, D'Agati V, Pirani CL. Myeloma cast nephropathy: Immunohistochemical and lectin studies. Washington D.C.: Proc Am Soc Nephrology 1987.
15. Bell ET. Renal lesions associated with multiple myeloma. Am J Path 1933; 9: 393—419.
16. Mizukami Y, Michigishi T, Kawato M, Matsubara F. Immunohistochemical and ultrastructural study of subacute thyroiditis, with special reference to multinucleated giant cells. Hum Path 1987; 18: 929—35.
17. Clyne DH, Kant KS, Pesce AJ, Pollak VE. Nephrotoxicity of low molecular weight protiens. Physicochemical interactions between myoglobin, hemoglobin, Bence Jones proteins and Tamm-Horsfall mucoproteins. Current Prob Clin Biochem 1979; 9: 299—308.
18. Costanza DJ, Smoller M. Multiple myeloma with the Fanconi syndrome. Study of a case, with electron microscopy of the kidney. Amer J Med 1963; 34: 125—33.
19. Clyne D, Brendstrup L, First MR, Pesce AJ, Finkel P, Pollak VE, Pirani CL. Renal effects of intraperitoneal kappa chain injection: Induction of crystals in renal tubular cells. Lab Invest 1974; 31: 131—42.
20. Koss M, Pirani CL, Osserman EP. Experimental Bence Jones cast nephropathy. Lab Invest 1976; 34: 579—91.
21. Clyne DH, Pesce AJ, Thompson RE. Nephrotoxicity of Bence Jones proteins in the rat: Importance of protein isoelectric point. Kid Intern 1979; 16: 345—52.
22. Preud'Homme JL, Morel-Maroger L, Brouet JC, Cerf M, Mignon F, Guglielmi P, Seligmann M. Synthesis of abnormal immunoglobulins in lymphoplasmacytic disorders with visceral light chain deposition. Am J Med 1980; 69: 703—10.
23. Wochner RD, Strober W, Waldmann TA. The role of the kidney in the catabolism of Bence Jones proteins and immunoglobulins fragments. J Exp Med 1967; 126: 207—21.
24. Tan M, Epstein W. Polymer formation during the degradation of human light chain and Bence Jones proteins by an extract of the lysosomal fraction of normal human kidney. Immunochemistry 1972; 9: 9—16.
25. Mogielnicki RP, Waldmann TA, Strober W. Renal handling of low molecular weight proteins I. L-chain metabolism in experimental renal disease. J Clin Invest 1971; 50: 901—9.
26. Clyne DH, Pollak VE. Renal handling and pathophysiology of Bence Jones proteins. Contrib Nephrol 1981; 24: 78—87.
27. Coward RA, Mallick NP, Delamore IW. Tubular function in multiple myeloma. Clin Nephrol 1985; 24: 180—5.

3. Monoclonal immunoglobulin deposition disease: Immunopathologic aspects of renal involvement

GLORIA GALLO & JOEL BUXBAUM

Introduction

Monoclonal light chain deposition disease, as distinguished from light chain amyloid (AL), was first noted in renal biopsies in 1973 [1]. Its immunohistology and systemic nature were detailed in 1976 [2]. Since then approximately 90 cases of these nephropathies associated with dysproteinemias have been reported from different institutions and countries, variously termed: nodular glomerulosclerosis, nodular glomerulopathy, nonamyloidotic light chain glomerulopathy, and kappa light chain nephropathy. More recently the realization that monoclonal deposits are of several types has led us to the use of the more inclusive term — Monoclonal Immunoglobulin Deposition Disease (MIDD) — to encompass a particular spectrum of renal lesions associated with the dysproteinemias.

The present report describes 12 patients in whom a diagnosis of MIDD was made by immunohistologic and/or electron microscopic examination of their kidneys at NYU Medical Center.

Materials and methods

Tissue was obtained from patients at NYU Medical Center or from referrals. Six of the patients reported elsewhere are included with the addition of new data [3—5]. Of the 12 patients, 2 of whom were examined at necropsy, 10 were identified by immunofluorescence microscopy with the routine parallel use of monospecific antisera to light and heavy chain isotypes and complement as previously described [3]. The 2 remaining patients were identified retrospectively by the presence of characteristic ultrastructural deposits, together with other evidence of plasma cell dyscrasia including a monoclonal light chain in the serum or urine. Renal tissue in all was examined by electron microscopy. In addition to serum

Minetti et al. (eds.), The kidney in plasma cell dyscrasias. ISBN 978-94-010-7085-0

and urine immunoelectrophoreses, in some patients bone marrow smears or biopsy sections were examined by immunofluorescence or immunoperoxidase, respectively, for determination of kappa/lambda ratio, and bone marrow cell cultures were radiolabelled for analysis of newly synthesized immunoglobulin as described [3, 6].

Diagnosis and classification

Since all but one of our patients presented with renal symptoms, the diagnosis of MIDD usually was made initially by renal biopsy examined by routine immunofluorescence microscopy, and subsequently confirmed by other evidence of plasmacytic dyscrasia. The detection of deposits of a single light chain class, noncongophilic and thus distinct from AL amyloid, was the major diagnostic criterion that identified the patients with MIDD, and served as the basis for inclusion in this series. In the 2 patients lacking immunofluorescence microscopic examination, characteristic electron-dense renal deposits, together with evidence of myeloma, was considered adequate for inclusion.

Immunofluorescence microscopy was the basis for further subclassification of deposits of different isotypes for analysis and comparison of our cases (Fig. 1). In this overall scheme of MIDD we have included AL

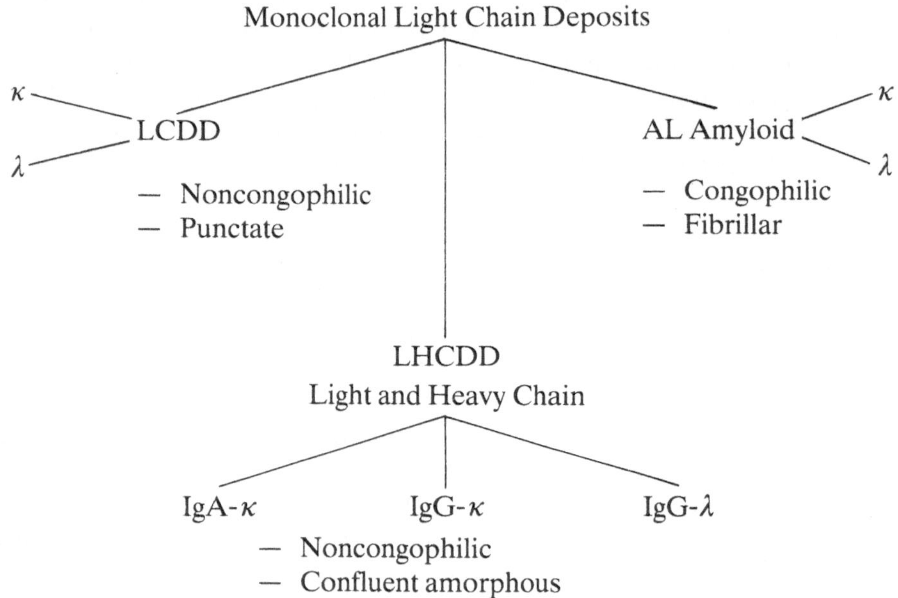

Fig. 1. Monoclonal immunoglobulin deposition disease, classification.

amyloid, as it relates to nonamyloidotic deposition disease, because it is clear from our study and those of others, that the 2 types of deposits (fibrillar and nonfibrillar) may exist concurrently in the same patient [7, 8]. Thus as we have used the terms, Light Chain Deposition Disease (LCDD) includes those with renal deposits of a single light chain isotype, either kappa or lambda, while Light and Heavy Chain Deposition Disease (LHCDD) includes those with deposits of both light and heavy chain of a single immunoglobulin isotype. These distinctions seem warranted until the full spectrum of morphologic, immunochemical, and clinical manifestations are apparent and the pathogenesis and mechanisms of deposition are better understood.

Results

Immunopathologic Features: Among the 10 patients classified by immunofluorescence microscopy, 4 different types of monoclonal deposits were found: 6 patients had only kappa light chain, 1 had only lambda light chain, 1 had IgA-kappa and 2 had IgG-lambda. The morphologic features of these groups differed as detailed in Table 1.

Light chain deposition disease

Kappa light chain. By light microscopy 4 of the 7 patients with kappa deposits had normal appearing glomeruli in H&E and silver-methenamine (PASM) stained sections. The glomeruli in the other 3 patients showed mesangial expansion, nodular with membranoproliferative features in 2 cases, due to amorphous fuchsinophilic deposits in sections stained with periodic acid-Schiff (PAS) and slight to moderate increased matrix shown in PASM stains. Five patients had eosinophilic refractile tubular casts with giant cell reactions typical of Bence Jones (B-J) casts in 3 of them together with a moderate to severe degree of tubular atrophy and dilatation, interstitial fibrosis and patchy leukocytic cell infiltration.

Immunofluorescence microscopy, similar in all, revealed bright diffuse linear staining of glomerular, capsular and tubular basement membranes, (GBM, CBM, TBM), mesangial nodules, and vessels for kappa, but not lambda light chain or any heavy chains, C_3 or Clq in all of the 6 patients from whom frozen sections of kidney were examined.

In the 5 of 7 examined by electron microscopy there were distinctive punctate clusters of quasi-regular-spaced electron-dense deposits in all layers of the GBM, and in mesangium, TBM, and vessel walls. The concentration gradients in GBM versus TBM differed. In the case of the

Table 1. Monoclonal immunoglobulin deposition disease, NYU series.

Morphologic features (n)	LCDD Light chain		LHCDD Light & heavy chain	
	κ (7)	λ (2)	IgA-κ (1)	IgG-λ (2)
Light microscopy				
Glomeruli				
Normal	4	2	0	0
Mesang/nodules	3	0	1	2
Confluent deposits	0	0	1	1
Tubules				
Bence-Jones casts	5	1	0	0
Vessels				
Amyloid	1	1	0	0
Immunofluorescence				
Deposits				
GBM	6/6	1/1	1	2
TBM	6/6	1/1	1	2
Vessels	6/6	1/1	0	1
Electron microscopy				
Clustered deposits				
GBM	5	1	0	0
TBM	7	2	0	0
Mesang	5	1	0	0
Vessels	5	1	0	0
Confluent deposits				
GBM & mesang	0	0	1	1
Fibrillar deposits				
Vessels	1	1	0	0
Extra renal parenchyma	1	1		

Fractions = number positive/number examined.

GBM, the deposits were denser along the luminal than subepithelial aspect while in the TBM the density was greater in the outer than inner aspect. In 2 patients in whom basement membrane deposits were seen by immunofluorescence microscopy, corresponding electron-dense deposits could not be demonstrated in the GBM but both had scanty clustered deposits in the TBM.

Lambda light chain. In the biopsies of 2 patients, there was minimal mesangial expansion but otherwise normal-appearing glomeruli; one of the

2 patients had prominent B-J casts and severe interstitial edema and leukocytic cell infiltration.

Immunofluorescence microscopy of the one examined revealed a pattern and distribution of staining in basement membranes and vessels similar to that seen for the kappa light chain deposition as described above.

Ultrastructurally, punctate deposits identical to those seen in kappa LCDD were found in one patient. The other had only slight finely granular electron densities in the TBM but not the GBM.

Coexistence of amyloid and light chain deposition disease

In 2 patients with LCDD (1 kappa, the other lambda) whose tissues were examined at necropsy, amyloid was found in some renal and systemic vessels. In the patient with kappa LCDD, amyloid was seen also in the myocardium and in the wall of the gastrointestinal tract; in the the other patient there was amyloid in the endocardium.

Heavy and light chain deposition disease

Three patients had both monoclonal light and heavy chain determinants in deposits that differed in the distribution and appearance from those with only light chain deposits.

IgA-kappa. Heavy and confluent deposits in peripheral capillary walls and in the mesangium produced enlarged lobulated glomeruli with focal duplication of peripheral basement membranes resembling membranoproliferative glomerulonephritis. In this patient the deposits were intensely fuchsinophilic in sections stained with Schiff (PAS) reagent. The reaction was diastase resistant indicating that glycogen was not responsible for the strong PAS staining. Blocking of the PAS staining reaction by acetylation of glycol groups was achieved by pretreatment with acetic anhydride, and positive staining restored by de-acetylation with a solution of NaOH. This reversible blocking reaction histochemically can be attributed to the presence of 1,2 glycol groups in the deposits that are responsible for the strong Schiff reaction [9].

Immunofluorescence microscopy demonstrated bright staining for both IgA heavy chain and kappa light chain in the same distribution in glomeruli. Some TBMs stained for IgA and kappa light chain; there was no staining of vessels, and other immunoglobulin isotypes and complement were not detected.

Ultrastructurally the massive deposits were dense, homogeneous, and confluent in the mesangial matrix and along the inner aspect of peripheral capillary walls, expanding the mesangium and the subendothelial space, often obliterating capillary lumens. Tubular basement membranes exhibited focal poorly defined densities suggestive of deposits.

IgG-lambda. In both patients there was mesangial expansion associated with deposits. One had pronounced nodules due to increased matrix and homogeneous deposits; the other had heavy confluent deposits in peripheral capillary walls as well as mesangium. The deposits in both were deeply stained with Schiff reagent. The increased mesangial matrix was variably silver-stained in a meshwork around eosinophilic deposits.

Immunofluorescence microscopy revealed bright staining for both IgG and lambda determinants in the same distribution in the mesangium and peripheral capillary walls. In one patient there was no extraglomerular staining for IgG or lambda light chain; in the other, there was smooth staining of TBMs for both IgG and lambda light chain, but no staining of vessel walls. One patient had trace staining of mesangial nodules for C_3 and the other had moderate to strong staining for Clq; other stains were negative.

By electron microscopy massive confluent homogeneous electron dense deposits were found predominantly in mesangial regions and in expanded subendothelial and occasionally subepithelial locations of peripheral capillary walls in only one of the patients. In the other patient with bright staining deposits in immunofluorescence microscopy and pronounced mesangial nodules, there were only slight but poorly defined densities that were difficult to distinguish from the mesangial matrix and GBM, but no discrete electron densities typical of deposits were observed. Neither had electron dense deposits in TBMs.

Clinical features

The age and sex distribution of the 12 patients in the subgroups were comparable: patients with LCDD ranged from 36 to 77 with a mean age of 59 years, and those with LHCDD ranged from 41—74 years with a mean age of 56 years. The male/female ratio was 2:1 in both groups.

The clinical features, biased by selection, were dominated by azotemia and proteinuria in all but one who had gastric bleeding.

Mode of presentation. (Table 2) Acute renal failure was the presenting feature in 6 patients all of whom had LCDD (5 kappa, the other lambda). Their levels of BUN ranged from 100 to 120 mg/dl and serum creatinine

Table 2. Monoclonal immunoglobulin deposition disease, NYU series.

Clinical features	LCDD		LHCDD	
	κ (7)	λ (2)	IgA-κ (1)	IgG-λ (2)
Mode of presentation				
Acute renal failure	5	1		
– BUN 100–120 mg/dl – S.Cr. 10–23 mg/dl – Proteinuria 0.5–5.7 g (mean 2.45 g/l)				
Proteinuria	1	1	1	2
– Maximal levels (3.0–8.9 g/l) – (mean 5.86 g/l) – BUN 14–54 mg/dl – S.Cr. 1.4–2.4 mg/dl				

from 10 to 23 mg/dl. All had prominent tubular casts, 4 with giant cell reactions, and varying degrees of tubulo-interstitial inflammation, edema, and fibrosis. The maximal urine 24 h protein excretion ranged from 0.5 to 5.7 g with a mean of 2.45 g/l. Glomeruli appeared normal in 4 of the patients and in the other 2 there was mesangial expansion with nodules in one.

Proteinuria was the presenting feature in 5 patients, 2 of whom had LCDD, one kappa and the other lambda. The other 3 patients had LHCDD. The maximal urine 24 hr protein excretion ranged from 3.0 to 8.9 g/l with a mean fo 5.0 g in LCDD and 6.43 g in LHCDD. One of the patients, with kappa LCDD, had mesangial nodules; the other had mild mesangial expansion by light microscopy. All of the 3 patients with LHCDD, had heavy glomerular deposits visible by light microscopy as detailed above.

Evidence of plasma cell dyscrasias. All of the patients for whom there was adequate information had hypogammaglobulinemia (Table 3).

A corresponding monoclonal Ig in serum or urine was found in all but 3 patients who had kappa LCDD. In 6 patients with LCDD, a monoclonal light chain was found either in the urine (3 patients) or in the serum (1 patient); in the other 2 patients, both had monoclonal H_2L_2 in the serum, one also had H_2L_2 in the urine, and both had B-J proteinuria. In the 3 patients with LHCDD, all had monoclonal H_2L_2 in the serum. Two had

Table 3. Monoclonal immunoglobulin deposition disease, evidence of plasma cell dyscrasia.

	LCDD		LHCDD	
	κ (7)	λ (2)	IgA-κ (1)	IgG-λ (2)
Hypogammaglobulinemia	6/6	1/1	1	2
Monoclonal Ig serum and/or urine	4/7	2	1	2
Myeloma	3/7	1/2		
Plasmacytosis (10—15%)	3/7		1	2
Increased κ/ratio	2/3		1	
Decreased κ/ratio				1

the same protein in the urine, and 2 had B-J proteinuria. Thus, the distinction between LCDD and LHCDD could not be drawn on the basis of the serum or urine monoclonal protein.

Four of the patients with LCDD (3 kappa, 1 lambda) and B-J casts had myeloma, and 6 patients (3 LCDD and 3 LHCDD) had 10—15% bone marrow plasmacytosis, without cytologic or clinical evidence of myeloma. The remaining 2 patients, both with LCDD, had normal numbers of plasma cells.

The kappa/lambda ratio was elevated in 2 patients with kappa LCDD (100:1, 50:1) and in one (30:1) with LHCDD (IgA-kappa); the ratio was decreased (1:27) in the patient with LHCDD (IgG-lambda) as determined by immunofluorescence microscopy of bone marrow smears and immunoperoxidase study of bone marrow biopsy.

Thus, all except two of the patients with MIDD had at least one other feature of a plasmacytic dyscrasia corresponding to the light chain isotype deposited in the kidney. In the other 2 patients, only biosynthetic studies of bone marrow cells in culture demonstrated production of a corresponding monoclonal protein.

Four of the 7 with kappa LCDD were analyzed using radiolabelling techniques. All synthesized polypeptides of approximately normal light chain size plus molecules which were precipitable with anti kappa serum but were smaller than normal. Cells from the patient with IgA-kappa deposits produced a smaller than normal alpha chain polypeptide while the cells from the patient with IgG lambda deposits synthesized normal and small gamma and lambda chains. Hence, of this group of patients, marrow cells obtained from all produced either intact light chains and light chain fragments or heavy and light chain fragments.

Discussion

The key to the diagnosis of MIDD is the detection of deposits of a single light chain isotype in tissues, usually by renal biopsy. In our experience, renal manifestations are the most frequent presenting features, although we recognize that a selection bias is introduced by the nature of our interest.

Recognition of MIDD is relatively recent, but it is not a new disease [3]. Earlier reports describing myeloma with renal deposits of 'Paraamyloid' that did not have the congophilic properties of amyloid, upon which the histopathological diagnosis depends, were likely examples of MIDD [10]. The routine use of monospecific antisera against each of the heavy and light chain isotypes now allows the identification and classification of monoclonal Ig deposits that are noncongophilic, and distinguishes them from immune complex deposits which are polyclonal. The most frequent MIDD in our series, and the experience of others, is kappa LCDD. Lambda LCDD is seen less commonly while deposits with monoclonal light and heavy chain determinants are seen in fewer than 10% of cases [4].

In LCDD the highly characteristic and pathognomonic finding is diffuse linear deposition of monoclonal light chain in all the basement membranes and vessel walls of the kidney as detected by immunofluorescence microscopy, and the ultrastructural electron-dense deposits arranged in regularly-spaced punctate clusters. Exceptions do occur: in some instances deposits, although present in TBMs, are not found in GBMs on immunofluorescence examination [11]. In other instances, as observed in 3 of our patients, deposits seen by immunofluorescence may not be sufficiently electron-dense to be distinguished from basement membranes or mesangial matrix. Occasionally, deposits seen by electron microscopy are not detectable by immunofluorescence microscopy [11].

The light microscopic features are heterogeneous and nondiagnostic in the absence of other data. The glomeruli may appear normal or exhibit mesangial widening or prominent nodules that resemble other diseases. Rarely proliferation and crescents are described [12]. In our series, in contrast to the prevalence of nodules in reported cases, two-thirds of the patients with LCDD had normal appearing glomeruli and only one-third had mesangial widening or nodules. The disparity may be a function of the mode of presentation of the disease since in most of our patients with normal appearing glomeruli the presenting feature was acute renal failure associated with cast nephropathy while in those with nodular mesangial lesions heavy proteinuria was more common. Furthermore, the evolution from normal to nodular glomerular lesions has been described, suggesting that nodules represent an accumulation of deposits over time [13].

In 2 of our cases of LHCDD, heavy confluent deposits were visible by light microscopy in peripheral capillary walls, resembling those in immune complex diseases, emphasizing the need for the routine use of antisera against each light and heavy chain isotype to identify MIDD.

Most of our patients with MIDD had serum or urine evidence of a monoclonal gammopathy. However, 3 with LCDD did not. In such patients, bone marrow smears, which are not diagnostic of myeloma with Wright's stain, may demonstrate a corresponding altered K:L ratio when studied by immunofluorescence using double labels, antikappa and anti-lambda. Biosynthetic studies of bone marrow cells in culture may also provide additional confirmatory data suggesting a plasmacytic dyscrasia. These tests are especially helpful in patients lacking overt evidence of myeloma or a monoclonal gammopathy by routine methods.

The similarities between AL amyloid and MIDD are apparent in their ability to deposit and replace the parenchyma of the kidney and other organs in the presence of an underlying plasma cell dyscrasia. They differ, however, in several ways. Amyloid is fibrillar and congophilic while deposits in MIDD are not. Additionally, no heavy chain has been found yet in amyloid in contrast to MIDD.

The relationship between fibrillar AL amyloid and nonfibrillar monoclonal light chain deposits is of interest in view of the fact that both forms of the light chain deposits may co-exist in individual patients. Whether these different forms are generated biosynthetically or by the action of various local tissue factors, e.g. enzymes, ionic strength, pH, or some combination of these is still unknown. Clearly the biochemical examination of tissues with both forms of deposits is likely to provide the information.

Continued studies in MIDD are necessary to obtain a complete description of the clinical and pathologic features and to gain more insight into the mechanism of tissue localization. Amyloid fibrils extracted from tissues have been examined immunochemically and in a single case compared with the synthesized Ig in bone marrow cell cultures [14], but this has not been accomplished thus far in MIDD. Such studies might reveal distinguishing features between MIDD and AL-amyloid and clues about the properties of the proteins leading to their accumulation in tissues.

Acknowledgement

Supported by The National Kidney Foundation, New York/New Jersey; the VA Merit Review Research Fund and NIH Grant AM 14031.

References

1. Antonovych T, Linc C, Parrish E, Mostofi K. Light chain deposits in multiple myeloma (Abstract). Am Soc Nephrol, 1973; Seventh Annual Meeting.

2. Randall RE, Williamson WC Jr, Mullinax F, Tung MY, Still WJS. Manifestations of systemic light chain deposition. Am J Med 1976; 60: 293–9.
3. Gallo GR, Feiner HD, Katz LA, Feldman GM, Correa EB, Chuba JV, Buxbaum JN. Nodular glomerulopathy associated with nonamyloidotic kappa light chain deposits and excess immunoglobulin light chain synthesis, Am J Pathol 1980; 99: 621–44.
4. Gallo GR, Feiner HD, Buxbaum JN. The kidney in lymphoplasmacytic disorders. In: Sommers SC, Rosen PI, eds. Pathology Annual, Part I. New York: Appleton-Century-Crofts, 1982: 291–317.
5. Bangerter AR, Murphy WM. Kappa light chain nephropathy. A pathologic study. Virchows Arch A 1987; 410: 531–9.
6. Zolla S, Buxbaum J, Franklin EC, Scharff MD. Synthesis and assembly of immunoglobulins by malignant human plasmacytes. I. Myelomas producing V-chains and light chains. J Exp Med 1970; 132: 148–62.
7. Ganeval D, Noel LH, Preud'homme JL, Droz D, Grünfeld JP. Light-chain deposition disease: Its relation with AL-type amyloidosis. Kidney Int 1984; 26: 1–9.
8. Jacquot C, Saint-Andre JP, Touchard G, Nochy D, D'Auzac de Lamartinie C, Oriol R, Druet P, Bariety J. Association of systemic light-chain deposition disease and amyloidosis: A report of three patients with renal involvment. Clin Nephrol 1985; 24: 93–8.
9. Pearse AGE. Histochemistry, Theoretical and applied. Vol. II: Analytical Technology, 4th ed. New York: Churchill Livingstone, 1985: 686.
10. Sanchez LM, Domz CA. Renal patterns in myeloma. Ann Intern Med 1960; 52: 44–54.
11. Pirani CL, Silva F, D'Agati V, Chander P, Striker L. Renal lesions in plasma cell dyscrasias: Ultrastructural observations. Am J Kid Dis 1987; X: 208–21.
12. Silva FG, Meyrier A, Morel-Maroger L, et al. Proliferative glomerulonephropathy in multiple myeloma. J Pathol 1980; 130: 229–36.
13. Colvin R. Case records of the Massachusetts General Hospital. Case 1–1981. N Engl J Med 1981; 304: 33–4.
14. Picken M, Gallo GR, Buxbaum J, Frangione B. Characterization of renal amyloid derived from the variable region of the lambda light chain subgroup II. Am J Pathol 1986; 124: 82–7.

4. The glomerulonephritis of essential mixed cryoglobulinemia

GIULIANO COLASANTI, FRANCO FERRARIO, ANTONIO TARANTINO, GIANNI BARBIANO DI BELGIOJOSO, RENATO SINICO, ROBERTO CONFALONIERI, LOREDANA RADAELLI, GIOVANNI BANFI & GIUSEPPE D'AMICO

In cryoglobulinemia there are immunoglobulins in the blood that precipitate reversibly in the cold. The most widely accepted classification, recognizes three types of cryoglobulinemia [1]. In type I cryoglobulinemia, the cryoprecipitable Ig is a single monoclonal Ig, usually a myeloma protein or a macroglobulin. Type II and type III are mixed cryoglobulinemias, containing a polyclonal IgG and an anti-IgG rheumatoid factor, most frequently of the IgM class. The IgM antiglobulin component in type III cryoglobulinemia is polyclonal, is probably antigen-driven and seems to be result of an abnormal overactivity of physiological immunoregulatory mechanisms. On the contrary, the IgM antiglobulin component in type II cryoglobulinemia is monoclonal, and since it is due to abnormal proliferation of a special clone of B lymphocytes, it probably is the consequence of a plasma cell dyscrasia.

This review will deal with the clinical syndrome of 'essential' cryoglobulinemia [2] (purpura, arthralgias and glomerulonephritis, with no other underlying diseases), which is almost exclusively observed in patients with type II IgG-IgMk cryoglobulinemia. Our personal experience is based on the analysis of a large population of patients observed in the Divisions of Nephrology of Cà Granda, Policlinico and San Carlo Hospitals [3, 4, 5].

The pathology of the disease is a variable combination of a number of histological lesions, but in the majority of patients the glomerular involvement can be classified as a *diffuse proliferative glomerulonephritis* (*GN*) *with marked thickening of the capillary wall* (Fig. 1). Unlike other types of proliferative GN the exudative component of the proliferation largely prevails in Essential Mixed Cryoglobulinemia-GN (EMC-GN). It consists of a massive infiltration of monocytes, as has been shown by the esterase method and by monoclonal antibodies (Fig. 2). In particular, data from the S. Carlo group [6, 7] indicate the large prevalence in these cases of activated monocytes, as shown by the massive infiltration of cells recognized by monoclonal antibodies FMC32 and A1—3 (anti-tissue factor procoagulant activity) [8].

Minetti et al. (eds.), The kidney in plasma cell dyscrasias. ISBN 978-94-010-7085-0

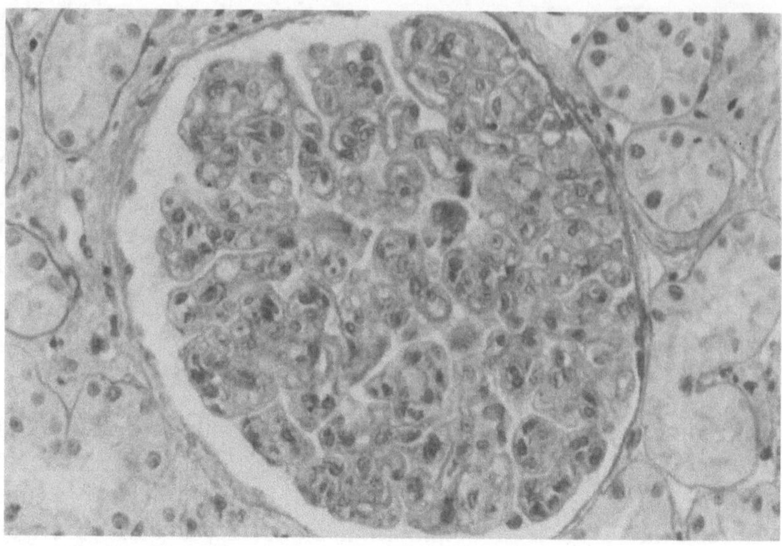

Fig. 1. Diffuse proliferative glomerulonephritis of essential mixed cryoglobulinemia. Endocapillary lumina appear filled by massive resident and blood-borne cells (Masson's thrichrome, × 225).

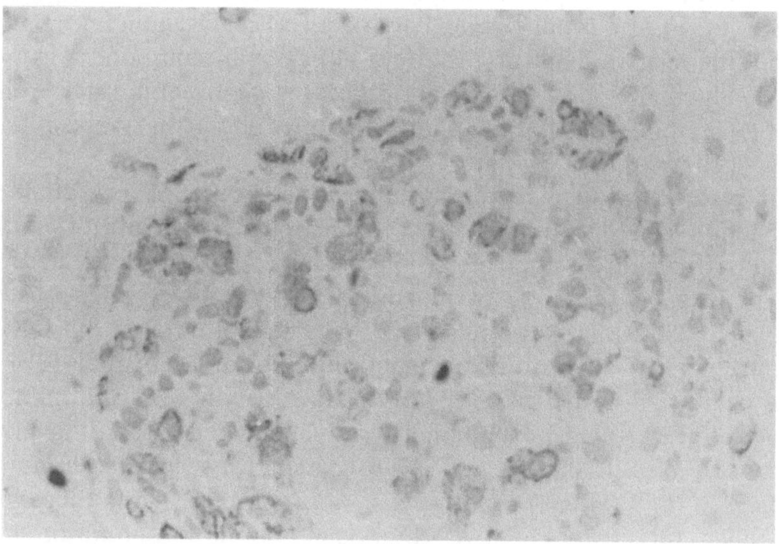

Fig. 2. Intraglomerular infiltration of FMC 32-positive cells (4-layer immunoperoxidase staining, × 225).

The thickening of the capillary wall and its double-contoured appearance, that are particularly diffuse and evident in this disease, are partly due to mesangial expansion and interposition, but mainly due either to the presence of monocytes within the capillary wall, or to the subendothelial deposition of immune complexes (Fig. 3).

In about one third of cases, especially in clinically active phases, intraluminal 'thrombi' of variable size and diffusion can be found (Fig. 4). That these are precipitated cryoglobulin is strongly indicated by their amorphous, eosinophilic, PAS-positive and Congo red-negative appearance, by their positivity for IgM and IgG at IF and by their peculiar fibrillar or crystalloid structure under the electron microscope [9].

In the kidney, as in other organs, vasculitis is particularly frequent in EMC, characterized by fibrinoid necrosis of the wall of small and medium size vessels, often with perivascular monocyte infiltration.

The clinical renal syndrome of persistent urinary abnormalities (proteinuria and hematuria) is observed in about half of the patients with EMC-GN. In the other cases, there may be either an acute nephritic syndrome, with macroscopic hematuria, hypertension and azotemia, or a typical nephrotic syndrome with massive proteinuria [4, 10].

The course of the renal disease is variable [3]: in about 2/3 of the patients, whatever the presenting syndrome, there is either remission of the renal symptoms or a chronic, indolent course with persistence of urinary abnormalities. In the remaining cases, one single or multiple episodes of reversible exacerbations, such as acute nephritic syndrome, take place during the course of the disease, sometimes associated with flare-ups of the systemic signs of the disease. Progression to end-stage renal failure is not a

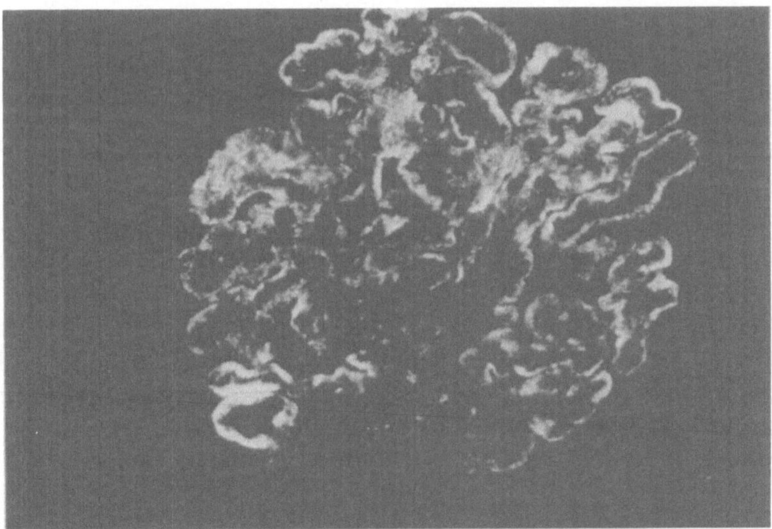

Fig. 3. Diffuse deposits of IgM along the subendothelial aspect of the capillary wall (× 200).

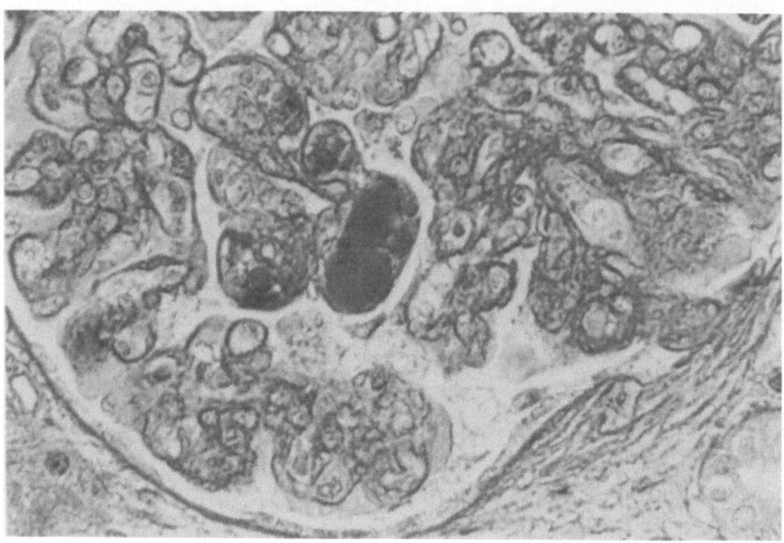

Fig. 4. Endoluminal thrombi in a case of glomerulonephritis associated with essential mixed cryoglobulinemia (PAS, × 360).

common event: it has been described for 10% of patients reported in the literature, while no more than 3% of patients required regular dialysis treatment [10—12]. The actuarial curve calculated for our patients showed 70% survival at ten years after the onset of the disease [12]. Patients with EMC die mainly because of extrarenal complications, such as infections, liver failure, cardiovascular and cerebrovascular accidents, the latter two certainly being favoured by the arterial hypertension, which is particularly frequent and severe in this disease [3].

The more common laboratory findings such as variable amounts of circulating cryoglobulins, serum titers of IgM rheumatoid factor, characteristic C_4 and C_1 hypocomplementemia, do not seem to correlate with the severity of the renal or extrarenal clinical symptoms.

There is consistent evidence that type II cryoglobulinemia is a consequence of an immunoproliferative disorder of selected clones of B lymphocytes that produce monoclonal IgMk with rheumatoid activity versus polyclonal IgG or versus IgG-containing immune complexes. The antigens in these immune-complexes have not as yet been identified, although HBs and coccidiomycosis have been advocated for a minority of cases [13]. More recently, we have shown that the EB virus genome is incorporated in bone-marrow cells of patients with type II- (but not with type III) cryoglobulinemia [15].

The mechanism of cryoprecipitation of the Igs involved in type II-EMC is still unclear. The intrinsic physico-chemical properties of the single components are not sufficient to explain the phenomenon, since it has been demonstrated that both Ig must be present for cryoprecipitation to take place. Factors such as the Ag-Ab ratio [16], Fc-Fc interactions [17], or reduced solubility due to hypocomplementemia [18], salt concentration, binding with fibronectin [19], hydrophobic properties [20] (largely due to aminoacid composition) and carbohydrate content of proteins, have all been taken into consideration.

The renal involvement in the patients with this disease is probably due to the deposition of serum cryoglobulins in the glomeruli. The evidence for this is the EM fibrillar appearance of intraglomerular deposits (Fig. 5) similar to 'in vitro' aspects [21], and the fact that these deposits have an antiglobulin activity similar to that of serum cryo-IgM [22]. Moreover, using monoclonal antibodies against cross-reactive idiotypes present on rheumatoid factors, we have recently shown that the IgM rheumatoid factor present in the kidney consists of the same IgM rheumatoid factor found both in the serum cryoglobulins and in the B lymphocytes from bone-marrow and from peripheral blood of the same patient [23].

Once deposited, in the glomerulus, there is evidence that cryoglobulins are immune complexes highly inflammatory, triggering endocapillary accumulation of activated monocytes from the bloodstream. These cells play the role of scavenger cells, as shown by their intimate contact with thrombi and deposits, and also appear to be mediators of tissue damage, through liberation of lytic enzymes and other inflammatory products.

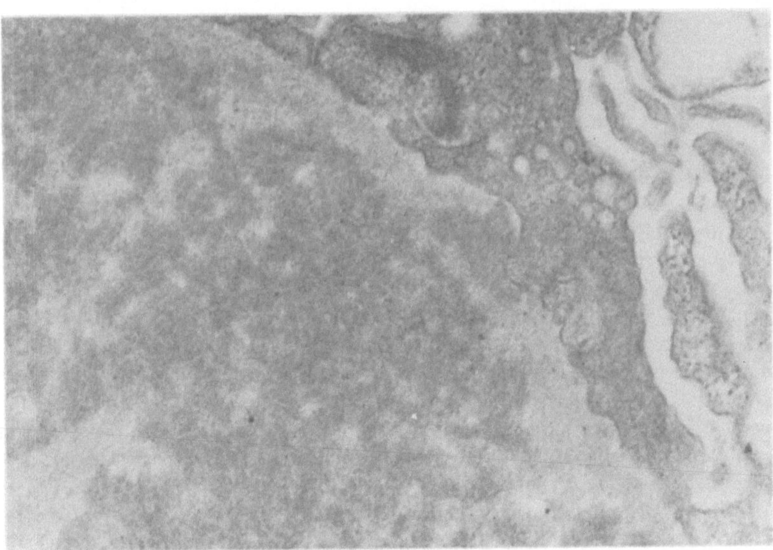

Fig. 5. Ultrastructural fibrillar appearance of endoluminal thrombi (× 13,200).

On the basis of detailed analysis of clinical, histological and immunohistological data for our patients and on the basis of current knowledge, we can hypothesize that in type II EMC-GN two distinct mechanisms can lead to kidney damage: the first is characterized by time-limited, sometimes recurrent, bouts of intraglomerular cryoglobulin precipitation which causes reversible exudative lesions and is associated with nephritic syndrome and with reversible renal failure. The second is characterized by continuous subendothelial deposition of cryoglobulins and of other immune-complexes which causes a specific type of membranoproliferative GN, with variable monocyte exudation and with a low tendency to progressive mesangial sclerosis, and which is associated with a clinical syndrome of persistent urinary abnormalities, sometimes with moderate chronic renal failure.

Acknowledgements

The Authors wish to thank Mrs Mascia Marchesini and Miss Viviana Baretto for skilled secretarial help. Part of this work has been supported by grant n° 86.00486.04, from Consiglio Nazionale delle Ricerche, Rome, Italy.

References

1. Brouet JC, Clauvel JP, Danon F, Klein M, Seligman M. Biological and clinical significance of cryoglobulins. A report of 86 cases. Am J Med 1974; 57: 775—88.
2. Meltzer M, Franklin EC, Elias K, McCluskey RY, Cooper N. Cryoglobulinemia — a clinical and laboratory study. II cryoglobulins with rheumatoid factor activity. Am J Med 1966; 40: 837—56.
3. Tarantino A, Montagnino G, Baldassarri A, Barbiano Di Belgioioso G, Colasanti G, Montoli A, Bucci A, Ponticelli C. Prognostic factors in essential mixed cryoglobulinemia nephropathy. In: Ponticelli C, Minetti L, D'Amico G, eds. Antiglobulins, cryoglobulins and glomerulonephritis. Boston: M. Nijhoff, 1986: 219—25.
4. Barbiano Di Belgioioso G, Montoli A, Tarantino A, Ferrario F, Maldifassi P, Baldassarri A, Minetti L. Clinical and histological correlations in essential mixed cryoglobulinemia (EMC) glomerulonephritis. In: Ponticelli C, Minetti L, D'Amico G, eds. Antiglobulins, Cryoglobulins and Glomerulonephritis. Boston: M. Nijhoff, 1986: 203—10.
5. Ferrario F, Colasanti G, Barbiano Di Belgioioso G, Banfi G, Campise R, Confalonieri R, D'Amico G. Histological and immunohistological features in essential mixed cryoglobulinemia glomerulonephritis. In: Ponticelli C, Minetti L, D'Amico G, eds. Antiglobulins, Cryoglobulins and glomerulonephritis. Boston: M. Nijhoff, 1986: 193—202.
6. Fiorini G, Bernasconi P, Sinico AR, Chianese R, Pozzi F, D'Amico G. Increased frequency of antibodies to ubiquitous viruses in essential mixed cryoglobulinemia. Clin Exp Immunol 1986; 64: 65—70.

7. Castiglione A, Bucci A, Fellin G, D'Amico G, Atkins RC. The relationship of infiltrating renal leucocytes to disease activity in lupus and cryoglobulinemic glomerulonephritis. Nephron (in press)
8. Monga G, Mazzucco G, Barbiano Di Belgioioso G, Busnach G. The presence and possible role of monocyte infiltration in human chronic proliferative glomerulonephritis. Am J Pathol 1979; 94: 271—84.
9. Feiner H, Gallo G. Ultrastructure in glomerulonephritis associated with cryoglobulinemia. Am J Pathol 1977; 88: 145—55.
10. Gorevic PD, Kassab HJ, Levo Y, Kohn R, Meltzer M, Prose P, Franklin EC. Mixed cryoglobulinemia: clinical aspects and long-term follow-up of 40 patients. Am J Med 1980; 69: 287—308.
11. D'Amico G, Ferrario F, Colasanti G, Bucci A. Glomerulonephritis in essential mixed cryoglobulinemia (EMC). In: Davison PJ, Guillon PJ, eds. Proceedings of the XXI Congress of the European Dialysis and Transplant Association. London: Pitman, 1985: 527—48.
12. Tarantino A, De Vecchi A, Montagnino G, Imbasciati E, Mihatsch MJ, Zollinger HU, Barbiano Di Belgioioso G, Busnach G, Ponticelli C. Renal disease in essential mixed cryoglobulinemia. Long-term follow-up of 44 patients. Quart J Med 1981; 50: 1—30.
13. Levo Y, Gorevic PD, Kassab HJ, Tobias H, Franklin EC. Association between hepatitis B virus and essential mixed cryoglobulinemia. N Engl J Med 1977; 296: 1501—4.
14. Gamble CN, Ruggles SW. The immunopathogenesis of glomerulonephritis associated with mixed cryoglobulinemia. N Engl J Med 1978; 299: 81—4.
15. Fiorini GF, Sinico RA, Winearls C, Custode P, De Giuli-Morghen C, D'Amico G. Persistent Epstein-Barr Virus infection in patients with type II essential mixed cryoglobulinemia. Clin Immunol Immunopathol (in press)
16. Griswold WR, Brady. Cryoglobulins in acute experimental immune complex glomerulonephritis. J Lab Clin Med 1978; 92: 423—8.
17. Moller NPH, Steensgaard J. Fc-mediated immune precipitation. II Analysis of precipitating immune complexes by rate-zonal ultracentrifugation. Immunology 1979; 38: 641—4.
18. Schifferli JA, Amos N, Pusey CD, Sissons JGP, Peters DK. Metabolism of IgG in type II mixed essential cryoglobulinemia-autologous precipitated and normal homologous IgG are incorporated into complexes and metabolized in vivo at similar rates. Clin Exp Immunol 1983; 51: 305—15.
19. Bartlow BG, Oyama JH, Ing TS, Miller AW, Economou SG, Rennie IDS, Lewis EJ. Glomerular ultrastructural abnormalities in a patient with mixed IgG-IgM essential cryoglobulinemic glomerulonephritis. Nephron 1975; 14: 309—16.
20. Wang A, Wang IY. Intrinsic properties inducing precipitation of cryoglobulins. In: Ponticelli C, Minetti L, D'Amico G, eds. Antiglobulins, cryoglobulins and glomerulonephritis. Boston: M. Nijhoff, 1986: 101—12.
21. Cordonnier D, Martin H, Groslambert P, Micouin C, Chenais F, Stoebner P. Mixed IgG-IgM cryoglobulinemia with glomerulonephritis. Immunochemical fluorescent and ultrastructural study of kidney and in vitro cyroprecipitate. Am J Med 1975; 59: 867—72.
22. Maggiore Q, Bartolomeo F, L'Abbate A, Misefari V, Martorano C, Caccamo A, Barbiano Di Belgioioso G, Tarantino A, Colasanti G. Glomerular localization of circulating antiglobulin activity in essential mixed cryoglobulinemia. Kidney Int 1982; 21: 387—93.
23. Winearls CG, Ono M, Sinico A, Fiorini G, Grennan D, D'Amico G, Sissons JGP. Identification of circulating MRF-producing cells in essential mixed cryoglobulinemia (submitted for publication).

5. Clinical spectrum of tubular disorders from light chains

GIACOMO COLUSSI, LUCIANA BARBARANO, CRISTINA AIRAGHI, PATRIZIA ROLANDO, ALBERTO MONTOLI, SIMONETTA GRANATA, FRANCESCO DE CATALDO & LUIGI MINETTI

Renal damage from light chains (LC) may result from a number of events, such as intratubular cast formation, interstitial fibrosis and tubular atrophy, amyloidosis and glomerular and peritubular deposition of LC granular deposits; in addition direct lympho-plasmacitic cell infiltration, hypercalcemia, hyperuricemia, hyperviscosity and infections may also contribute to renal damage [1—2]. 'Functional' disturbances of the renal tubule (both proximal and distal) have widely been described in patients with LC proteinuria both in isolated case reports [3—16] and in large, unselected series [17—22], and might simply be a consequence of the aforesaid anatomical lesions. However, both clinical and experimental evidence would suggest a direct effect of at least some LC on renal tubule cell metabolism and function, independently from any concomitant anatomical tissue damage: tubular function was found abnormal in many patients with normal GFR [12, 15, 17, 20] and with normal, or almost normal, renal biopsies [11, 12, 17]. In addition, when renal biopsy was performed in patients in whom severe tubular disfunctions coexisted with different degrees of GFR impairment, anatomical lesions (tubular atrophy, interstitial fibrosis and intratubular casts) did not differ from those seen in the majority of patients with classical 'myeloma kidney' [4—7, 9, 16]. Intracellular crystal-like inclusions, possibly LC aggregates, were seen in some patients with abnormal tubular function [4—6, 9, 16], but not in other ones [11, 12, 7, 17], thus the link between this anatomical finding and tubule disfunctions, if any, remains unclear.

Experimentally, incubation of renal tissue slices with Bence Jones proteins in vitro, at similar concentrations as those supposed to exist in proximal tubule fluid of patients with plasma cell dyscrasias (PCD), was shown to inhibit tubule cell metabolic processes and transmembrane solute fluxes, such as gluconeogenesis, PAH uptake [23, 24] and Na/K-ATPase enzyme activity [25]. Thus, it is believed that LC may play a 'toxic' effect on renal tubule cell function which is not simply the consequence of any coexistent anatomical renal damage [11, 12].

Minetti et al. (eds.), The kidney in plasma cell dyscrasias. ISBN 978-94-010-7085-0

Abnormal tubular function in patients with PCD might be of great clinical relevance, because of sistemic metabolic consequences (chronic acidosis, hypophosphatemia, fluid and electrolyte abnormalities) and possible enhancement of renal damage from LC: reduced proximal tubule competence would reduce the catabolism of filtered LC, thus allowing increased amounts of LC to be delivered to the distal nephron where they might induce cast formation. It has also been suggested that functional disturbances of the renal tubule might be an early sign of chronic LC toxicity on tubule cells, which eventually will ensue in tubule atrophy, cell death and chronic renal failure [17]. Many questions still remain open concerning the tubular effects of LC, including the pattern(s) of functional abnormalities, the mechanism(s) of toxicity, the relative importance of the degree of LC overproduction and/or of some still unknown physicochemical characteristics of individual LC, the relation of tubular abnormalities with the presence of global renal impairment.

In the present paper we have evaluated the prevalence of functional tubular abnormalities in 87 patients with PCD (of whom 37 had significant LC proteinuria): a large series of proximal and distal tubule parameters were chosen as indices of tubular function in order to better understand the specificity and sensitivity of each of them, and disclose any possible 'pattern' of tubular disfunction. All the result were correlated with quantitative LC urine excretion and the GFR.

Patients and methods

Between November 1985 and January 1987, 87 consecutive patients with known or newly discovered PCD were enrolled for this study; inclusion criteria were the presence of a urine and/or plasma monoclonal peak by immunofixation and no previous citotoxic and/or steroid therapy; only 5 patients had previously been treated, but were included because treatment had been stopped for at least one month before the study. Two patients were treated with local X-ray therapy (not involving lumbar regions) at the time of the study. Forty eight patients were males, and 39 females; mean age was 62 years (range 30—82). Clinical diagnosis and monoclonal peak in plasma and urine are shown in Table 1: overall 37 patients had a detectable Bence Jones (BJ) protein (i.e. monoclonal free LC) in urine. This was a κ LC in 20 and a λ LC in 17 patients. These 87 patients will be defined as 'prospective' patients.

Three additional patients who had previously been studied because of widespread tubular disfunction, which was eventually shown to be related

Table 1. Clinical diagnosis and immunological characterization of plasma and urine monoclonal peaks in the 87 patients (number of cases in parenthesis).

Clinical diagnosis	Plasma M-peak		BJ protein*	
Myeloma (n = 34)	IgG κ	(n = 11)	κ	(n = 7)
	IgA κ	(n = 4)	κ	(n = 4)
	IgM κ	(n = 1)	/	
	κ	(n = 1)	κ	(n = 1)
	/	(n = 2)	κ	(n = 2)
	IgG λ	(n = 7)	λ	(n = 3)
	IgA λ	(n = 3)	λ	(n = 2)
	IgM λ	(n = 2)	/	
	IgD+ λ	(n = 1)	λ	(n = 1)
	/	(n = 2)	λ	(n = 2)
MGUS** (n = 44)	IgG κ	(n = 18)	/	
	IgA κ	(n = 2)	κ	(n = 2)
	IgM κ	(n = 4)	κ	(n = 1)
	IgG λ	(n = 17)	λ	(n = 4)
	IgA λ	(n = 1)	/	
	IgG κ + IgA λ	(n = 1)	/	
	IgG λ + IgA λ	(n = 1)	λ	(n = 1)
Waldenström	IgM κ	(n = 2)	κ	(n = 1)
Macroglobulinemia (n = 3)	IgM λ	(n = 1)	λ	(n = 1)
Lymphoma (n = 3)	IgG κ	(n = 1)	κ	(n = 1)
	IgG λ	(n = 1)	/	
	IgM λ	(n = 1)	λ	(n = 1)
1° Amyloidosis (n = 2)	IgG λ	(n = 2)	λ	(n = 2)
Mixed 'essential' cryoglobulinemia	IgM κ	(n = 1)	κ	(n = 1)
Total		n = 87	κ + λ = 37 (κ = 20; λ = 17)	

* BJ protein = monoclonal free LC in urine (κ and λ in serum indicate free monoclonal LC's).
** MGUS = monoclonal gammopathy of undetermined significance.

to BJ proteinuria, are also included in this study. These 3 patients, here defined as 'Fanconi' patients (FS), will not be included in the evaluation of the prevalence of tubule disorders in our series, and will only be taken into account for defining the 'pattern' of tubular abnormalities. The first patient (FS_1) was a 56-year old female with IgAλ 'smoldering' myeloma and λBJ proteinuria; the second one (FS_2) was a 76-year old male with 'idiopathic' BJλ proteinuria and the third (FS_3) was a 6-year old male with a BJκ myeloma. Thirty-five sex and age-matched healthy subjects (20 males and 15 females, aged 42—81 years, mean 54) served as controls: results in the patients were considered abnormal when outside ± 2SD from the mean in these controls.

Renal function studies

'Static' parameters. All the patients underwent this study. Drugs, such as diuretics and non steroidal anti-inflammatory drugs (but not allopurinol, digitalis, antihypertensives, insulin and oral antidiabetics), were stopped at least 3 days before the study. A 24 h urine collection was made at home or in the hospital under mineral oil and kept at 4°C during all the collection period; no other preservative was used. At the end of the collection, a fasting 'spot' urine sample and fasting venous and arterial blood samples were also taken in the hospital.

Evaluated parameters included:

- creatinine clearance (CCr, 24-hour urines), taken as an index of GFR, and BJ proteinuria (24-hour urines).
- β_2 microglobulin fractional excretion (24-hour urine: $FE\beta_2M = C\beta_2M/CCr \times 100$, i.e. β_2M and creatinine clearance ratio). $FE\beta_2M$, instead of quantitative excretion ($U_{\beta 2M}V$) or urine concentration ($U\beta_2M$) of β_2M, was chosen because in patients with PCD both β_2M production and plasma levels may be increased [26] and could potentially increase urine excretion independently from any change in tubular reabsorption. Available knowledge of renal handling of microproteins, as shown by lysozime [27], indicates that urine excretion rapidly increases when filtered load increases only a few times above 'physiologic' filtered load, but fractional excretion remains constant until a saturation limit (i.e. a Tm) is reached, at levels about 20 times greater, for lysozime, than 'physiologic' filtered loads. Thus $FE\beta_2M$ is expected not to change as a sole consequence of increased plasma levels and/or glomerular hyperfiltration, at least until saturation is not exceeded. However saturation limit for β_2M is not known, and might differ from that of lysozyme.
- Total aminoacid excretion (AA, 24-hour urines).
- Urine glucose excretion (U_GV, 24-hour urines); only normoglycemic, nondiabetic patients were considered for this test.
- Uric acid (Ua) fractional excretion (fasting urines: $FEUa = CUa/CCr \times 100$, i.e. uric acid and creatinine clearance ratio). This parameter of tubular urate reabsorption is known to change little with varying degrees of uric acid production and plasma levels [28].
- Renal phosphate threshold (TmP/GFR, fasting urines) (Walthon and Bijvoet nomograms) [29].
- Arterial blood pH, P_{CO2} and calculated HCO_3 (Stat Profile, Nova Biomedica), and fasting urine pH (PHM82 pHmeter, Radiometer).

'Dynamic' parameters. In some patients one or more of the following evaluations were randomly performed:

- Renal glucose threshold (TmG/GFR): 18 patients (3 FS and 15 'prospective' patients) underwent this study. Glucose (2 g/Kg bw as a 30% solution) was infused over a 60-min period, and blood and urines were collected every 10 minutes. From the regression line ($y = bx + a$) between all plasma glucose values (X, mg/dl) outside the 'splay' region (chosen by visual inspection) and corresponding urine excretion rates (y, mg/dl GFR), TmG/GFR (mg/dl GFR) was calculated as the $|a|/b$ ratio.

- Renal bicarbonate threshold ($TmHCO_3/GFR$): 12 patients (3 FS and 9 'prospective' patients) underwent this study. $NaHCO_3$ (4.5 mmol/Kg bw as a 1M solution) was infused over a 180-min period, and venous blood and urines were collected every 30 minutes. Regression line was calculated between every plasma HCO_3 levels (X, mM) outside the 'splay' and corresponding urine excretion rates (y, mmol/l GFR), and $TmHCO_3/GFR$ (mmol/l GFR) was calculated as the $|a|/b$ ratio.
- Lithium clearance (CLi): this test was performed in the course of maximal water-induced diuresis as previously described [30] in 30 patients (28 'prospective' patients and 2 FS). CLi (as percent of creatinine clearance) is a measure of the 'distal delivery', i.e. of the percent of glomerular filtrate which escapes reabsorption along the proximal tubule. 'Distal' reabsorption of Na (DRNa, as percent of CLi), is calculated as $[(CLi - CCl)/CLi \times 100]$, i.e. as the difference of Li and chloride clearances divided by Li clearance.

  Minimal urine osmolality ($UOsm_{min}$, $mOsm/KgH_2O$) and CH_2O (ml/dl GFR) were also measured as an index of maximal dilution capacity.
- Maximal acidification capacity. Fifty five patients (52 'prospective' patients and 3 FS) were evaluated. Arterial blood pH and bicarbonate and fasting urine pH were first measured; if UpH was ≤ 5.3, normal urine acidification capacity was considered to be present. If UpH was > 5.3, an oral acid load (NH_4Cl 0.1 g/Kg bw) was given. This was performed in 12 patients (11 'prospective' and 1 FS). Minimal urine pH over the 5 hours following the load was taken as an index of maximal acidification capacity.

Analytical methods and statistical analysis

Characterization of individual components of urine and plasma M-peaks was performed by immunofixation [31], after that a standard cellulose-acetate ELF (urines were previously 100-fold concentrated by B-15 Minicon® membranes) disclosed the presence of a likely monoclonal band. Immunofixation was run on agarose gel (Titan Gel Immunofix, Helena Lab., Beaumont, Texas): sera were diluted 1/5 to 1/20 (usually 1/10) and urines were concentrated 20 to 50 times (rarely unconcentrated urines or the 100-fold concentrated samples were selected) in order to reach an optimal Ab/Ag concentration ratio. For quantitative assessment of BJ proteinuria, total protein excretion was measured by the biuret reaction, and a densitometric profile of the 100-fold concentrated urine cellulose acetate ELF was used to indicate which fraction of total protein content was accounted for by the monoclonal band. The high sensitivity of immunofixation technique in detecting small amounts of monoclonal bands has been emphasized [31]; its resolution limit is likely to be in the order of only a few mg/l. β_2M in plasma and urines was measured by turbidimetry [32]; phosphorus by enzymatic-colorimetric method (Inorganic Phosphorus Sera Pak, Ames Div., Miles Lab. Inc.); glucose by glucose oxidase; uric acid [33] and creatinine [30] as reported. Bicarbonate in urines was calculated according to the Henderson—Hasselbach equation, where $pK = 6.33 - 0.5\sqrt{UNa + UK}$ [34].

AA in urines were measured by the colorimetric reaction with dinitrofluorobenzene. After acidification with 0.1N HCl, samples were first filtered through a Dowex cationic exchange resin and then eluted with Na-borate. A glycine solution was used as a standard. With this reaction, involving the amino group of aminoacids, there may be a slight overestimation as regards as dibasic aminoacids. In 37 patients urine aminoacids were measured with both colorimetric method and gas-cromatography: there was a very good correlation between the results of the two methods ($y = 8.04X - 1689, r = 0.85, p < 0.001$).

Statistical analysis was performed by use of unpaired Student's t test for the comparison of parametric data and the Mann-Witney U test for non parametric data; the χ^2 test with Yeates correction was used for evaluating statistical significance of any difference in the prevalence of tubule disorders in patients with or without BJ proteinuria; linear correlation analysis (after log transformation of data if necessary) was performed for the evaluation of any correlation between pairs of data.

Results

Patients with detectable BJ proteinuria had lower GFR than either BJ-negative patients and the controls (C) (Table 2). CCr was not correlated with BJ excretion (mg/g Cr) either in BJκ ($r = 0.35$, p = NS) or in BJλ ($r = 0.08$, p = NS).

Out of all BJ-positive patients, 18 patients (11 BJκ and 7 BJλ) had GFR > 70 ml/min: BJ excretion was in these patients 570 ± 1064 mg/g Cr (ranges 50—3644), not statistically different than in 19 BJ-positive patients with GFR < 70 ml/min (951 ± 1087, ranges 50—3848). Plasma

Table 2. Biochemical data in controls and 'prospective' patients (mean ± SD).

	CCr ml/min	$PHCO_3$ mM	PCa mg/dl	TmP mg/dlGF	FEUa %	$P\beta_2M$ $\mu g/ml$	$U_{\beta 2M}V$ $\mu g/day$	$FE\beta_2M$ %	AA/Cr mg/g	U_GV mg/day	BJ/Cr mg/g
C (n = 35)	106 ± 39	24.2 ± 2.9	9.0 ± 0.5	3.20 ± 0.5	8.4 ± 3.2	1.8 ± 0.6	142 ± 172	0.04 ± 0.05	707 ± 232	10 ± 34	—
BJ-neg (n = 50)	94 ± 32	24.9 ± 2.2	8.9 ± 0.5	3.01 ± 0.65	9.2 ± 6.4	2.3 ± 1.4	272 ± 424	0.08 ± 0.1	738 ± 296	27 ± 126	—
BJκ (n = 20)	73 ±• 32	23.7 ± 2.8	8.8 ± 0.7	2.95 ± 0.97	10.5 ± 7.1	6.2 ±¶ 8.0	4739 ±* 6731	3.5 ±° 7.9	986 ±§ 558	91 ± 279	823 ± 111
BJλ (n = 17)	72 ±• 47	24.7 ± 2.8	8.8 ± 0.7	2.96 ± 1.04	8.5 ± 7.8	7.0 ±# 7.3	14351 ±# 26385	4.6 ±° 9.4	862 ±§ 359	351 ± 1195	687 ± 1070
$\kappa + \lambda$ (n = 37)	73 ±* 39	24.2 ± 2.8	8.8 ± 0.7	2.96 ± 0.98	9.5 ± 7.4	6.2 ±¶ 7.7	9133 ±* 18800	4.1 ±• 8.5	926 ±§ 470	221 ± 864	760 ± 1079

vs controls (C), p <: § = 0.05; ° = 0.02; • = 0.01; ¶ = 0.005; # = 0.002; * = 0.001

calcium levels were not different in the patients from the controls. No patient had plasma calcium values > 10.2 mg/dl, 2 were hypocalcemic (n° 45: 7.1 mg/dl, he was later disclosed to have primary hypoparathyroidism; n° 81: 6.9 mg/dl, he was uremic with a GFR at 8.4 ml/min).

β_2M *excretion.* BJκ and BJλ but not BJ-negative patients had significantly higher plasma levels (Pβ_2M), urine excretion ($U_{\beta 2M}V$) and FEβ_2M than C (Table 2); overall 20/35 BJ-positive patients (12 BJκ and 8 BJλ) but only 4/48 BJ-negative patients, had FEβ_2M values higher than the upper normal limit of 0.2% ($p < 0.0001$) (Table 3). FEβ_2M was inversely correlated with CCr (log FEβ_2M = −0.013 CCr + 0.18, $r = 0.53$, $p < 0.001$).

Moreover GFR in patients with increased FEβ_2M (89.8 ± 32.3 ml/min) was not significantly different than that in patients with normal FEβ_2M (74.9 ± 42.9 ml/min). Pβ_2M levels were lower in patients with FEβ_2M < 0.2 (2.36 ± 1.3 μg/ml, ranges 1.2—8.8) than in patients with FEβ_2M > 0.2 (8.27 ± 8.8, ranges 1.54—32, $p < 0.01$), however there was a large overlap of values for many patients of the two groups. Considering only patients with GFR > 70 ml/min, FEβ_2M was higher in 18 BJ-positive patients (0.87 ± 2.57%, ranges 0.005—11.1) than in 39 BJ-negative patients (0.086 ± 0.1, ranges 0.003—0.503, $p < 0.01$) and controls ($p < 0.002$); Pβ_2M did not differ in these 18 BJ-positive patients (2.7 ± 1.0 μg/ml, ranges 1.46—5.39, $p < 0.01$ vs controls) from those in the 39 BJ-negative patients (2.1 ± 1.09, ranges 1.2—4.65, $p < 0.001$ vs controls).

Aminoacid excretion. BJκ and BJλ had significantly higher AA urine excretion than C and BJ-negative patients (Table 2); in 7/37 BJ-positive patients, but only in 1/49 BJ-negative patients, AA were higher than the upper normal limit ($p < 0.01$) (Table 3). In all the patients AA excretion was slightly correlated with GFR ($y = -2.59X + 1029$, $r = 0.24$, $p < 0.05$). In 26 patients with GFR < 70 ml/min AA were 816 ± 470 mg/g Cr vs 778 ± 337 in 60 patients with GFR > 70 ml/min (p = NS). Since AA excretion decreases in patients with renal insufficiency [9], increased excretion is likely to indicate tubular damage for any level of GFR.

Phosphate excretion. There were no significant differences in TmP/GFR between the patients and controls (Table 2). TmP/GFR was lower than control limits in 9/37 BJ-positive (GFR 8.4 to 93 ml/min) and in 5/20 BJ-negative patients (GFR 71 to 131 ml/min) (Table 3) (p = NS). TmP/GFR was not correlated with GFR ($r = 0.06$, p = NS). Only in 2 patients with reduced TmP/GFR and GFR of 23.5 (n° 65) and 8.4 ml/min

Table 3. Prevalence and patterns of tubular transport disorders observed in patients with or without BJ proteinuria.

	Pt n°	β_2M	AA	GLUC°	P	Ua	RTA II[&]	RTA I	GFR
BJ-neg	8	–	+	–	+	+	–•	–	74
	11	–	–	–	–	+	–	N.I.	73
	12	–	–	–	–	+	–	–	83
	17	+	–	–	–	+	–	N.I.	75
	21	+	–	–	–	–	–	N.I.	109
	26	+	–	–	+	–	–	N.I.	72
	27	–	–	–	+	–	–	–	84
	28	+	–	–	–	–	–	N.I.	97
	29	–	N.I.	–	+	–	–	–	179
	33	–	–	+	–	–	–	–	158
	46	N.I.	–	+	–	–	–•	–	83
	49	–	–	–	+	–	–	N.I.	131
	12/50	4/48	1/49	2/45	5/50	4/49	0/50	0/32	101 ± 36
BJ κ	54	+	+	–	–	–	–	N.I.	76
	55	+	+	–	–	–	–	N.I.	31
	56	+	+	+	–	–	–	N.I.	71
	58	+	–	–	–	–	–	–	43
	59	+	–	–	+	–	–	N.I.	81
	61	+	–	–	–	–	–	N.I.	18
	62	+	–	–	–	+	–	+	5
	64	+	–	–	+	–	–	–	77
	65	+	+	+	+	+	–•	N.I.	24
	66	+	–	–	+	–	–•	+*	61
	69	+	–	–	+	+	–	–	94
	70	+	–	–	–	–	–	–	134
	12/20	12/19	4/20	2/17	5/20	3/20	0/19	2/11	60 ± 37

Table 3. (*Continued*)

	Pt n°	β_2M	AA	GLUC°	P	Ua	RTA II[&]	RTA I	GFR
BJλ	71	–	–	+	+	–	–	N.I.	67
	73	+	–	–	–	–	–	–	39
	75	+	–	–	–	–	–	N.I.	7
	77	–	+	–	–	–	–	–	130
	79	+	+	–	–	–	–	N.I.	137
	81	+	–	+	+	+	+•	+	9
	83	+	+	–	+	–	–	N.I.	46
	84	+	–	–	–	–	–	N.I.	84
	85	+	–	+	+	+	–	–	42
	86	+	–	–	–	–	–	–	54
	10/17	8/16	3/17	3/17	4/17	2/17	1/17	1/8	61 ± 44
($\kappa + \lambda$)	22/37	20/35	7/37	5/34	9/37	5/37	1/36	3/19	60 ± 39
BJ-neg vs BJ-pos: χ^2 or t, $p <$	0.001	0.0001	0.01	N.S.	N.S.	N.S.	N.S.	0.05	0.001
BJ-neg vs BJ-pos:	⩾2 disorders: 3/50 vs 14/37							$\chi^2 = 13.7$,	$p < 0.0005$
	⩾3 disorders: 1/50 vs 8/37							$\chi^2 = 8.83$,	$p < 0.005$
	⩾4 disorders: 0/50 vs 3/37							$\chi^2 = 4.20$,	$p < 0.05$
	GFR > 70 ml/min, ⩾2 disorders: 1/43 vs 6/18							$\chi^2 = 12.01$,	$p < 0.01$

[&] Normal plasma pH and HCO_3 levels (in the absence of alkali therapy) were considered to exclude RTA II; • indicates patients in whom a bicarbonate titration curve was performed.

°: Diabetic patients were excluded.

*: 'Incomplete' RTA I.

N.I.: Not investigated.

(n° 81), respectively (Table 3), PTH was increased to 14.8 and 31.3 pmol/ml (n.v. < 8.4) while it was normal in the remaining 12 patients.

Uric acid excretion. FEUa was not significantly different in the patients and the controls (Table 2). In 5/37 BJ-positive and 4/48 BJ-negative patients it was higher than control limits (p = NS) (Table 3). There was a significant inverse correlation between FEUa and GFR ($y = -0.064X + 14.7$, $r = 0.35$, $p < 0.01$); however FEUa in patients with GFR > 70 ml/min (8.7 ± 6.1) did not differ from values in patients with GFR < 70 ml/min (10.8 ± 7.9). Overall 5/37 BJ-positive and 4/49 BJ-negative patients had increased FEUa: GFR was higher than 70 ml/min in 5 of these patients (Table 3). No 'prospective' patient had hypouricemia (PUa < 2.2 mg/dl).

Glucose excretion. Glucose excretion was not statistically higher than in controls in 45 BJ-negative and 34 BJ-positive nondiabetic patients (Table 2); 2 BJ-negative and 5 BJ-positive patients had glucose excretion higher than 200 mg/day (207 to 4960 mg/day); GFR was > 70 ml/min in 3 out of them (Table 3).

TmG/GFR was evaluated in 15 patients (8 BJ-negative and 7 BJ-positive) without 'spontaneous' glicosuria (GFR 94 ± 30 ml/min, 61 to 155 ml); results in the patients did not differ from normal values (BJ-negative : 272 ± 64 mg/dl GFR; BJ-positive: 272 ± 73; 16 controls: 292 ± 45, p = NS). In 4 patients with normoglycemic glicosuria (n° 46 and the 3 'Fanconi' patients) the glucose titration curve was typical of 'type A' glicosuria in 2 (FS1 and FS3, TmG/GFR 168 and 154 mg/dl GFR respectively, n.v. 195—385) and of 'type B' glicosuria in 2 (n° 46 and FS2, TmG/GFR 361 and 347 mg/dl, respectively).

Renal acidification and acid base parameters. Plasma HCO_3 levels were not different in the patients from the controls (Table 2). Only 2 'prospective' patients (n° 62 and n° 81, with GFR 5 and 9.4 ml/min, respectively), and 2 'Fanconi' patients (FS1 and FS2, with GFR 24 and 38 ml/min) were acidotic (n° 62: $PHCO_3$ 15 mM; n° 81: 17.3; FS1: 17; FS2: 19.5; n.v. 21—28). $TmHCO_3$/GFR was low in the 3 patients in whom it was performed (n° 81: 19.7 mmol/lGFR; FS1: 19.2; FS2: 20; n.v. 23—31) confirming a type II RTA (Table 4). $TmHCO_3$/GFR was evaluated in 7 additional nonacidotic 'prospective' patients (4 BJ-negative and 3 BJ-positive, GFR 25 to 113 ml/min) and in FS3: in all it was normal (23.5 to 28.5). Distal acidification was evaluated randomly in 52 patients (32 BJ-negative and 20 BJ-positive) and in the 3 'Fanconi' patients. Forty patients had urine pH of 5.3 or less on 'basal' urine sample, and, in

Table 4. Clinical and biochemical data in 5 patients with abnormal acid-base homeostasis.

Pt n°	BJ	Ig g/l	$PHCO_3$* mM	min UpH	$TmHCO_3$ mmol/l	AG mM	GFR ml/min	Diagnosis
62	κ	48	15	6.87	/	8.4	5	RTA I; ?RTA II
66	κ	41	24.8	5.92°	28.6	10	61.3	RTA I, incomp.
81	λ	20	17.3	5.71°	19.7	14	9.4	RTA I + II
F.S.1	λ	21	17	6.5	19.2	12	24	RTA I + II
F.S.2	λ	11	19.5	5.07°	20	13	38	RTA II
n.v.		<20	21—29	<5.3	21—31	8—18	>80	

* = 'Basal' plasma HCO_3; ° = minimal UpH after oral acid load; AG = plasma anion gap.

the absence of acidosis, were considered to have 'normal' acidification capacity. Eleven patients with fasting urine pH > 5.3 underwent a NH_4Cl acid load: only in 2 patients urine pH did not fall below 5.3: n° 81 (min UpH 5.71 with plasma HCO_3 14.2 mM, GFR 9 ml/min) and n° 66 (min UpH 5.92 with plasma HCO_3 20.5 mM, basal 24.8, and GFR 61.3 ml/min): thus the latter patient had 'incomplete' type I RTA. A last patient (n° 62) had both acidosis and abnormally high urine pH (6.87) and was considered to have complete type I RTA (Table 4). Of the 3 'Fanconi' patients, FS3 had normal acid base status ($PHCO_3$ 24 mM, urine pH 5.05, $TmHCO_3$/GFR 26.5); FS1 had acidosis with abnormally high urine pH (6.5) and was considered to have combined type I and II RTA; FS2 had 'basal' urine pH of 5.65 ($PHCO_3$ 19.5 mM) which fell to 5.07 after acid load ($PHCO_3$ 14.5 mM): this response was considered to be consistent with pure type II RTA (in which increased distal delivery of HCO_3 might have prevented maximal acidification of basal urines despite systemic acidosis) (Table 4). Overall only 5 patients (3 'prospective', FS1 and FS2) had abnormal acid-base metabolism (Table 4): all but one (n° 66) had a severe reduction of GFR; type I and II RTA were associated in 3 patients and only in one patient there was an isolated type II RTA. Hyperglobulinemia (> 40 g/l) was present in 2 patients with type I RTA (n° 62 and n° 66); other 3 patients with hyperglobulinemia (n° 24, 35 and 75) had normal acidification, while in additional 5 hyperglobulinemic patients (n° 11, 56, 61, 63, 65) distal acidification was not evaluated. In no one of them was $PHCO_3$ reduced.

Segmental Na reabsorption and maximal urine dilution capacity. Both CLi and DRNa were higher in 10 BJ-positive than in 18 BJ-negative patients, but not than in 13 young (not age-matched) healthy controls (Table 5). However, since no age-matched controls were available for this study,

Table 5. Lithium clearance (CLi), distal Na reabsorption (DRNa), minimum urine osmolality ($UOsm_{min}$) and maximal free water clearance (CH_2O) in patients and controls.

	CLi ml/dl GFR	DRNa ml/dl GFR	$UOsm_{min}$ mOsm/Kg H_2O	CH_2O ml/dl GFR	GFR ml/min
Controls (n = 13)	21.2 ± 6.7	18.8 ± 6.6	66 ± 13	7.7 ± 2.2	98 ± 16
p <	NS	NS	NS	NS	0.02
BJ-neg (n = 18)	16.5 ± 5.8	15.9 ± 4.1	74.4 ± 16.5	6.9 ± 2.3	78 ± 24.2
p <	0.05	0.05	0.01	0.02	NS
BJ-pos (n = 10)	22.7 ± 8.1	22.4 ± 7.3	55.1 ± 10.3*	9.4 ± 1.6*	91 ± 46.9

*: vs C, $p < 0.05$.

comparison with these 'normal' values might not be correct, since renal parameters are known to change consistently in elderly people. GFR was > 50 ml/min in all but one BJ-positive patient (n° 81, Table 3).

DRNa was highly correlated with CLi ($y = 0.92X - 0.31$, $r = 0.98$, $p < 0.001$). During maximal water diuresis, BJ-positive patients had lower $UOsm_{min}$ and higher CH_2O than BJ-negative patients and controls (Table 5). Both FS2 and FS3 had increased CLi (49 and 52, 8 ml/dl GFR respectively, n.v. in young healthy people 16—32) and DRNa (46.4 and 49 ml/dl GFR, n.v. 10—28); UOsm and CH_2O were 61 and 45.3 mOsm/Kg H_2O (n.v. 40—90) and 16.5 and 19.8 ml/dl GFR (n.v. 4—11) respectively.

Thus these data suggest increased Na reabsorption along distal nephron in BJ-positive patients as a consequence of increased distal Na delivery out of the proximal tubule.

Prevalence and pattern of tubule disorders

As shown in Table 3, 12/50 BJ-negative (24%) and 22/37 BJ-positive (60%) patients had 1 or more tubule transport abnormality: the higher prevalence in BJ-positive patients was statistically significant ($p < 0.001$). BJ-positive patients also had a significantly higher prevalence of reduced tubular reabsorption of β_2M and AA, and of type I RTA. No difference was shown in the prevalence of tubule disorders between BJκ and BJλ. The prevalence of more than one tubule disorder (up to more than 4) was still significantly higher in BJ-positive than in BJ-negative patients. GFR in 53 patients with normal tubule function (86.2 ± 35.6 ml/min) was not different than in 34 patients with one or more tubule disorders (81.5 ± 37.6). Bence Jones proteinuria in 22 BJ-positive patients with abnormal tubular function (906 ± 1107 mg/g Cr) was not different than in 15 BJ-positive patients with normal tubular function (548 ± 1037).

To exclude any effect of reduced GFR on renal tubule function, the prevalence of tubule disorders was evaluated in patients with GFR > 70 ml/min (43 BJ-negative and 18 BJ-positive): again there was a significantly higher prevalence of tubular disorders in BJ-positive patients (Table 3). The pattern of tubular disorders was highly variable in each patient; increased excretion of β_2M was the most frequently observed event (29% of all cases, 59% of BJ-positive patients); reabsorption of phosphorus (16 and 24% respectively), uric acid (10.5 and 13.5%), aminoacids (9.5 and 19%), glucose (8 and 15%), bicarbonate (1.2 and 2.8%) were much less frequently abnormal.

Only in 9 patients (1 BJ-negative) 3 or more transport disorders were associated, and in only 3 (i.e. 8% of BJ-positive patients) there were more than 3 disorders. In all BJ-positive patients, BJ proteinuria (mg/g Cr) was not correlated with GFR (r = 0.16), FEβ_2M (r = 0.07), AA (r = 0.16), FEUa (r = 0.001), TmP/GFR (r = 0.17).

Discussion

This study confirms the significant association of BJ proteinuria with both renal damage (as assessed by reduced GFR) and tubular function abnormalities. In effect patients with detectable BJ proteinuria, but not BJ-negative patients, had significantly reduced GFR; in addition the former had a significantly higher prevalence of tubular abnormalities than the latter. Though GFR impairment (< 70 ml/min) and tubular disfunctions were frequently associated, there was still a higher prevalence of tubule abnormalities in BJ-positive patients when only patients with well preserved GFR (i.e. > 70 ml/min) were considered. Thus, abnormal tubular function does not appear to be simply a consequence of reduced GFR, but instead may precede the appearance of significant GFR impairment. κ or λ BJ proteins had similar effects on both GFR and tubular function, confirming previous reports [18, 20, 21]. On the other hand even the amount of urine excretion of BJ protein was not correlated with tubular effects: some patients with small amounts of BJ protein had severe and widespread tubular disfunction (as our patients FS1 and FS2), while other patients with very high BJ proteinuria had normal GFR and tubular function.

The detection of tubular abnormalities in patients with BJ proteinuria appears to be critically dependent upon the type and sensitivity of each individual analyte and/or test of tubular function: Cooper et al. [20] have shown that urine excretion of α_1-microglobulin and α_1-acid glycoprotein is increased in almost all the patients with significant LC proteinuria. Other microproteins, instead, such as retinol-binding protein [20, 21] and lysozime [21], appear to increase only in patients with reduced GFR. In our patients β_2M excretion was increased in about half BJ-positive patients, with or without GFR impairment.

This different behaviour of each microprotein might indicate either a different severity of tubular lesions, or instead might simply be related to different mechanism(s) of proteinuria. 'Tubular' proteinuria may result either from reduced tubular reabsorption of microproteins or from increased glomerular filtration above a tubular 'threshold' for reabsorption (so-called 'overflow' proteinuria) [27]. Competition for reabsorption of each microprotein is also exercised either by other microproteins as well as by more simple molecules, such as aminoacids [27]. Inhibition of cell metabolism also results in reduced tubular reabsorption, indicating that microprotein reabsorption is an energy-dependent cellular process. 'Overflow' microproteinuria occurs in renal failure because plasma levels of microproteins increase, due to reduced renal catabolism [27, 35]; hyperfiltration in the remaining glomeruli is also likely to contribute in a still unpredictable manner to increased filtered load per single nephron of each microprotein above tubular threshold. Moreover, maximal reabsorption capacity (in relation to 'normal' filtered load) is likely to vary for each different microprotein, though little information on this point is as yet available.

Available evidence suggest that tubular threshold of α_1-microglobulin (one of the biggest microproteins, with a molecular weight of 33.000) is very near to physiologic filtered loads: its plasma levels and fractional excretion increase very early in chronic renal disease, when GFR is still near to 80 ml/min [35]. Maximal reabsorptive capacity for lysozime, a much smaller protein (m.w. 14.000), is instead about 20 times higher than physiologic filtered loads [27]. Thus increased excretion of α_1-microglobulin in the context of BJ proteinuria might simply result from competition for reabsorption and/or subtle reductions of renal parenchimal mass, or both, while increased urine excretion of lysozime and retinol-binding protein might indicate a sufficiently severe renal damage to increase plasma levels and filtered load for single glomerulus above a rather high tubular threshold. However it has to be stressed that even increased plasma levels above tubular threshold do not exclude a concomitant reduction of tubular reabsorptive capacity (if urine excretion were higher than expected for any degree of plasma levels and GFR), and that increased urine excretion of one microprotein does not necessarily indicate reduced tubular reabsorptive capacity (if plasma levels are not known). These informations, however, are not generally available in most published series of patients with BJ proteinuria.

In our patients, FEβ_2M showed a significant inverse correlation with GFR, confirming the influence of decreasing GFR on renal handling of microproteins. However in patients with GFR > 70 ml/min, BJ-positive patients, but not BJ-negative patients, had significantly increased FEβ_2M, despite similar Pβ_2M values. Thus BJ proteinuria 'per se', in the absence of any significant GFR impairment, appeared to be able to reduce tubular reabsorptive capacity for β_2M. Similar results as ours were reported by Engström et al. [36], who showed increased β_2M urine excretion in some myeloma patients despite normal GFR and only slightly increased plasma levels. Since FEβ_2M and BJ proteinuria were not correlated, increased excretion of β_2M was unlikely to be related to competition for tubular reabsorption with light chains. The significantly higher prevalence, in patients with BJ proteinuria in comparison with BJ-negative patients, of specific tubular transport abnormalities other than reduced β_2M reabsorption suggests instead that tubule reabsorptive processes were more widely disrupted in patients with BJ proteinuria. BJ-positive patients had significantly increased aminoacid excretion; they also had a significantly higher CLi (i.e. distal delivery of glomerular filtrate) than BJ-negative patients, even though an absolute increase was seen only in a few patients. Abnormal proximal reabsorption of Na/fluid in patients with BJ proteinuria was more clearly shown by the increased free water generation, and a lower UOsm attained during maximal water diuresis, which were clearly indicative of increased delivery of Na/fluid to post-proximal segments of the renal tubule.

Thus, one possible explanation of the mechanism(s) of light chain toxicity on renal tubule cells is inhibition of Na reabsorption, which would also impair the reabsorption of all Na-cotrasported solutes. Experimental evidence would support this possibility, since in vitro BJ proteins from patients with multiple myeloma were able to inhibit the activity of the ouabain-sensitive Na/K-ATPase enzyme [25].

It has to be remembered, however, that the pattern of tubular abnormalities we have observed in our patients was quite variable (Table 3); in particular a generalized tubular disfunction was by no means the rule, and only in 3 'prospective' patients more than 3 transport abnormalities were seen. The meaning of this variability remains unclear, and might possibly indicate different degrees of 'toxicity' of each individual BJ protein.

Despite distal tubule abnormalities have frequently been described in patients with BJ proteinuria [3, 4, 6, 7, 9, 10, 12, 13, 15, 17] we were unable to confirm this finding: distal Na reabsorption and free water generation were perfectly normal in the patients studied, and only in 3/52 'prospective' patients acidification capacity was abnormal. Almost all the patients with abnormal acid-base homeostasis had also advanced renal failure (Table 4). Also in our patients, when tubular acidification was abnormal both proximal and distal tubule acidosis most often coexisted (Table 4), as widely reported [3, 4, 6, 7, 9, 10, 12, 13, 15].

An important question is which the clinical consequences of abnormal tubular function in the context of BJ proteinuria might be. Osteomalacia (secondary to hypophosphatemia, acidosis and possibly abnormal renal vitamin D metabolism) [15, 37] and chronic metabolic acidosis are two well documented, though rather rare, possibilities. Predisposition to dehydration might result from reduced concentration capacity [17, 21] as well as from abnormal tubular handling of Na, as observed in our patients. It has been suggested [20, 21] that reduced proximal tubular competence might be associated with decreased tubular catabolism of light chains and thus to increased BJ proteinuria and a greater risk of cast formation along the distal nephron. However we did not show any statistical difference either in BJ proteinuria or in GFR levels between patients with normal or abnormal tubular function. Thus our data do not allow to confirm enhanced nephrotoxicity of light chains in patients with tubular abnormalities.

References

1. Bradley JR, Thiru S, Evans DB. Light chains and the kidney. J Clin Pathol 1987; 40: 53—60.
2. Ganeval D, Jungers P, Noel LH, Droz D. La néphropathie du myélome. Actualités Néphrologique de l'Hopital Necker. Paris: Flammarion, 1977: 309—41.
3. Sirota JH, Hamerman D. Renal function studies in an adult subject with the Fanconi syndrome. Am J Med 1954; 16: 138—52.
4. Engle RL, Wallis LA. Multiple Myeloma and the Adult Fanconi Syndrome. Report of a case with crystal-like deposits in the tumor cells and in the epithelial cells of the kidney. Am J Med 1957; 22: 5—12.
5. Costanza DJ, Smoller M. Multiple myeloma with the Fanconi syndrome. Study of a case, with electron microscopy of the kidney. Am J Med 1963; 34: 125—33.
6. Dedmon RE, West JH, Schwartz TB. The adult Fanconi syndrome. Report of two cases, one with multiple myeloma. Med Clin North Am 1963; 47: 191—206.
7. Harrison JF, Blainey JD. Adult Fanconi syndrome with monoclonal abnormality of immunoglobulin light chain. J Clin Pathol 1967; 20: 42—8.
8. Horn ME, Knapp MS, Page FT, Walker WHC. Adult Fanconi syndrome and multiple myelomatosis. J Clin Pathol 1969; 22: 414—6.
9. Lee DBN, Drinkard JP, Rosen VJ, Gonick HC. The Adult Fanconi syndrome. Medicine 1972; 51: 107—38.
10. Finkel PN, Kronenberg K, Pesce AJ, Pollak VE, Pirani CL. Adult Fanconi syndrome, amyloidosis and marked K-light chain proteinuria. Nephron 1973; 10: 1—24.

11. Maldonado JE, Velosa JA, Kyle RA, Wagoner RD, Holley KE, Salassa RM. Fanconi Syndrome in adults. A manifestation of a latent form of myeloma. Am J Med 1975; 58: 354—64.
12. Smithline N, Kassirer JP, Cohen JJ. Light chain nephropathy. Renal tubular disfunction associated with light chain proteinuria. N Engl J Med 1976; 294: 71—4.
13. Lazar GS, Feinstein DI. Distal renal tubular acidosis in multiple myeloma. Arch Intern Med 1981; 141: 655—7.
14. Sewell RL, Dorreen MS. Adult Fanconi syndrome progressing to multiple myeloma. J Clin Pathol 1984; 37: 1256—8.
15. Rao DS, Parfitt AM, Villanueva AR, Dorman PJ, Kleerekoper M. Hypophosphatemic Osteomalacia and adult Fanconi syndrome due to light-chain nephropathy. Another form of oncogenous osteomalacia. Am J Med 1987; 82: 333—8.
16. Chan KW, Ho FCS, Chan MK. Adult Fanconi syndrome in κ light chain myeloma. Arch Pathol Lab Med 1987; 111: 139—42.
17. De Fronzo RA, Cooke CR, Wright JR, Humphrey RL. Renal function in patients with multiple myeloma. Medicine 1978; 57: 151—66.
18. Dahlstrom U, Martensson J, Lindstrom FD. Occurrence of adult Fanconi syndrome in benign monoclonal gammopathy. Acta Med Scand 1980; 208: 425—9.
19. Scarpioni L, Ballocchi S, Bergonzi G, Cecchettin M, Dall'Aglio, Fontana F, Gandi U, Pantano C, Poisetti PG, Zanazzi MA. Glomerular and tubular proteinuria in myeloma relationship with Bence Jones proteinuria. Contr Nephrol 1981; 26: 89—102.
20. Cooper EH, Forbes MA, Crockson RA, Maclennan ICM. Proximal renal tubular function in myelomatosis: observations in the fourth Medical Research Council Trial. J Clin Pathol 1984; 37: 852—8.
21. Coward RA, Mallick NP, Delamore IW. Tubular function in multiple myeloma. Clin Nephrol 1985; 24: 180—5.
22. Fermin EA, Johnson CA, Eckel RE, Bernier GM. Renal removal of low molecular weight proteins in myeloma and renal transplant patients. Lab Clin Med 1974; 83: 681—94.
23. Preuss HG, Hammack WJ, Murdaugh HV. The effect of Bence Jones protein on the in vitro function of rabbit renal cortex. Nephron 1967; 5: 210—6.
24. Preuss HG, Weiss FR, Iammarino RM, Hammack WJ, Murdaugh HV. Effects on rat kidney slice function in vitro of proteins from the urines of patients with myelomatosis and nephrosis. Clin Sci Mol Med 1974; 46: 283—94.
25. McGeoch J, Ledingham J, Smith JF, Ross B. Inhibition of active-transport sodium-potassium ATPase by myeloma protein. Lancet 1978; i: 17—8.
26. Poulik MD. Structural, biological and clinical aspects of β_2-microglobulin. Am Ass Clin Chem (Prot.) 1984; 1: 1—10.
27. Maack T. Renal handling of low molecular weight proteins. Am J Med 1975; 58: 57—64.
28. Puig JG, Antón FM, Sanz AM, Gaspar G, Lesmes A, Ramos T, Vázquez JO. Renal handling of uric acid in normal subject by means of the pyrazinamide and probenecid tests. Nephron 1983; 35: 183—6.
29. Walton RJ, Bijvoet OLM. Nomogram for derivation of renal threshold phosphate concentration. Lancet 1975; ii: 309—10.
30. Rombolà G, Colussi G, De Ferrari ME, Surian MM, Malberti F, Minetti L. Clinical evaluation of segmental tubular reabsorption of sodium and fluid in man: lithium vs free water clearances. Nephrol Dial Transplant 1987; 2: 212—8.
31. Ritchie FR, Smith R. Immunofixation. Applications to the study of monoclonal proteins. Clin Chem 1976; 22: 1982—5.

32. Bernard AM, Lawerys RR. Comparison of turbidimetry with particle counting for the determination of human $\beta_2$microglobulin by latex immunoassay (LIA). Clin Chim Acta 1982; 119: 335—9.
33. Colussi G, Rombolà G, De Ferrari ME, Rolando P, Surian M, Malberti F, Minetti L. Pharmacological evaluation of urate renal handling in humans : pyrazinamide test vs combined pyrazinamide and probenecid administration. Nephrol Dial Transpant 1987; 2: 10—6.
34. Roscoe JM, Goldstein MB, Halperin ML, Wilson DR, Stinebaugh BJ. Lithium-induced impairment of urine acidification. Kidney Int 1976; 7: 344—50.
35. Kusano E, Suzuki M, Asano Y, Ifoh Y, Takagi K, Kawai T. Human alfa 1 microglobulin and its relationship with renal function. Nephron 1985; 41: 344—50.
36. Engstrom W, Hyldahl L, Wahregren P. Urinary excretion of $\beta_2$microglobulin in myeloma patients. Clin Chim Acta 1980; 108: 369—74.
37. Colussi G, De Ferrari ME, Surian M, Malberti F, Rombolà G, Pontoriero G, Galvanini G, Minetti L. Vitamin D metabolites and osteomalacia in the human Fanconi syndrome. Proc EDTA-ERA 1984; 21: 756—60.

6. Renal amyloidosis — Retrospective collaborative study

G. BANFI, M. MORIGGI, R. CONFALONIERI, E. MINETTI, F. FERRARIO, A. BUCCI, S. PASQUALI, U. DONINI, E. SCHIAFFINO, G. BARBIANO DI BELGIOJOSO, T. BERTANI, C. POZZI, M. RAVELLI, L. FURCI, A. LUPO, C. COMOTTI, A. VOLPI & E. P. SCHENA

Renal amyloidosis

The kidney frequently contains amyloid deposits in the so-called 'imunocyte dyscrasia-associated systemic amyloidosis' (IDSA) and renal abnormality is the main presenting feature in most patients [1]. In the literature renal abnormality has been reported for 40—80% of the cases with primary (AL) amyloidosis and it is even more frequent in patients with myeloma associated (MAL) amyloidosis [1, 2, 3]. Progressive renal failure, which is almost invariable in renal amyloidosis, has bad prognostic significance and is one of the main causes of death. In this study we retrospectively analyzed the morphologic and clinical features of 99 patients with AL or MAL renal amyloidosis.

Patients and methods

Eighty-five patients with clinical diagnosis of primary and 14 with myeloma-associated amyloidosis had biopsy-proven renal amyloidosis, as seen by light microscopy of Congo Red stained material observed under polarized light or by electron microscopy. Patients were excluded from the study if their diseases were considered secondary to hereditary factors or chronic inflammatory disease or to cancer other than myeloma. Biopsy samples adequate for a semiquantitative evaluation were obtained from 63 patients. The amount of amyloid in the interstitium and vascular tree, the tubular atrophy, and the interstitial fibrosis were all scored from 0 to 3+. Both entity and pattern of distribution of glomerular amyloid were evaluated; three degrees of intensity were scored and a 'nodular' or 'diffuse' pattern was identified. Sixty-five AL patients were followed for 25 ± 29 and 12 MAL patients for 11 ± 12.5 months. Statistical analysis has been performed by the 't' Student and Chi-square tests. Survival curves were

Minetti et al. (eds.), The kidney in plasma cell dyscrasias. ISBN 978-94-010-7085-0

calculated starting from histologic diagnosis by the methods of Peto [4] and statistically evaluated by the Log-Rank test.

Results

Clinical features at presentation

The main clinical variables at time of referral are shown in Table 1. Nephrotic syndrome (urinary protein excretion $\geqslant$ 3 g/l and plasma albumin < 2.5 g/dl) was the most common renal syndrome in both AL and MAL patients. In both groups it was associated with renal insufficiency of variable degrees (plasma creatinine > 1.5 mg/dl) in a considerable number of cases, with a slight prevalence in MAL patients. Isolated proteinuria (<3 g/l) was rare and found only in AL patients. Acute renal failure was observed in few and comparable numbers of cases in both groups: it was favoured mostly by infection, dehydration or antibiotic administration, preceding the presentation. Twenty-eight (33%) AL and 7 (50%) MAL patients had had signs of nephropathy, mainly proteinuria, for 15 ± 7.7 and 18 ± 5 mos, respectively, before biopsy. Among the extra-renal manifestations of heart involvement, arrhythmias, branch block, low-

Table 1. Clinical features at presentation in 99 patients with renal AL or MAL amyloidosis.

	AL	MAL
N° patients	85	14
Male/female	40/45	8/6
Mean age (y)	57 ± 12	60 ± 7
Renal syndrome (n° pts %)		
Nephrotic syndrome	85	78
Renal insufficiency	41	57
Acute renal failure	5.5	7
Isolated proteinuria	4.5	—
Extrarenal-syndromes		
Cardiomyopathy	50	60
Hypertension	23	25
Hepatomegaly	57	77
Splenomegaly	15	23
Gastrointestinal tract abnormalities	13	—
Macroglossia	7	—
Neuropathy	12	18

voltage electrocardiogram, hypertrophic cardiomyopathy without hypertension were the most common and worrying in both groups of patients. Gastrointestinal tract (GIT) symptoms and macroglossia were rare and found exclusively in AL patients. About 25% of both groups had severe hypotension (SP ⩽ 100 mm Hg). Fifty percent of the AL patients had had sporadic non-specific manifestations from few months to two years before the onset of nephropathy. Fatigue, weight loss, fever, GIT symptoms and purpura were most commonly reported. The mean values for the usual laboratory variables were comparable in the two groups. Severe anemia and/or leukopenia were exceptional and thrombocytopenia was never found, even in MAL patients, nor was severe hypercalcemia (> 11 mg%).

Twenty-seven of 75 (37%) AL patients had a paraprotein in the serum: IgA in 5, IgG in 13, IgM in 2 and isolated light chain in 4. In 10, the Bence Jones (BJ) protein was also found in urine. Seven cases had only a urinary paraprotein making the 45% of patients in whom it was sought with a monoclonal protein in serum and/or urine. The lambda chain was more frequent than kappa both in urine and serum. Eight MAL patients had IgG-lambda and 1 lambda light chain type monoclonal protein; 6 out of 14 also had BJ protein. The "M" component was found in most cases at the same time or after the diagnosis of AL amyloidosis was made. In contrast, 7 patients were known to have myeloma 12 to 36 months before renal amyloidosis was demonstrated. There were increased number of plasma cells from 10 to 30% in 9 out of the 38 bone marrow needle aspirations obtained from the AL patients.

Pathology

In the early stages of glomerular involvement, two distinct patterns of amyloid deposition were evident: nodular, with scattered almost exclusively mesangial location, and uniform or diffuse, characterized by parietal distribution with slight regular thickening of the capillary wall. As the amyloid deposition increased, the nodular pattern became rarer and uniform, and mesangial and parietal involvement was predominant. MAL cases had preferential distribution of these patterns or stages, and the only distinctive feature was seen in 1 case, who had a few myeloma casts.

The degree of tubular damage was comparable in both groups and was more pronounced in cases with acute renal failure. Inflammatory mononuclear cell infiltrate was rarely prominent and usually paralleled the entity of the tubulo-interstitial damage. It was severe only in 2 cases with acute renal failure and patchy tubular necrosis. In Table 2 some morphologic features are correlated. The amount, but not the pattern, of glomerular amyloid seemed to be correlated with the entity of interstitial fibrosis and

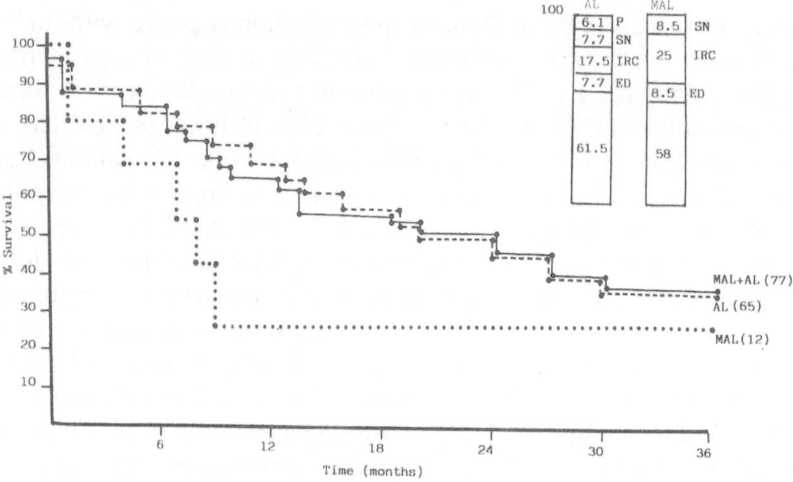

Fig. 1. Survival from time of diagnosis and clinical status at the end of follow-up of patients with primary (AL) and myeloma associated (MAL) amyloidosis. Number of patients in parenthesis.

tubular atrophy, with that of vascular amyloid and, less significantly, with the amount of interstitial amyloid. Interstitial fibrosis was significantly correlated with the amount of interstitial but not of vascular amyloid. The entity of glomerular, vascular and interstitial amyloid was not correlated with the percentage of hyaline glomeruli. Among clinical parameters at time of referral, only the plasma creatinine level was correlated with the amount but not with the pattern of glomerular amyloid. There were no differences between the actuarial survival rates of patients with nodular or diffuse glomerular pattern or those with different stages of glomerular involvement, although there seemed to be a trend towards a better renal survival for patients with early stages of glomerular amyloid.

Outcome

Sixty-five patients with AL amyloidosis were followed for 25 ± 29.4 months (0.5—120). By the end of follow-up, 40 (61%) patients died and 25 (39%) were alive, 5 with nephrotic syndrome, 4 with proteinuria and plasma creatinine ⩽ 1.5 mg/dl, 11 with renal insufficiency of variable degrees; 5 were on regular dialysis. Twelve MAL patients were followed for 11 ± 12.6 months. At the end of follow-up, 7 (58%) were dead and 5 (42%) were alive, 1 on regular dialysis, 3 with renal insufficiency and 1 with nephrotic syndrome and pl. creatinine ⩽ 1.5 mg/dl. In Fig. 1 the actuarial survival curves of AL and MAL patients are reported; 70% of

Table 2. Morphologic correlations in 63 patients with renal AL or MAL amyloidosis.

	Hyaline glomeruli (%)	Tubular atrophy and interstitial fibrosis	Interstitial amyloid	Vascular amyloid
Glomerular amyloid				
1–2 vs 3	ns	0.001	0.02	0.05
Nodular vs uniform	ns	ns	ns	ns
Interstitial amyloid				
0 vs 1–2–3	ns	0.001	–	–
0–1 vs 2–3	ns	0.02	–	–
Vascular amyloid				
1 vs 2–3	ns	ns	–	–
1–2 vs 3	ns	0.05	–	–

AL patients and only 30% of MAL patients were alive 12 months after diagnosis. At 24 months, however, the two curves approached each other, and survivals of AL and MAL patients at that time were 50 and 30% respectively. Even earlier the two curves did not differ significantly. The mean cumulative survival for AL and MAL patients was 24 months. It has to be pointed out that about 30% of the patients died within the first 12 months of observation, accounting for the steep decline of the initial part of the survival curve.

We analyzed the clinical features of patients who died within 6 months after diagnosis and those of patients who died or survived after this period (Table 3), in attempt to identify factors that might have influenced the outcome. Only the incidence of acute renal failure and the degree of renal insufficiency were significantly higher in patients who died within 6 months. Two patients who died, one within and one after 6 months had irreversible ARF that developed after i.v. contrast media infusion. No differences were found in other variables, such as extra-renal involvement, paraprotein in serum or urine, severity of proteinuria, either between MAL patients who died within 6 months and those who died after this time, or between the latter and those alive 6 months after diagnosis.

The main causes of death were cardiac accident (40%), uremia (15%), sepsis (8%), vascular accident (8%) and cachexia (8%); the cause of death remained unknown in 11%, with the same incidences in patients who died within and after 6 months.

It is worth noting, however, that more than 60% of the patients who died had some degree of renal insufficiency. While the majority of patients alive after 6 months developed terminal uremia, some of them after several

Table 3. Clinical and laboratory features of 71 patients with renal AL or MAL and different outcomes.

	Patients dead ≤ 6 mos	Patients dead > 6 mos	Patients alive > 6 mos
N° of patients (MAL)	21 (4)	26 (3)	24 (3)
Mean follow-up (mo)	3.2 ± 2.4	21 ± 12.7	39 ± 35.7
Plasma creatinine mg/dl (excluded ARF)	4.1 ± 3.7*	2.0 ± 1.7	1.6 ± 1.3
Urine protein g/l	8.0 ± 5.0	5.2 ± 3.2	5.3 ± 3.8
'M' component n° pts (%) (serum/urine)	9 (42%)	8 (30%)	9 (37%)
Acute renal failure (ARF)	6 (28%)**	1 (4%)	1 (4%)
Hypertension	4 (20%)	7 (27%)	4 (16%)
Extrarenal involvement	18 (85%)	21 (91%)	16 (70%)
Cytotoxic therapy	3 (14%)	11 (44%)	9 (24%)

* $p < 0.02$.
** $p < 0.01$.

months of stable renal function, 9 patients unexpectedly have maintained normal or slightly abnormal renal function over the entire follow-up period, most of them without receiving any cytotoxic drug. A minority of patients (32%) was given cytotoxic and/or anti-inflammatory drugs, but the evaluation of therapeutic efficacy was impossible because of the great differences in the treatment regimens of each patient.

Twelve patients in this series were submitted to regular dialysis. The overall follow-up was 17.6 ± 15.7 (3—60) months. Eight patients did not have any clinical problem during this time, 4 had chronic hypotension, in 1 associated with episodes of GIT bleeding. Six patients died, 3 with cachexia, 2 with sepsis and 1 with a cardiac arrhythmia, after 8 ± 7.7 months. Six patients were still alive after 27.3 ± 15.7 months. The presence of signs of extra-renal involvement before and after initiation of dialysis apparently did not influence the outcome. The surviving patients had had a longer duration of their disease before terminal uremia than the patients who died (30.3 ± 35.4 months vs 7.5 ± 6.8 months).

Discussion

At onset, primary (AL) amyloidosis has in most of the cases minimal and non specific manifestations, making early diagnosis very difficult. Signs of renal involvement are the most common and earliest clinical manifestations [1, 5] and amyloidosis is one of the diseases one should keep in mind when a nephrotic or proteinuric patient, especially if elderly, is seen. In this series of patients with AL and myeloma-associated (MAL) amyloidosis, renal abnormalities were the first sign of the disease in about 50% and led to correct diagnosis for all of them. While the majority of MAL patients were older than 60 years, about two-thirds of the AL patients were less than 50 years old, a relatively younger age than that reported in other series [5]. Nephrotic syndrome was the most common renal syndrome at presentation, with the same incidence in AL and MAL. In most of them it was accompanied by some degree of renal insufficiency. These findings are comparable to those reported by others [1, 6] but not with those of Kyle [5], who reported a higher incidence of non-nephrotic proteinuria and of Jassen [3], who reported a higher incidence of renal insufficiency in AL and MAL patients not selected for the presence of nephropathy. In our series, signs of cardiomyopathy, hepatomegaly and hypotension were found in a number of cases comparable to those of Jassen [3], but at variance with those of Browning [1] and Kyle [5], who reported a lower incidence of these syndromes. However, unlike these investigators, we rarely observed cases with overt congestive heart failure or with macroglossia.

According to the literature [7, 8, 2, 6], monoclonal protein was found in serum and/or in urine of 20—100% AL patients, probably depending on the sensitivity of the methods or whether or not it was looked for. We found a paraprotein in only 45% of AL patients, versus 100% of MAL patients. As in Kyle's series [5], there was a bone marrow plasmacytosis of more than 10% in 23% of our AL patients, none of whom had evidence of osteolytic lesions, which in contrast were present in one-third of our MAL patients.

In our study as in those of other groups [5], MAL patients did not differ from AL patients in clinical or laboratory features. Because of the common immunochemical characteristics of the fundamental amyloid proteins, in both conditions, the histologic features also could not differentiate AL from MAL cases. Nodular and diffuse or uniform glomerular patterns were equally frequent, the diffuse pattern being more common in advanced stages. The glomerular pattern, at variance with Nakamoto [9], was not correlated with any of the histologic parameters evaluated nor with the degree of proteinuria, of renal insufficiency or of patient survival, while unlike Dikman [10] the amount of glomerular amyloid was correlated with that of vascular and interstitial deposits.

Few renal diseases have an outlook as bad as that for renal amyloidosis associated with immunocyte dyscrasia (IDSA). The mean survival time for IDSA patients ranges from 6 to 28 months [1, 3, 5, 11, 12], not so different from the 4 to 17 months observed for patient with renal AL amyloidosis [5, 6]. Some investigators report a shorter mean survival period for MAL patients than for AL patients without myeloma [4—13], but others do not [11, 12]. In our study the mean survival times for MAL and AL patients respectively were 8 and 24 months, but at 30 months they were 25 and 35%. For the overall series the mean survival was about 24 months, substantially better than the 4 months in Ogg's series [6]. In Browning's study [1], all AL patients died within 3 years of diagnosis. In his recent series, numerically comparable to ours, Kyle [5] reported 17 months median survival in 81 AL patients with nephrosis, with 9 patients surviving more than 4 years, 2 on hemodialysis (HD). Although more than 50% of our patients died by the end of the follow-up, 12 survived more than 3 years, 7 with normal renal function and 4 on HD, and 6 of them more than 5 years, 2 on HD. Hence, we share Kyle's experience [5] that some AL patients may have a surprisingly longer survival than the average. Among the clinical factors, we found that only the severity of renal impairment when first seen seemed to negatively influence the prognosis. Six out of 8 patients with oliguric acute renal failure at referral died within 6 months. Only a minority (30%) of patients were given different types of cytotoxic or anti-inflammatory drugs for variable periods of time. Two out of 23 patients seemed to benefit from therapy, with partial remission of the nephrotic syndrome, but another 2 patients did so spontaneously. In our series, as in most others, cardiac involvement was the main cause of death, but in the large majority of patients who died there were variable degrees of renal insufficiency, which was the major contributing factor to death.

In this study only 12 patients among those who developed terminal uremia were submitted to regular dialysis. Their mean survival was 24 months, comparable to that reported in the EDTA registry [14] for patients with all types of amyloidosis. Therefore, these patients too, although they have systemic disease, should not be denied the benefits of substitutive treatment programs.

References

1. Browning MJ, Banks RA, Tribe CR, Hollingworth P, Kingswood C, MacKenzie JC,

Bacon PA. Ten years' experience of an amyloid clinic. A clinicopathological survey. Q J Med 1985; 54: 213—27.
2. Kyle RA, Bayard ED. Amyloidosis: review of 236 cases. Medicine 1975; 54: 271—99.
3. Janssen S, Van Rijswijk MH, Meijer S, Ruinen L, Van der Hem GK. Clinical evaluation of AA an AL amyloid disease. In: Marrink J, Van Rijswijk MH, eds. Amyloidosis. Dordrecht, The Netherlands: Martinus Nijhoff Publishers, 1986: 61—72.
4. Peto R, Dike MC, Armitage P. Design and analysis of randomized clinical trials requiring prolonged observation of each patient. II Analysis and examples. Br J Cancer 1977; 35: 1—39.
5. Kyle RA, Greipp PR. Amyloidosis (AL). Clinical and laboratory features in 229 cases. Mayo Clin Proc 1983; 58: 665—83.
6. Ogg CS, Cameron JS, Williams DG, Turner DR. Presentation and course of primary amyloidosis of the kidney. Clin Nephrol 1981; 15: 9—13.
7. Barth WF, Willerson JT, Waldmann TA, Decker JL. Primary Amyloidosis. Am J Med 1967; 47: 259—63.
8. Isobe T, Osserman EF. Patterns of amyloidosis and their association with plasma-cell dyscrasia, monoclonal immunoglobulins and Bence-Jones proteins. N Eng J Med 1974; 290: 473—7.
9. Nakamoto Y, Hamanaka S, Akihama T, Miura AB, Uesaka Y. Renal involvement patterns of amyloid nephropathy: a comparison with diabetic nephropathy. Clin Nephrol 1984; 22: 188—94.
10. Dikman SH, Churg J, Kahn T. Morphologic and clinical correlates in renal amyloidosis. Hum Pathol 1981; 12: 160—9.
11. Alexanian R, Fraschini G, Smith L. Amyloidosis in multiple myeloma or without apparent cause. Arch Intern Med 1984; 144: 2158—60.
12. Pruzanski W, Katz A. Clinical and laboratory findings in primary generalized and multiple-myeloma-related amyloidosis. Can Med Assoc J 1976; 114: 906—9.
13. Stone MJ, Frenkel EP. The clinical spectrum of light chain myeloma: a study of 35 patients with special reference to the occurrence of amyloidosis. Am J Med 1975; 58: 601—19.
14. EDTA Registry: personal communication.

7. Kidney involvement in light chain deposition disease

D. GANEVAL

Among the systemic diseases associated with plasma cell dyscrasia is Light Chain Deposition Disease, identified only recently. In fact, the glomerular lesions of this disease were described as early as the sixties in patients with myeloma, but remained unelucidated. The most typical glomerular lesion had a lobular aspect similar to that of the glomerulosclerosis or Kimmelstiel-Wilson, observed in diabetic patients. The precise nature of this glomerulopathy only became apparent with the availability of immunofluorescence techniques which allowed the demonstration of monoclonal light chain determinants in the glomerular nodules [1, 2]. The presence of monoclonal light chains — usually kappa — was also observed on the tubules, the vessels, and the interstitium. Electron microscopy demonstrated the nonamyloid, nonfibrillar nature of the deposits which appeared finely granular and electron dense [3—7].

Such deposition of light chains in the kidneys was first reported by Antonovych in 1973 [1] but its real significance only appeared in 1976 with the report by Randall and colleagues [8] of two patients with these lesions. In this report, the main characteristics of what is usually called Light Chain Deposition Disease (LCDD), were already present, i.e., the possibility of the disease occurring either in patients with myeloma or in patients without detectable malignant disease; the widespread deposition of light chains, making the nephropathy a part of a systemic disease; the prominent place of the kidneys among the affected organs.

We now have ten years' experience of the disease since the description of Randall et al. [8] and the present report will summarize how LCDD has been further characterized.

Frequency

About a thousand cases have now been reported in the literature; however,

Minetti et al. (eds.), The kidney in plasma cell dyscrasias. ISBN 978-94-010-7085-0

the actual frequency of the disease is certainly very much higher since numerous cases are no longer published, and many others are still undiagnosed. In Necker Hospital, 17 patients with LCDD have been seen since 1975. In our experience, LCDD is as frequent as amyloidosis in patients with multiple myeloma and kidney involvement. This incidence, for each type of disease, is five per cent in our series.

The plasma cell clone

A patient reported by Randall [8] had no convincing evidence of underlying plasma cell dyscrasia that might account for the light chain deposition. Similar patients have been reported since that time, and the total percentage of patients who have no detectable myeloma or other malignancy at diagnosis of LCDD is about 25 per cent. Some of these patients may have a small amount of monoclonal light chains in serum and/or urine, but others do not, and only the presence of monoclonal light chains in tissues suggests the existence of a lymphoplasmacytic disease; however, bone marrow cell study by immunofluorescence confirms this hypothesis showing a monoclonal population of cells producing light chains of the same type as those found in renal deposits [5, 12].

A follow-up has been obtained for many of these patients. It is interesting since it appears that most of them do not evolve to myeloma, at least during the time they have been followed-up. Five out of our 17 patients had no initial malignancy (Table 1). Two of them have died, 2 and 4 years after diagnosis. The 3 others are alive after 6 months, and 4 and 10 years. In none did myeloma or other malignancy occur. The patient with the ten year-follow-up never received chemotherapy. Thus, experience has confirmed that the plasma cell clone, responsible for LCDD, may be either malignant or controlled, an eventuality already known for AL amyloidosis.

Table 1. Evolution in 5 patients with LCDD and no detectable myeloma at presentation.

Pt No.	Chemotherapy	Follow-up years	Outcome	Occurrence of myeloma
1	no	2.2	dead	no
2	no	4.2	dead	no
3	no	0.6	alive	no
4	yes	6.1	alive	no
5	no	10.1	alive	no

Kidney lesions

The most striking kidney lesion is glomerular and first reports emphasized mesangial nodules with resulting nephrotic syndrome as characteristics of the disease. However, more numerous cases, and histological data obtained in patients with LCDD and mild proteinuria, have shown that mesangial nodules are not as frequent as previously thought. Their actual incidence is about 30—50% of cases [4—6, 9]. Most other patients have mild glomerular lesions with thickening of glomerular capillary walls, with or without moderate enlargement of the mesangium. Finally, ten per cent of patients have near normal glomeruli by light microscopy study. In contrast, the tubular lesions still appear to be constant lesions in LCDD.

During last years, studies have been made to evaluate the nature of the mesangial nodules. Indeed, mesangial nodules in LCDD appear composed of two parts: first, light chains containing deposits, which have an electron dense ultrastructure and fix the monoclonal anti-light chain antisera; and second, a nonimmunological material, finely granular and nonelectron dense at electron microscopy. On light microscopy, this mesangial material is PAS positive and argyrophilic, and closely similar to nodular glomerulosclerosis observed in diabetes. Recent studies [10, Noël L. H., unpublished results] using antibodies to collagenic and non-collagenic components of basement membranes, have demonstrated the membrane-like nature of the enlarged mesangial area (presence of collagen IV, laminin, fibronectin, heparan-sulfate proteoglycan, and absence of collagens I and III), identical to that of diabetic glomerulosclerosis. In diabetics, it has been proposed [11] that the presence of hyperglycosylated proteins in such patients could be responsible for the synthesis of excess membrane proteins by mesangial cells, leading to the mesangial nodules. A similar hypothesis could be suggested in LCDD, in which hyperglycosylated light chains have been demonstrated [5, 12].

Why some patients have mesangial nodules and others do not is unclear. Nodules do not appear to represent a late stage of the disease, and near normal glomeruli may be observed after LCDD has been present a number of years. They probably rather reflect the peculiar properties of certain monoclonal light chains.

Evolution of LCDD nephropathy

Most cases, if not all, present as a nephropathy [3, 5, 6, 8, 9, 13]. Two distinct patterns may be observed (Table 2): the first is that of the nephrotic syndrome, and typical nodular glomerulosclerosis is found in

Table 2. Presenting renal symptoms in LCDD. Relation with presence of mesangial nodules.

Presenting symptom	% Patients	Mesangial nodules
Nephrotic syndrome	30%	in one-half
Mild proteinuria, Plus rapidly progressive Renal Failure	65%	in one-quarter
Other	5%	

about half of such patients. Thus, nephrotic syndrome which, in patients with myeloma, was for a long time synonymous with amyloidosis, must also suggest LCDD. The second pattern is that of mild proteinuria without hematuria or hypertension, and with the peculiarity of being associated with rapidly progressive renal failure. Such a presentation, in our experience, is highly suggestive of LCDD, and 12 out of our 17 patients presented in this form. It must be stressed that, in the absence of renal biopsy, such cases of LCDD would remain undiagnosed.

As a whole, and although some patients have been reported without or with mild renal insufficiency, the severity of the nephropathy remains indisputable, with most patients reaching end-stage renal failure in a few months in the absence of therapy.

Extrarenal deposits

Randall et al. [8] emphasized the role of extrarenal deposits in LCDD, their two patients having multiorgan deposits of light chains (Table 3), with organ dysfunction contributing to death. Observation of more numerous patients has both confirmed the systemic character of the disease and shown the variability of its clinical consequences. In our series (Table 3), light chains were found in every patient in whom they were sought (i.e., liver deposits were found in all 11 of our patients in whom the liver was examined [14], and widespread tissular deposition of light chains was demonstrated by autopsy in 3 patients [5]. The deposition could be discrete, confined to the vascular areas without associated parenchymal lesions, or massive with severe alteration of organs. The clinical counterpart showed the same variability. Some patients died of early and severe extrarenal manifestations of LCDD, mainly cardiac and hepatic (Table 4). In many, however, light chains deposits remain few or asymptomatic, even after a long time. This variability of evolution makes estimating results of treatment difficult.

Table 3. Extra renal deposition of light chains.

	Randall et al. 2 pts	Necker's series 17 pts	related death
Liver	2	11/11	1 moderate liver function tests abnormalities in others
Lung		0/1	
CNS	2		
PNS	1		
GI tract	2		
Bone marrow		1/3	
Thyroid	1		
Lymph nodes	1		
Muscle	2		
Skin	2	1/4	
Pancreas	2	3/3	
Heart	2	3/3	2 silent in the third pt
Abdominal vessels		3/3	

Table 4. Principal cause of death in 13 patients with LCDD.

Myeloma		4
LCDD		3
Cardiac	2	
Hepatic	1	
Renal		2
Renal failure	1	
Complication of dialysis	1	
Unknown		2

Treatment

Since the disease is linked to the production of light chains by one plasma cell clone, chemotherapy — whether myeloma is present or not — is the logical treatment of LCDD, and most patients now receive such therapy. Available data show that chemotherapy (i.e., melphalan or cyclophosphamide associated with prednisone) has a favourable effect on the course of renal insufficiency. In our series, of the 6 patients who were treated with chemotherapy early after diagnosis, only one had reached end-stage renal failure at the end of follow-up. In contrast, all 8 patients untreated, or

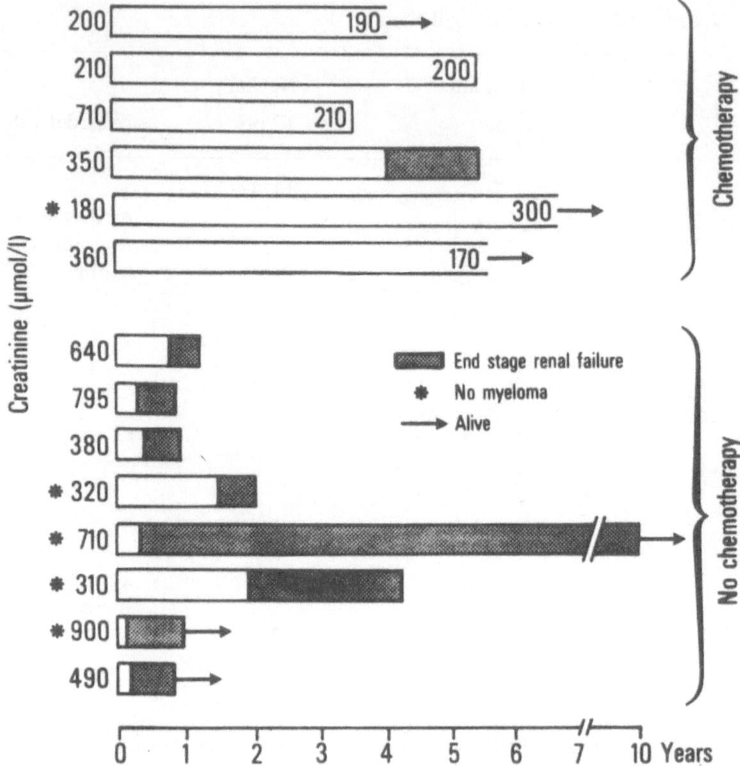

Fig. 1. Influence of chemotherapy on evolution of renal function in 14 patients with LCDD.

treated late, did so (Fig. 1). The effect of chemotherapy on extrarenal deposits is more difficult to assess given the uncertainties mentioned above with regard to its natural history.

In the absence of myeloma, survival in LCDD may be of more than ten years in some patients.

Regular dialysis treatment has been utilised in patients with LCDD and end-stage renal failure. Nine out of our 17 patients were treated by hemodialysis, 3 of them for more than one year, one of these 3 being alive and on dialysis for more than nine years. Kidney transplantation has been performed in a few patients with LCDD. Recurrence of the disease is usually observed [15, 16].

Mechanisms of light chain deposition. Relationship to AL amyloidosis

The mechanisms of tissue precipitation of light chains and the possible role of abnormalities of immunoglobulin synthesis are analysed elsewhere in this volume, and will not be discussed in the present chapter.

The various abnormalities demonstrated in LCDD [3—5, 17, 18] have also been found in some patients with AL amyloidosis [6, 19, 20], which represents an other aspect of light chain deposition in tissues. Thus, similar mechanisms probably can lead to LCDD and to amyloidosis, and this could explain the finding of the two types of lesions in the same patient, as recently reported [13, 21, 22]. In our series, two patients had LCDD and AL amyloidosis, simultaneously in one, and successively in the other one. Such an association is increasingly recognized, and probably five to ten per cent of LCDD patients have associated amyloid deposits.

References

1. Antonovych T, Lin C, Parrish E, Mostofi K. Light chain deposits in multiple myeloma, in Abs. 7th Annu. Mtg Soc Nephrol 1973; No. 3.
2. Noël LH, Droz D, Ganeval D, Jungers P. Glomérulosclérose nodulaire du myélome, in Abs. Montreal: VIIth Int Congr Nephrol, 1978: L16.
3. Preud'homme JL, Morel-Maroger L, Brouet JC, Cerf M, Mignon F, Guglielmi P, Seligmann M. Synthesis of abnormal immunoglobulins in lymphoplasmacytic disorders with visceral light chain deposition. Am J Med 1980; 69: 703—10.
4. Gallo GG, Feiner HD, Buxbaum JN. The kidney in lymphoplasmacytic disorders. In: Sommers SC, Rosen PP, eds. Pathology Annual, Vol. 17, part 1. Norwalk Connecticut: ACC (Appleton-Century-Crofts), 1982; 306—7.
5. Ganeval D, Mignon F, Preud'homme JL, Noël LH, Morel-Maroger L, Droz D, Brouet JC, Mery JPh, Grunfeld JP. Visceral deposition of monoclonal light chains and immunoglobulins: a study of renal and immunopathologic abnormalities. In: Hamburger J, Crosnier J, Grunfeld JP, Maxwell MH, eds. Advances in Nephrology. Chicago: Year Book Medical Publishers Inc. 1982; 11: 25—63.
6. Ganeval D, Noël LH, Preud'homme JL, Droz D, Grunfeld JP. Light-chain deposition disease: its relation with AL-type amyloidosis. Kid Int 1984; 26: 1—19.
7. Noël LH, Droz D, Ganeval D, Grunfeld JP. Renal granular monoclonal light chain deposits: morphological aspects in 11 cases. Clin Nephrol 1984; 21: 2163—9.
8. Randall RE, Williamson WC Jr, Mullinax F, Tung MY, Still WJS. Manifestations of systemic light chain deposition. AM J Med 1976; 60: 293—9.
9. Tubbs RR, Gephardt GN, McMahon JT, Hall PM, Valenzuela R, Vidt RG. Light chain nephropathy. Am J Med 1981; 71: 263—9.
10. Bruneval P, Foidard JM, Nochy D, Camilleri JP, Bariety J. Glomerular matrix proteins in nodular glomerulosclerosis in association with light chain deposition disease and diabetes mellitus. Hum Pathol 1985; 16: 477—84.
11. Martinez-Hernandez A, Amenta PS. The basement membrane in pathology. Lab Invest 1983; 48: 656—77.
12. Preud'homme JL, Mihaesco E, Guglielmi P, Morel-Maroger L, Ganeval D, Danon F, Brouet JC, Mihaesco C, Seligmann M. La maladie des dépôts de chaînes légères ou d'immunoglobulines monoclonales: concepts physiopathogéniques. Nouv Presse Med 1982; 11: 3259—63.
13. Seymour AE, Thompson AJ, Smith PS, Woodroffe AJ, Clarkson AR. Kappa light chain glomerulosclerosis in multiple myeloma. Am J Pathol 1980; 101: 557—80.
14. Droz D, Noël LH, Carnot F, Degos F, Ganeval D, Grunfeld JP. Liver involvement in nonamyloid light chain deposits disease. Lab Invest 1984; 50: 683—9.

15. Case records of the Massachusetts General Hospital (Case 1—1981). New Engl J Med 1981; 304: 33—43.
16. Gerlag PGG, Koene RAP, Berden JHM. Renal transplantation in light chain nephropathy: case report and review of the literature. Clin Nephrol 1986; 25: 101—4.
17. Solling K, Askjaer SA. Multiple myeloma with urinary excretion of heavy chain components of IgG and nodular glomerulosclerosis. Acta Med Scand 1973; 194: 23—9.
18. Preud'homme JL, Morel-Maroger L, Brouet JC, Mihaesco E, Mery JPh, Seligmann M. Synthesis of abnormal heavy and light chains in multiple myeloma with visceral deposition of monoclonal immunoglobulin. Clin Exp Immunol 1980; 42: 545—53.
19. Buxbaum JN, Hurley ME, Chuba J, Spiro T. Amyloidosis of the AL type. Clinical, morphologic and biochemical aspects of the response to therapy with alkylating agents and prednisone. Am J Med 1979; 67: 867—78.
20. Buxbaum J. Aberrant immunoglobulin synthesis in light chain amyloidosis. Free light chain and light chain fragment production by human bone marrow cells in short-term tissue culture. J Clin Invest 1986; 78: 798—806.
21. Jacquot CC, Saint-Andre JP, Touchard G, Nochy D, D'Auzac de Lamartinie C, Oriol R, Druet P, Bariety J. Association of systemic light-chain deposition disease and amyloidosis: a report of three patients with renal involvement. Clin Nephrol 1985; 24: 93—8.
22. Kirkpatrick CJ, Curry A, Galle J, Melzner I. Systemic kappa light chain deposition and amyloidosis in multiple myeloma: novel morphological observations. Histopathology 1986; 10: 1065—76.

8. Some aspects of kidney involvement in plasma cell dyscrasias: A forum

A. SOLOMON, R. A. COWARD, J. L. PREUD'HOMME, R. A. KYLE, P. W. SANDERS, C. L. PIRANI, G. COLASANTI, C. PONTICELLI, G. COLUSSI, L. MINETTI, J. S. CAMERON, G. BANFI, J. N. BUXBAUM & D. GANEVAL

SOLOMON: The first point for the nephrologists is to maintain a high level of suspicion. In other words, in a patient with unexplained proteinuria or some manifestation of renal dysfunction it is necessary for the clinician to keep the possibility in mind that this patient may have a some type of light chain related renal disease. This is very often overlooked. Secondly, I would like to reiterate the importance of recognizing the presence of Bence Jones proteinuria, especially in patients with nephrotic syndrome. Immunofixation on urine concentrated 50—100 fold is the preferable method of analysis. In a patient with nephrotic syndrome there is so much serum protein in the urine (especially transferrin, albumin, etc.), that the monoclonal light chain component is often very difficult to detect. Not infrequently the diagnosis of amyloidosis responsible for the nephrotic syndrome is not made until a renal biopsy is done. In retrospect a careful analysis of the urine using serological techniques will disclose the presence of Bence Jones protein. The antisera that the hospital laboratory uses is also very important. Many of the commercial anti-light chain antisera are not very satisfactory (particularly for the detection of lambda chains). For example, to detect the lambda VI Bence Jones proteins requires a special antiserum; this antiserum is not commercially available as yet, however the identification of Bence Jones proteins of this subgroup indicates with high probability amyloidosis.
COWARD: We routinely measure the amounts and ratios in the urine for free kappa and lambda light chains by radioimmunoassay and found this a sensitive and useful technique to identify paraproteins, especially when there is also a lot of other proteins in the urine which may make it difficult interpreting the electrophoresis. It is very sensitive with low levels of light chain.
PREUD'HOMME: Dr Solomon showed that to detect light chains in serum and urine immunofixation is a much more sensitive and accurate procedure than immunoelectrophoresis. I would like to point out that in

Minetti et al. (eds.), The kidney in plasma cell dyscrasias. ISBN 978-94-010-7085-0

our laboratory we have now developed an assay which is close to immunofixation. The principle is the following: we take the serum or urine, which do not need to be concentrated and we submit them to thin layer agarose electrophoresis, which is then transferred to nitrocellulose sheets; the sheets are revealed by peroxidase or alkaline phosphatase-coupled antibodies (classical western blot). This turns out to be much more sensitive than immunofixation and also much more specific, because in commercial immunofixation kits you have anti-bodies that are not specific and when you control every step yourself you have something which is specific. And using such a procedure you have a very good way to assess the presence of monoclonal immunoglobulins. When doing so in myeloma and lymphoma or any kind of immunoproliferative disorders, biclonal or triclonal proliferations are not rare.

The study of the urine during light chain deposition disease does not help very much. When a deposited immunoglobulin (either heavy of light chain) is structurally abnormal, it is usually indetectable in serum and urine.

KYLE: I think that when considering amyloidosis one should look at the more easily obtainable tissue first, that is subcutaneous fat, rectal biopsy, and then go to the appropriate organ that is involved. In our experience, bleeding and other complications from renal biopsies is no greater than in patients with renal disease of other types. In our experience biopsy of the liver has been associated with bleeding in four of our 85 patients. None of the patients had to be explored in order to stop bleeding. Endomyocardial biopsy is a very good source for tissue. We have biopsied about 40 patients with primary systemic amyloidosis and have found amyloid in the heart in every instance. It has been associated with no mortality and virtually no morbidity. Occasional patients will have a mild arrhythmia but it has not been serious. Subcutaneous fat aspiration was first described by Per Westermark, in Sweden. Dr Shirahama's group in Boston had had a lot of experience with it, and we, too, have had a good deal of experience. We find that 80% of the patients with AL will have a positive subcutaneous fat biopsy.

SANDERS: In three patients with nephrotic syndrome and minimal changes on light microscopy we were able to demonstrate by immunoelectronmicroscopy subendothelial deposits of L-chains. The dark electron-dense material was not seen by routine electronmicroscopy. So I think that this could be considered the earliest manifestation of light chain nephropathy.

PIRANI: The evidence strongly suggests that the crystallization of the light chain in the cast is responsible or is possibly responsible for the so-called fractured appearance of the cast. We also have found that when there were crystals, not in all the casts (probably in ten per cent only — and you have to look very carefully for them) invariably there were giant cells. When there were no crystals usually there were no giant cells. So I think the crystals act as a foreign body. Now, what induces crystallization? We know that in vitro normal light chain will crystallize and are also refractile. To the best of my knowledge there is only a single case report in which refractility was shown to be present in tissue light chains crystals. In vitro crystals of normal light chains are refractile but in our cases we are looking to crystals of abnormal light-chains. The other problem is that crystals do not stain for either kappa or lambda. This is not really surprising again because we are dealing with abnormal light chains.

SOLOMON: The identification of light chains in the crystals using commercial anti-light chain antisera may be difficult, especially if the crystals contain only variable region-related fragments of the light chain. Such antisera will not react with such fragments. To recognize these fragments requires special antisera. The best would be those with idiotype specificity-prepared against the Bence Jones proteins.

Certain Bence Jones proteins cleave readily with variable and constant half fragments. This cleavage can be obtained with many types of enzymes including uropepsin. The constant half is very susceptible to proteolysis and will eventually be digested into very small peptides, while the variable half remains intact. The light chain variable fragment is relatively easy to crystallize in vitro as compared to the intact protein. Thus it is likely that crystals represent variable half fragments.

COLASANTI: We have seen one case in which the morphology of the glomerular lesions was very suggestive for cryoglobulinemia, and the pathologist said to look for cryoglobulins, but we could not find them. I think that cryo-precipitability is a laboratory finding which reflects a particular property of such complexes, and this is not the only biological property. Furthermore it has been described that methods for detecting cryoglobulins should be changed and hypotonic solutions used to detect very small amounts. C4 hypocomplementemia is a characteristic pattern of the disease, and we found it about in 100% of cases with no correlation with the activity of the disease; it means that C4 hypocomplementemia persists also during remission.

PONTICELLI: I wonder whether the difference in the evolution between idiopathic membrano-proliferative glomerulonephritis, and cryoglobulinemic nephritis, might be the result of the different therapeutic attitudes adopted in the two diseases. In fact, in cryoglobulinemic nephritis there are frequent exacerbations that we use to treat either with corticoids or cytotoxic agents, and it seems that in flare-ups the therapy can work, while in idiopathic membranoproliferative nephritis most of us do not give any treatment at all.

COLUSSI: Alpha-1 microglobulin is a more sensitive index of reduced reabsorption of microproteins than beta-2 microglobulin. Maybe these two proteins could indicate different mechanisms of impairment of reabsorption. I think that alpha-1 microglobulin might compete with light chains for reabsorption, so that what we see when alpha-1 microglobulin increases is competition for reabsorption. What the meaning of beta-2 microglobulin is I don't know well. I think that microglobulins are not a very useful tool in the study of tubule function in patients with renal failure at least until we know more about their saturation limit for reabsorption. What we know about renal handling of microproteins suggests that there is a saturation limit for reabsorption, which may be overwhelmed. Now it may be that different microproteins have different saturation limits for reabsorption. Thus, when plasma levels are increased because of renal failure, one cannot easily determine whether increased urine excretion is due to reduced tubular reabsorption or saturation of tubular reabsorption capacity.

MINETTI: Tubular disfunction, expressed by high urinary concentration of alpha-1 microglobulin and other microproteins, could be due to a competitive effect of light chain proteinuria per se. But the tubular functional abnormalities in your cases seem to suggest that also minor, subtle cellular abnormalities could be responsible of this impairment of tubular reabsorption.

COLUSSI: Theoretically there might exist different mechanisms of lesion. A first mechanism may be simple competition between the reabsorption of one microprotein, i.e. light chains, and other microproteins. A second possibility is that reabsorption of huge amounts of one microprotein may be limited by cell-membrane availability: since microprotein reabsorption occurs mainly by endocytosis, I wonder whether there might be a limit in the synthesis of new cell membrane and thus in the formation of endocytotic vescicles. As a third possibility, there are experimental data showing that light chains may interfere with metabolic processes of the cells and in particular with Na^+/K^+-ATPase. Now some inhibition of sodium reabsorption may be a good explanation for reduced reabsorption of all sodium co-transported solutes such as aminoacids, glucose, phosphate and bicarbonate.

CAMERON: In two patients with nephrotic syndrome, renal biopsy on optical microscopy appeared entirely normal, and the Congo red stain was, even when repeated, negative. They had torrential proteinuria and we treated these patients as though they had minimal change. When they did not respond we went back and looked again, with electron microscopy, and also saw very minor amyloidosis and on the silver stains we could see little 'spike-like' areas. Similar patients to this have been reported by the Japanese recently. One of these patients was only thirty five years old, so we had no suspicion at all that he had primary amyloid. He died of cardiac failure within eighteen months.

BANFI: Our youngest patient was twentynine years old and a few of these patients had a very initial form of amyloid deposition which at the routine staining were overlooked and recognized only after careful searching for amyloid with specific staining. The spiky appearance of capillary wall is a diagnostic feature of initial amyloidosis, and we observed these early spike formation in two or three cases. Sometimes we observed normal glomeruli, but in further sections we found that some arterial vessels were involved, so we reached the diagnosis by the vessel lesions in the biopsy and not from the glomerular morphology.

BUXBAUM: With respect to diagnosis, we have looked at twenty five patients with AL amyloid disease. Using our biosynthetic techniques they all have monoclonal light chains, regardless of what is in the serum or in the urine. If they have a monoclonal protein in the serum, that has both heavy and light chains, and no free light chains in the serum or urine, we find free light chains inside the cells. So I think that in these particular cases, where there is an issue of diagnosis, and the patient has nephrotic syndrome and hypogammaglobulinemia, biosynthetic analysis is a sensitive technique to identify these patients and to determine the nature of the amyloid precursor.

GANEVAL: In our series, two patients with light chain deposits disease (LCDD) had evidence of amyloid. In one of them, who had amyloid a few years after the diagnosis of LCDD, in the first biopsy there was no amyloid. Afterwards this patient had a relapse of the myeloma, and on this point subcutaneous nodules and carpal tunnel syndrome occurred. Biopsies of nodules and of carpal tunnel showed amyloid. We did not have for this patient serial kidney specimen.

Part IV. The therapeutic approach

1. Controlled trial of plasma exchange in rapidly progressive renal failure

P. ZUCCHELLI, S. PASQUALI, F. LOCATELLI & C. POZZI

Introduction

More than 50% of patients with multiple myeloma (MM) have renal failure at the time of diagnosis with uremia being the second most common cause of death in the MM population [1, 2]. Although the pathophysiology of this disease is still unclear, the strong association between light chain excretion and renal failure suggests that the former plays a primary pathogenetic role in producing kidney damage [2, 3]. In recent years plasma exchange (PE) has been considered to be the most rational way of rapidly removing large amounts of light chains and it has been recommended in the treatment of severe myeloma nephropathy. However, clinical works so far published are based on uncontrolled studies of very small patient series as shown in Table 1 [4—8]. This fact has prompted us to examine 35 patients with rapidly progressive renal failure due to MM in a controlled study so as to assess the effectiveness of PE in treating severe myeloma nephropathy.

Patients and methods

Patients

From 1980 to 1987, thirty-five consecutive patients were referred to the above-mentioned Renal Services with rapidly progressive renal failure caused by previously or subsequently recognized MM. They included 24 males and 11 females who were 48 to 74 years old, with a mean age of 63 years. The MM diagnosis was based on the presence of marrow-plasmacytosis in sheets or clusters involving more than 15% of the cells and on the discovery of monoclonal paraprotein in the serum and/or urine. No patient took any nephrotoxic or chemotherapeutic drugs for at least 2

Minetti et al. (eds.), The kidney in plasma cell dyscrasias. ISBN 978-94-010-7085-0

Table 1. Plasma exchange therapy in multiple myeloma.

Reference	Year	Number of patients	Reversible renal failure	Survival (months)
Feest et al.	1976	1	1	9
Sieberth et al.	1979	2	0	—
Misiani et al.	1979	3	3	—
Locatelli et al.	1980	4	4	14.2
Cohen et al.	1984	1	—	—

months prior to renal failure. In other words, the acute nature of renal failure was defined by:

(a) a rapid rise in serum creatinine to 5 mg/dl or more *not reversible* by a correction of volume status, urinary tract obstruction or any other extra-renal abnormalities;
(b) previous findings of normal or near-normal serum creatinine or blood urea nitrogen (BUN);
(c) normal or increased kidney size [11].

None of the patients had any severe infections, dehydration, hyperviscosity or worsening of renal function following intravenous urography. Clinical stratification of MM was done according to Durie and Salmon's method [9] and with the serum β_2-microglobulin level (β_2M).

Renal biopsies were performed on 23 patients and the renal histologic patterns were classified as outlined in our previous study [10].

Methods

Complete blood counts, coagulation studies, uric acid, creatinine and BUN concentrations were evaluated using standard laboratory methods. Serum protein electrophoresis was performed on the cellulose acetate membrane. Immunoelectrophoresis with monospecific antisera to gamma, alpha, mu, kappa and lambda chains was also carried out.

Electrophoresis and immunoelectrophoresis were performed on urine concentrated 5 to 100 times by ultrafiltration and then quantitated with the biuret method. Tumor cell mass was calculated for each case using the clinical staging system introduced by Durie and Salmon [9].

The quantitative determination of serum β_2M was done by solid phase enzyme immunoassay (Behring, Ingelheim, West Germany). The normal ranges for this assay in subjects 40—79 years old ranged from 1.2 to 3.0 mg/l.

Treatment protocol

Immediately after diagnosis the patients were treated with furosemide 500—1,500 mg/daily, 2 to 5 litres daily of intravenous saline and oral sodium bicarbonate to render the urine neutral. When renal function did not rapidly improve and/or a high fluid intake was not tolerated, the patients were randomly allocated from a table to random numbers to group I (PE, corticosteroids, cytotoxic drug and hemodialysis when needed) or group II (peritoneal dialysis, corticosteroids and cytotoxic drug).

Acute treatment consisted of methylprednisolone pulse (20 mg/Kg/day) given intravenously for 20—30 mins on 3 consecutive days followed by a course of oral prednisone at a dosage of 20—30 mg/m^2/day for 7 days together with cyclophosphamide 200 mg/m^2/day given intravenously for 5 days. In the event of myelotoxicity a one-day reduction in the cyclophosphamide course was permitted. In every group I patient, 5 PE sessions were performed on 5 consecutive days, while in some cases an additional PE was performed on 7th and 10th days, using the femoral veins for vascular access. Polypropylene plasma filters were used (Plasmex PF 20, 0.2 m^2) and about 3 to 4 litres of each patient's plasma was removed at each session. This plasma was replaced by saline solution, albumin and fresh frozen plasma in equal parts.

Sixteen out of the 18 patients in group I required dialytic treatment consisting of thrice-weekly, 4—5 hour hemodialysis sessions performed using the same femoral vein and with a plate hemodialyzer. The blood flow rate was maintained at ~250 ml/min. Thirteen out of the 17 group II patients required dialytic therapy consisting of intermittent peritoneal dialysis (40 litres every other day for at least 10 days). The other 4 group II patients underwent 2 or 3 peritoneal dialysis sessions during the chemotherapy week and high fluid intake was maintained.

A low protein, high caloric diet, antiacids and furosemide were administered to each patient both during treatment and in the follow-up period.

Follow-up treatment. After a 4 to 6 week interval, prednisone 60 mg/m^2/day and cyclophosphamide 100 mg/m^2/day were given orally for 4 days. This treatment was continued every month in all the surviving patients for at least 6—9 months regardless of renal function recovery.

Responder Patients were those who recovered renal function, evaluated as a fall in serum creatinine by at least 25%, and those who were able to suspend the dialytic treatment. If serum creatinine had significantly increased during the follow-up period and/or Bence-Jones proteinuria (BJP) had risen more than 50% over the level reached by the end of acute treatment, then group I responder patients would have received 2 PE session (with or without hemodialysis) while group II patients would have undergone 2 peritoneal dialysis sessions.

Non-responder patients were the ones whose serum creatinine did not improve or who still required dialysis about one month after starting treatment. They were subsequently treated by CAPD or put on maintenance hemodialysis.

Statistical analysis

Student's t test and Fisher's exact test were used to assess the differences between the 2 groups. $P < 0.05$ was regarded as significant. All values are expressed as arithmetical mean ± SD.

Results

The main clinical and laboratory data upon admission are summarized in Table 2.

There were no statistically significant differences between the PE group (group I) and the control group (group II) as regards as sex, age, initial serum creatinine, or the severity of the disease.

Twenty-two patients (62.8%) had light chain myeloma (13 kappa and 9 lambda) while 10 had IgG myeloma (7 kappa and 3 lambda) and 3 IgA (lambda). BJP was present in all cases and ranged between 1.2 and 13 g/day. Sixteen of the 35 patients were oliguric (daily diuresis < 500 ml) at admission, 4 others became oliguric shortly after admission so oliguria was present in approximately 57% of the cases. None of the patients showed any clinical signs of severe dehydration or hyperviscosity.

Serum calcium levels were < 12 mg/dl in all cases except in 3 group I patients and in 2 group II patients (12.5, 13.1, 17, 13.4, 13.9 mg/dl).

Total myeloma cell mass was very high (Stage III) in 74.2%. Renal biopsy was performed in 23 cases with all but one showing a myeloma cast nephropathy pattern. One group I patient presented protein crystalloid within the proximal tubular epithelial cells and the tubular lumina [10].

Short-term study

During the first 2 months of treatment (short-term period) 13 out of the 16 group I patients who required hemodialysis improved renal function (Table 3). In most of these patients serum creatinine fell to level ⩽ 2.5 mg/dl. The remaining 2 non-dialysis treated patients in group I improved renal function, reaching a serum creatinine level < 2.5 mg/dl during follow-up. Only 2 group I patients died within the first 2 months of therapy.

Thirteen out of the 17 control patients (group II) required dialysis. Two

Table 2. Clinical and laboratory data upon admission.

	Cases N°	Sex	Age (Yrs)	Monoclonal serum Class	Protein urine Type	g/day	Diuresis (ml/day)	Serum creatinine (mg/dl)	Clinical stage
Group I									
	1	M	73	K	K	1.2	100	17	III B
	2	M	73	λ	λ	4.0	50	10	III B
	3	M	48	λ	λ	10	2000	10	III B
	4	M	68	K	K	1.2	1200	11	III B
	5	M	68	K	K	1.6	2000	8.1	I B
	6	F	68	K	K	1.2	300	10	III B
	7	M	72	λ	λ	3.0	100	16	III B
	8	F	58	K	K	13	1500	9.7	III B
	9	M	61	λ	λ	3.5	1500	13	III B
	10	M	62	IgG K	K	3.8	1000	15.1	III B
	11	F	53	K	K	1.8	300	15	III B
	12	F	54	λ	λ	9.5	1000	8.9	III B
	13	F	58	K	K	6.5	400	9.9	II B
	14	M	58	IgG λ	λ	3.0	1800	5.1	III B
	15	M	69	IgG K	K	3.2	1500	8.7	II B
	16	M	65	IgG K	K	2.5	100	20.7	III B
	17	F	74	K	K	2.7	1500	11.5	II B
	18	F	72	IgA λ	λ	1.6	300	14.7	III B
Group II									
	1	F	50	λ	λ	2.1	200	11	I B
	2	M	58	K	K	1.8	100	13	II B
	3	M	61	K	K	5.7	3000	10	III B
	4	M	55	K	K	5.0	200	10.5	II B
	5	M	61	K	K	4.3	1800	8.8	III B
	6	M	63	λ	λ	3.4	100	3.5	III B
	7	F	72	IgG K	K	1.5	2000	9.6	III B
	8	M	55	IgG K	K	9.0	3000	3.8	III B
	9	F	73	IgG λ	λ	1.9	1000	9.5	III B
	10	M	64	IgG K	K	1.2	2000	5.5	III B
	11	M	70	K	K	1.7	200	10.6	III B
	12	M	67	IgA λ	λ	2.0	1500	5.0	II B
	13	M	65	IgG λ	λ	3.5	2000	5.4	III B
	14	M	71	λ	λ	2.2	200	11	III B
	15	F	73	IgA λ	λ	2.7	1350	22.3	II B
	16	M	59	IgG K	K	4.0	100	15.3	III B
	17	M	51	λ	λ	10.0	2500	5.2	III B

Table 3. Short-term effects of therapy in the 2 groups of patients.

	Group I	Group II	p
Number in group	18	17	
Number of patients requiring dialysis	16	13	ns
Number of patients interrupting dialysis	13	2	$p < 0.001$
Number of patients who died within the first 2 months	2	7	$p < 0.05$
Serum creatinine at the end of the 2nd month mean ± SD (mg/dl)	2.8 ± 2.1	7.7 ± 1.8	$p < 0.001$

of these patients recovered renal function well enough to stop dialytic treatment (serum creatinine 5.0 and 6.1 mg/dl respectively). Three patients died within one month and 4 more within 2 months despite continued dialysis. The remaining 4 patients required long-term dialysis. Thus by the end of the first 2 months (Table 3) only 2 of the 13 group II patients had recovered renal function sufficiently to stop dialysis (46 and 37 days after admission). Among the remaining 4 patients, who did not require dialysis, 3 maintained a stable serum creatinine level while in 1 renal failure was impaired without needing to start dialysis.

In group I BJP decreased dramatically (4.07 g/day at the beginning of the study vs 0.82 on the 30th day of the study; $p < 0.01$) while mean urine output increased significantly (0.92 l/day at the beginning of the study vs 1.92 l/day on the 30th day of the study; $p < 0.001$). In Group II we observed a slight and not significant reduction in light chain excretion (3.64 g/day at the beginning of the study vs 3.35 g/day on the 30th day of the study) without a significant increase in daily diuresis (1.25 l/day vs 1.44 l/day).

Long-term study

After the first 2 months of therapy 16 patients in group I survived and 10 in group II (Table 4). Among the 4 group II patients who did not require dialysis, one case (N° 13) became progressively oliguric 6 months after admission. Thus, after the initial 2 month period, 5 of the 10 surviving group II patients required maintenance dialysis until death for 3, 9, 10, 14 and 16 months after admission. The remaining 5 (2 of whom were

Table 4. Long-term effects of therapy in the 2 groups of patients.

	Group I	Group II	p
Number in group	16	10	
Number of patients requiring dialysis	1	5	$p < 0.05$
Number of patients interrupting dialysis	13	2	$p < 0.005$
Alive at the end of the follow-up period	6	2	ns
Deaths during the follow-up period	10	8	ns
Mean sruvival time (months)	26.6 ± 18.9	10.6 ± 5.7	$p < 0.05$

responders) continued conservative treatment for a period ranging from 5 to 21 months. The 2 responder patients were both treated with one further cycle of 2 peritoneal dialysis sessions required by a significant increase in BJP.

There was 13 responders in the 14 patients who had required dialysis out of the 16 surviving group I patients. None of the responders presented any fresh deterioration in renal function during follow-up. Serum creatinine stabilized at a level ⩽ 2.5 mg/dl in all but 4 responder patients. In 5 cases 2 PE sessions were repeated once (N°s 10 and 14), twice (N° 13) or three times (N°s 5 and 8) because of a significant increase in BJP from 3 to 12 months following admission. One non-responder patient was treated on maintenance hemodialysis for 7 months. Mean survival time was significantly higher in group I than in grou II ($p < 0.05$). The most frequent causes of death were infections (12 cases) and cancer cachexia or overwhelming tumor (10 cases). Other causes of death were gastrointestinal bleeding (2 cases), myocardial infarction (2 cases) and liver insufficiency (1 case). Peritonitis developed in only 1 group II patient and was resolved after antibiotic therapy. Side-effects related to PE were rare and mild: 3 patients (N°s 2, 8, 12) presented transient circumoral paraestesiae, while 1 case (N° 5) showed a brief episode of muscle twitching together with nausea and vomiting.

Discussion

Renal failure complicating MM has been associated with a very poor prognosis [1, 11]. Recently PE and peritoneal dialysis have been recommended in managing severe myeloma nephropathy because of their effective removal of circulating light chains that are thought to play a major causal role in renal damage due to MM [4—7, 15, 16]. However, although the rate of renal failure reversibility has been improving over the last few years, renal failure recovery is unlikely to occur when serum creatinine exceeds 5 mg/dl, in the presence of oliguria or in those patients with light chain myeloma type [12, 14].

Our study consisted of 35 patients with MM, 22 of whom had light chain myeloma and with 29 requiring dialytic therapy. Oliguria was present in 57% of the cases while tumor mass was classed has high in 74.2% according to Durie and Salmon's grading. Our experience in accordance with Cohen et al. [8] and Russell et al. [17], shows that in severe and acute renal failure due to MM a recovery of renal function is rarely achieved with chemotherapy and peritoneal dialysis. In fact, only 2 out of 13 group II patients requiring dialysis recovered renal function well enough to stop treatment. Moreover, mortality was very high in this group with 7 patients dying during the first 2 months of therapy.

As regards the PE group patients, 13 out of the patients requiring dialysis recovered adequate renal function with serum creatinine falling to a level $\leqslant$ 2.5 mg/dl in the majority. The effect of PE and chemotherapy on renal function persisted for a long time with no patient requiring further therapeutic PE as a result of a significant increase in serum creatinine. Mean survival time in PE-treated patients was significantly higher than survival in group II patients. Finally, in both groups BJP behaviour was always correlated to renal outcome in accordance with the pathogenetic hypothesis that light chains play a primary role in producing renal damage.

In conclusion, this controlled PE trial for the treatment of severe myeloma nephropathy shows that PE rapidly removes large amounts of light chains and is thus clearly superior to peritoneal dialysis in recovering renal function and improving long-term survival expectancies.

References

1. Kyle RA. Multiple myeloma-review of 869 cases. Mayo Clin Proc 1975; 50: 29—40.
2. De Fronzo RA, Cooke CR, Wright JR, Humphrey RL. Renal function in patients with multiple myeloma. Medicine 1978; 57: 151—66.
3. Fang LST. Light-chain nephropathy. Kidney Int 1985; 27: 582—92.
4. Feest TG, Burge PS, Cohen SL. Successful treatment of myeloma kidney by diuresis and plasmapheresis. Br Med J 1976; 1: 503—4.
5. Sieberth HG, Glockner W, Boberg H, Fohlmeister J. Plasmaseparation in Goodpasture's syndrome and multiple myeloma. Proc Eur Dial Transplant Ass 1979; 16: 528—34.

6. Misiani R, Remuzzi G, Bertani T, Licini R, Levoni P, Crippa A, Mecca G. Plasmapheresis in the treatment of acute renal failure in multiple myeloma. Am J Med 1979; 66: 684–8.
7. Locatelli F, Pozzi C, Pedrini L, Marai P, Di Filippo S, Ponti R, Costanzo R. Steroid pulses and plasmapheresis in the treatment of acute renal failure in multiple myeloma. Proc. Europ Dial Transpl Assoc 1980; 17: 690–4.
8. Cohen DJ, Sherman WH, Osserman EF, Appel GB. Acute renal failure in patients with multiple myeloma. Am J Med 1984; 76: 247–56.
9. Durie BGM, Salmon SE. A clinical staging system for multiple myeloma. Cancer 1975; 36: 842–54.
10. Pasquali S, Zucchelli P, Casanova S, Cagnoli L, Confalonieri R, Pozzi C, Banfi G, Lupo A, Bertani T. Renal histological lesions and clinical syndromes in multiple myeloma. Clin Nephrol 1987; 27: 222–8.
11. Woodruff R. Treatment of multiple myeloma. Cancer Treat Rev 1981; 8: 225–70.
12. Cosio FG, Pence TV, Shapiro FL, Kjellstrand CM. Severe renal failure in multiple myeloma. Clin Nephrol 1981; 15: 206–10.
13. Lazarus HM, Adelstein DJ, Herzig RH, Smith MC. Long-term survival of patients with multiple myeloma and acute renal failure at presentation. Am J Kidney Dis 1983; 2: 521–5.
14. Medical Research Council. Analysis and management of renal failure in fourth MRC myelomatosis trial. Br Med J 1984; 288: 1411–6.
15. Rosansky SJ, Richards FW. Use of peritoneal dialysis in the treatment of patients with renal failure and paraproteinemia. Am J Nephrol 1985; 5: 361–5.
16. Yium J, Martinez-Maldonado M, Eknoyan G, Suki WN. Peritoneal dialysis in the treatment of renal failure in multiple myeloma. South Med J 1971; 64: 1403–5.
17. Russell JA, Fitzharris BM, Corringham R, Darcy DA, Powles RL. Plasma exchange peritoneal dialysis for removing Bence-Jones protein. Br Med J 1978; 2: 1397.

2. Prevention and treatment of hyperviscosity syndrome

GHIL BUSNACH, ANNA CAPPELLERI, AUGUSTA DAL COL, MARIA LUISA PERRINO, BRUNO BRANDO, LUCIANA BARBARANO, SIMONETTA GRANATA & LUIGI MINETTI

Introduction

The clinical manifestations of hyperviscosity syndrome respond, at least transiently, to plasma exchange (PE). Once control of symptoms has been achieved, however, PE must be repeated since its effects are temporary [1].

PE is therefore indicated whenever benefit might be expected from an acute removal of paraprotein [2—4]. It can be performed either as a symptomatic therapy for the immediate control of symptoms due to circulating paraprotein, during the period of chemotherapy induction, or as a maintenance therapy for those patients where it may be impossible to control paraprotein levels with chemotherapy alone: it may, in these cases, offer the patient a reasonable quality of life for a prolonged period [5]. Although the optimal balance between PE and cytostatics need is not known, long-term PE may have a sparing effect on chemotherapy [6,7].

For the last 5 years we have treated hyperviscosity syndromes of various degrees with one or more intensive courses of PE, associated whenever possible with chemotherapy. In a few instances, a chronic PE treatment has been undertaken in selected cases of Waldenström macroglobulinemia. We have therefore performed a retrospective analysis of 29 treated patients, separated according to immunoglobulin class paraprotein, in order to evaluate PE need and its possible effect in the acute (or chronic) management of hyperviscosity syndrome.

Patients, materials and methods

For the past 10 years, the admissions in the Department of Hematology for plasma cell dyscrasias approximately accounted for 17.1 new patients/year with multiple myeloma, for 25.5 with monoclonal gammopathy of unknown significance (MGUS), and for 4.3 with Waldenström macro-

Minetti et al. (eds.), The kidney in plasma cell dyscrasias. ISBN 978-94-010-7085-0

globulinemia. Moreover, 4.7, 1.1 and 0.8 new patients/year respectively, with plasma cell dyscrasias and a predominant associated renal failure were admitted in the Department of Nephrology. Out of all these cases, during the last 5 years, a total number of 29 paraproteinemic patients have been referred to our Plasma Exchange Unit because of signs and symptoms of hyperviscosity. The underlying dyscrasia was an IgG myeloma in 5 cases, an IgA myeloma in 9, and a macroglobulinemia in 15 patients. Hyperviscosity syndrome therefore accounted for approximately 6 new cases/year, and more than 50% of these were due to Waldenström macroglobulinemia.

The circulatory disturbances, caused by the increased resistance of blood to flow, had as main targets ocular fundi, with hemorrages and exudates, neurologic manifestations (as a result of intracerebral vascular occlusions), peripheral neuropathies and hematologic complications such as a bleeding tendency. Patients became eligible for PE after the appearance of hyperviscosity symptoms, in some cases years after the diagnosis of the primary disease: their data at the beginning of the PE course are illustrated in Table 1.

IgG myeloma patients had neurologic signs of hyperviscosity in 5 cases out of 5, and altered fundi in 4 cases. Three patients received one PE course, and 2 out of 5 had a presenting renal failure.

In 9 IgA myeloma patients presenting symptoms of hyperviscosity (more than one per patient) were bleeding in 6 cases, neurologic manifestations in 5 cases, one peripheral neuropathy and 4 ocular hemorrages and exudates. In 6 patients only one PE course was undertaken. Renal failure was present in 6 patients.

In 15 patients with Waldenström macroglobulinemia the main presenting symptoms were bleeding in 8 cases, neurologic manifestations in 6, ocular disturbances with altered fundi in 8, and a peripheral neuropathy in one case. Only 4 patients were treated with one PE course: the other patients required 2 or more treatments, sometimes with months of interval. Renal failure was present in 4 cases.

A total number of 388 PE procedures have been performed, generally with the following schedule: one PE every other day for the first week, followed by 2 or 3 procedures during the second week. According to renal failure and hematologic status, chemotherapy was instituted immediately after the first PE, and prosecuted whenever possible with low dosages in cases with a concomitant renal failure. Another PE course was repeated after 7 to 15 days when the symptoms persisted, or when chemotherapy could not be continued because of intolerance or deleterious side effects. In selected cases of Waldenström macroglobulinemia, where chemotherapy had to be withdrawn or was unable to control the IgM over-

Table 1. Patients, primary plasma cell dyscrasia and presenting symptoms of hyperviscosity syndrome.

Disease	# Pts.	Sex M/F	Age M ± SEM	Presenting symptoms Bleed	Neurol	Ocular	Periph neurop	S creat > 2 mg/dl
IgG myeloma	5	3/2	65.6 ± 8.2	—	5 (100%)	4 (80%)	—	2 (40%)
IgA myeloma	9	7/2	66 ± 9.2	6 (66.6%)	5 (55.5%)	4 (44.4%)	1 (11.1%)	6 (66.6%)
Waldenström macroglob.	15	9/6	58.2 ± 10.2	8 (53.3%)	6 (40%)	8 (53.3%)	1 (6.6%)	4 (26.6%)

production, a chronic PE treatment was undertaken with one procedure per week, slowly tapered to one every 4 to 6 weeks.

A continuous flow centrifuge has been used (Vivacell®, Dideco, Mirandola Italy) with antecubital veno-venous access, and continuous heparin as anticoagulant. The exchanged volume per procedure was as much as possible equivalent to the patient's plasma volume, calculated, in defect, according to body weight and hematocrit (Table 2).

Albumin 3 to 4% w/v diluted in saline or Ringer solution was used as reinfusion. Saline was used in a few instances at the beginning of the procedure.

During the last two years, chronic PE treatment in patients with macroglobulinemia has been achieved with the cascade filtration technique, with high flow rate recirculating plasma on the secondary filter, as described elsewhere [8]. The selective removal of IgM macromolecules permitted to reduce and abolish the need for a reinfusion solution.

Among the usual laboratory data of the patients, the following have been collected:

(1) serum protein electrophoresis: the monoclonal band has been quantitated, and used as the 'paraprotein immunoglobulin (Ig) class', as confirmed by immunoelectrophoresis; immunonephelometric Ig serum concentration has not been employed because of the erratic results that have been so far obtained in paraproteinemic disorders;
(2) plasma viscosity: it was measured with a modified Ostwald viscosimeter, and plasma flow was compared to water flow. This 'relative viscosity' ranged in the normal between 1.4 and 1.8;
(3) plasma creatinine, as a marker of renal function: basal levels above 2 mg/dl were indicative of renal failure.

The statistical analysis was performed by the 't' test for unpaired data.

Results

Following PE, hyperviscosity symptoms improved in 22 out of 29 treated patients (75.8%): 4/5 IgG myeloma, 7/9 IgA myeloma and 11/15 macroglobulinemic patients. The improvement in neurologic manifestations and bleeding was very fast, within the first PE course; the effect was less evident on fundi alterations. There was no immediate apparent benefit on the peripheral neuropathy.

The initial elevated serum proteins concentration was directly related with the increased monoclonal paraprotein. Total proteins and paraprotein concentration correlated in a linear way with a regression coefficient (R-squared) of 0.56 for IgA, 0.62 for IgG and 0.45 for IgM.

Table 2. Plasma exchange requirement and volumes of exchange/procedure. Chemotherapy association with PE.

Disease	Exchange vol/ procedure ml	# Procedures /PE course	min max	PE Requirement 1 course	> 1 course	Associated cytostatic treatment	
IgG myeloma	2564 ± 598	4.4 ± 2.3	1 7	3	2	5	(100%)
IgA myeloma	2740 ± 689	5 ± 2.9	2 11	6	3	6	(66.6%)
Waldenström macroglob.	2853 ± 450	21.4 ± 22.6	2 86*	4	11	9	(60%)

* Long-term treatment.

As previously described [9], a nonlinear relationship was observed between paraprotein concentration and plasma viscosity. At any time (first and subsequent PE) paraprotein concentration at the beginning of PE correlated with the logarithm of the relative viscosity, with wide variations from patient to patient, presumably related with the physico-chemical structure of the immunoglobulin: R-squared was 0.32 for IgA, 0.53 for IgG and 0.50 for IgM (Fig. 1).

According to the quantity of plasma processed during PE, paraproteins and relative viscosity decreased exponentially (Fig. 2), and confirmed previous observations of a 50% reduction of intravascular IgM with an exchange volume equivalent to 100% plasma volume [11].

Unless otherwise indicated, the following data were obtained from the pre-exchange values of the first and of the last procedure of every patient.

IgG myeloma: initial total proteins level was 12.1 ± 2.6 g/dl, and 8.9 ± 1.4 g/dl at the last PE ($p < 0.025$). IgG monoclonal band decreased from 8.4 ± 2.5 to 5.3 ± 1.7 g/dl ($p < 0.05$), and plasma relative viscosity from 4.8 ± 2.7 to 2.2 ± 0.4 ($p < 0.01$).

Initial and final plasma creatinine respectively were 3.6 ± 3.3 and 1.6 ± 0.8 mg/dl. Two patients of this group required a temporary renal replacement therapy because of acute renal failure. Out of the 5 patients, 3 patients died within days, and 2 were lost to PE follow-up: no chronic renal failure developed (Table 3).

IgA myeloma: total proteins and paraprotein respectively decreased from 9.9 ± 1.7 to 8 ± 1.5 g/dl ($p < 0.01$), and from 5.7 ± 1.4 to 2.9 ± 1.2 g/dl ($p < 0.005$). Relative viscosity declined from 6.2 ± 4.6 to 4 ± 3.5 ($p < 0.01$). Initial plasma creatinine was 2.7 ± 1.2 mg/dl and final

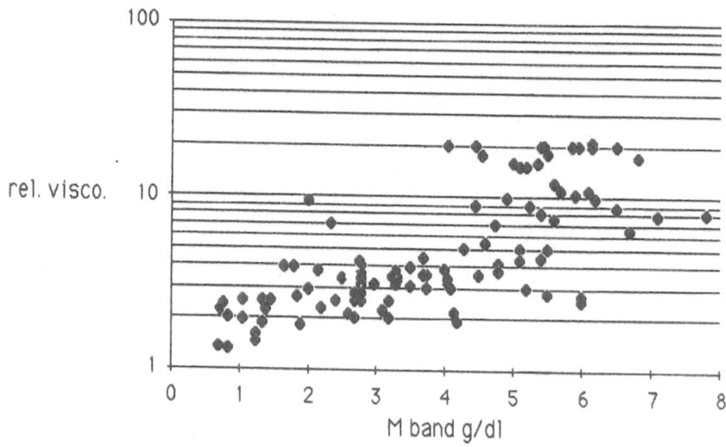

Fig. 1. Relationship between monoclonal paraprotein concentration (abscissa: M band, g/dl) and plasma relative viscosity (ordinate: log). Blood samples collected before PE.

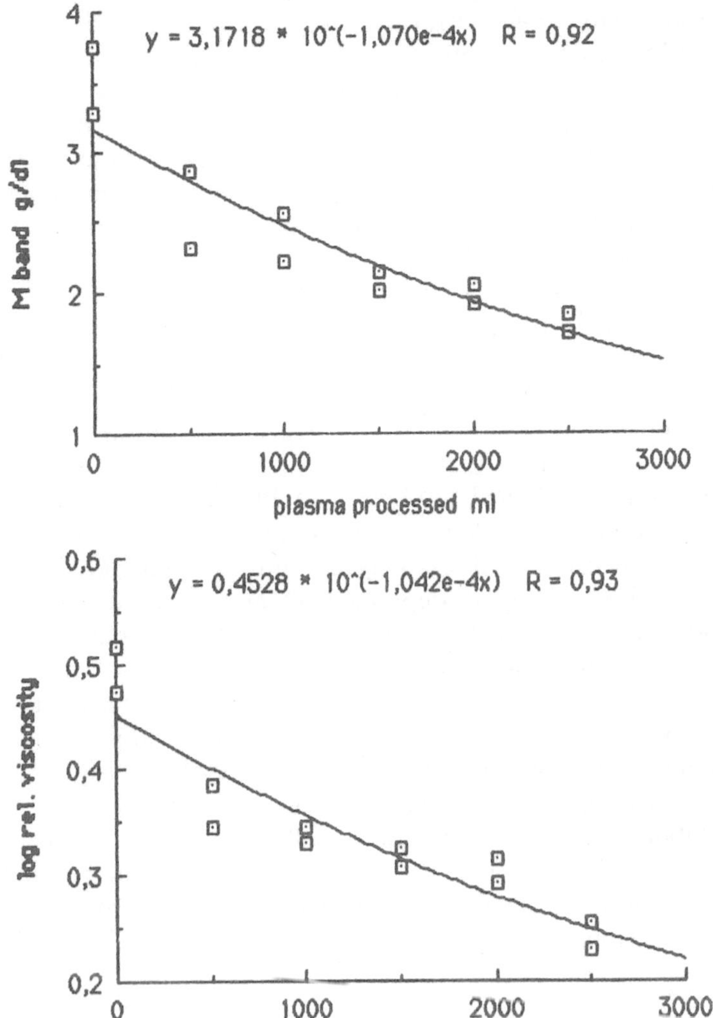

Fig. 2. (upper) Paraprotein (g/dl), and (bottom) relative viscosity (log) behaviour according to the quantity of plasma processed (ml), during 2 consecutive PE procedures, in a patient with Waldenström macroglobulinemia.

value was 2 ± 1.3 mg/dl: renal failure never required hemodialysis. Early death followed treatment in 5 out of 9 patients, without any evident relationship with PE procedures; 2 patients had a survival longer than 6 months after the end of PE (22.2%), and 2 patients were lost to follow-up.

Waldenström macroglobulinemia: out of 15 patients, 3 early deaths were seen, 1 patient was lost to follow-up, and 11 patients (73.3%) had a follow-up longer than 6 months after hyperviscosity syndrome appearance: 3 of them required only one PE course at the beginning of treatment, and

8 were repeatedly treated with chronic PE courses, in 5 cases with an associated low-dose chemotherapy. In 3 cases chemotherapy had been completely withdrawn, and PE has been the only supportive treatment respectively for 36, 52 and 60 months (Table 3). One patient presented with acute renal failure, and required a short hemodialysis period: afterwards, he recovered a nearly normal renal function. Renal biopsy, at the time of acute failure, disclosed a tubulo-interstitial nephropathy, with an interstitial mononuclear infiltrate.

Initial total proteins and paraprotein respectively were 9.7 ± 1.7 and 4.3 ± 1.5 g/dl; before the last procedure (either acute or chronic courses), they decreased to 6.5 ± 0.9 and 1.6 ± 0.7 g/dl ($p < 0.0005$). The initial viscosity of 6.7 ± 4.5 decreased to 2.1 ± 0.4 ($p < 0.005$).

Plasma creatinine was 2.4 ± 2.5 mg/dl (range 0.4—9.8) and was reduced to 1.4 ± 0.6 ($p < 0.05$).

As far as the technical modalities of PE are concerned, data were analyzed of continuous flow centrifuge procedures (CF), with plasma completely discarded and exchanged with albumin solutions, and of cascade filtration (DF), with depurated plasma reinfused into the patient, when both procedures were performed in the same patient: in 6 CF and 9 DF procedures, the ratio of processed plasma volume to patient's plasma volume was higher in DF (1.1 ± 0.1 vs 0.9 ± 0.1), presumably because the reduced need for reinfusion solution permitted a larger exchange. As a consequence, with cascade filtration there was also a slight increase in post-procedure paraprotein reduction (1.1 ± 0.4 vs 0.8 ± 0.2 g/dl; p: NS). Albumin reduction was significantly higher with DF than with CF (0.9 ± 0.3 vs 0.4 ± 0.3 g/dl; $p < 0.025$), but it has to be pointed out that in DF procedures a maximum amount of 10 g exogenous albumin was given as reinfusion solution.

Discussion

Paraproteins increase the risk of vascular complications, and some of the clinical features of paraproteinemic diseases result from the increased resistance to blood flow associated with hyperviscosity. Blood viscosity is affected by the paraprotein concentration; it increases logarithmically with each of the three main Ig classes, but it is also influenced by the hematocrit value [9]. The low hematocrit, that is generally found in those patients having a higher paraprotein concentration, may be partly a result of plasma hypervolemia, and resulting anemia can therefore be considered of dilutional origin [10, 12].

The nonlinear dependence of the blood viscosity on both the protein

Table 3. Follow-up of paraproteinemic patients with hyperviscosity syndrome, treated with plasma exchange.

Disease	Hyperviscosity syndrome		Follow-up				
	Improved	Unchanged/ worsened	M ± SEM (months)	min max	> 6 months	Chronic PE	Chronic PE + cytostatic drugs
IgG myeloma	4 (80%)	1 (20%)	1.4 ± 0.4	1 2	—	—	—
IgA myeloma	7 (77.7%)	2 (22.2%)	2.3 ± 2.6	1 8	# 2	—	—
Waldenström macroglob.	11 (73.3%)	4 (26.6%)	18.4 ± 21	1 60	# 11	# 8	# 5
Total	22 (75.8%)	7 (24.1%)					

concentration and the hematocrit value has to be taken into account for a rational therapeutic approach to the management of paraproteinemic patients. On one side, overtransfusion may precipitate hyperviscosity syndrome, on the other side PE, even with small reductions in circulating paraproteins, may transiently exert a considerable drop in blood viscosity. PE effect is corresponding to an increased paraprotein catabolic rate, and it induces an improvement in clinical and rheological conditions, at least until the monoclonal overproduction is overcome [5, 13]. The most frequently reported clinical complications of hyperviscosity are moreover influenced by many modifying factors, such as a primary vessel wall disease, the local temperature, the pressure gradients and the tendency of the paraprotein to cryoprecipitation: the clinical syndrome of hyperviscosity appears therefore at variable levels of paraprotein concentration, depending also on the unique stereochemical composition of the paraprotein [14, 15].

Cytostatics are still the milestone in the treatment of paraproteinemic disorders, but they often require a long time to obtain satisfactory results [3, 16]. PE therefore has a clear-cut indication when an immediate paraprotein removal is required in order to control hyperviscosity symptoms, and in the cases here reported over 75% had a symptomatic benefit on bleeding tendency and neurologic manifestations. With very limited exceptions, due to real intolerance to drugs or side effects, the association of PE and chemotherapy is mandatory, in order to inhibit as much as possible the overproduction of the malignant cell clone [4].

In most of the cases here reported, an intensive PE course, over 10 to 14 days, with each exchange procedure equivalent to one plasma volume, could overcome the immediate complications of hyperviscosity. All the patients had already been previously treated with cytostatics, lately withdrawn or reduced: at the time of PE, drugs were often added or increased after the first procedure.

PE treatment failed in about 25% of cases. The analysis of presenting laboratory data (mainly increased serum proteins) and the early deaths following PE suggest however that in some instances PE was regarded as an ultimate procedure in terminally ill patients.

A plasma relative viscosity above 3.5—4 seems to be the threshold for the appearance of hyperviscosity symptoms [15] and it is therefore reasonable to monitor patients with repeated viscosimetry controls. PE indications in plasma cell dyscrasias seem to be limited to those cases in which chemotherapy alone cannot control anymore the paraprotein production, or drugs have to be withdrawn because of serious side-effects (pancytopenia, infections).

As far as Waldenström macroglobulinemia is concerned, the long-term follow-up of patients, and the timely combined use of cytostatics and PE, has shown that both the tapering of drugs maintenance dose and the reduced need for PE could be obtained, in order to control and prevent the frequent occurrence of hyperviscosity syndrome.

References

1. Fahey JL, Barth WF, Solomon A. Serum hyperviscosity syndrome. JAMA 1965; 192: 120—3.
2. Editorial. Hyperviscosity syndrome in multiple myeloma. Lancet 1973; 1: 359—60.
3. Waldenström JG. Plasmapheresis. Bloodletting revived and refined. Acta Med Scand 1980; 208: 1—4.
4. Avnstorp C, Nielsen H, Drachmann O, Hippe E. Plasmapheresis in hyperviscosity syndrome. Acta Med Scand 1985; 217: 133—7.
5. Russell JA, Powles RL. The relationship between serum viscosity, hypervolaemia and clinical manifestations associated with circulating paraprotein. Br J Haematol 1978; 39: 163—75.
6. Pihlstedt P. Plasma exchange and moderate dose of cytostatics in advanced macro(cryo)globulinemia. Acta Med Scand 1982; 212: 187—90.
7. Busnach G, Dal Col A, Brando B, Perrino ML, Brunati C, Minetti L. Efficacy of a combined treatment with plasma exchange and cytostatics in macroglobulinemia. Int J artif Organs 1986; 9: 267—70.
8. Busnach G, Dal Col A, Perrino ML, Brando B, Brunati C, Minetti L. Performance evaluation of cascade filtration with high flow rate recirculating plasma on the secondary filter. Int J artif Organs 1987; 10: 121—8.
9. McGrath MA, Penny R. Paraproteinemia. Blood hyperviscosity and clinical manifestations. J Clin Invest 1976; 58: 1155—62.
10. MacKenzie MR, Brown E, Fudenberg HH, Goodenday L. Waldenström's macroglobulinemia: correlation between expanded plasma volume and increased serum viscosity. Blood 1970; 35: 394—408.
11. Orlin JB, Berkman EM. Partial plasma exchange using albumin replacement: removal and recovery of normal plasma constituents. Blood 1980; 56: 1055.
12. Kramer GC, Harms BA, Dodai BI, Demling RH, Renkin EM. Mechanisms for redistribution of plasma protein following acute protein depletion. Am J Physiol 1982; 243: H803.
13. Russell JA, Toy JL, Powles RL. Plasma exchange in malignant paraproteinaemias. Exp Hemat 1977; 5S: 105—16.
14. Alexanian R. Blood volume in monoclonal gammopathy. Blood 1977; 49: 301.
15. Beck JR, Quinn BM, Meier FA, Rawnsley HM. Hyperviscosity syndrome in paraproteinemia managed by plasma exchange; monitored by serum tests. Transfusion 1982; 22: 51—3.
16. Solomon A, Fahey JL. Plasmapheresis therapy in macroglobulinemia. Ann Intern Med 1963; 58: 789.

3. Implications of renal failure in multiple myeloma

RAYMOND ALEXANIAN & BART BARLOGIE

Implications of renal failure in multiple myeloma

Renal failure represents one of the major complications of multiple myeloma. Azotemia provides a clue to the diagnosis, poses a major management problem when severe, and has been considered an ominous prognostic factor. This presentation summarizes the frequency, pathogenesis and prognostic implications of renal failure in a large number of previously untreated patients with advanced myeloma who received a standard program of chemotherapy. Results indicated that hypercalcemia and/or moderate Bence Jones proteinuria from advanced disease explained the azotemia in most of our patients. Because renal failure was often reversible, the disease stage and the sensitivity of the myeloma to chemotherapy were more important prognostic factors than the presence or degree of azotemia.

Methods

Between September 1974 and November 1986, 495 consecutive, previously untreated patients received one of 9 different chemotherapy programs. Because treatments that consisted of an alkylating agent-glucocorticoid — vincristine — doxorubicin combination provided a higher and more consistent response rate than other therapies, only the 389 patients treated with one of 6 similar doxorubicin programs were included in the analysis. Dose regimens have been described elsewhere [1]. The plasma cell tumor mass of each patient was defined as high, intermediate, or low according to standard criteria. Clinical response was defined by a greater than 75% reduction of serum myeloma protein and disapearance of Bence Jones protein excretion [2]. Survival was measured from the start of treatment

Minetti et al. (eds.), The kidney in plasma cell dyscrasias. ISBN 978-94-010-7085-0

and remission time was measured from the onset of a 75% reduction of tumor mass to the first evidence of relapse. Short-term hemodialysis was used in several patients but none was maintained on chronic dialysis.

Frequency of renal failure

Azotemia was defined by a serum creatinine above 1.7 mg/100 ml and occurred in 21% of our patients (Table 1). Only 8 patients with low tumor mass had azotemia, constituting 10% of all patients with renal failure. Since our primary goal was to assess the prognostic impact of renal failure on response and survival, all 110 patients with such early disease and more favorable outcome were excluded from further analysis. Thus, 26% of the remaining patients with high or intermediate tumor mass had a pretreatment creatinine above 1.7 mg/100 ml (Table 1). Median age and gender distribution were similar among patients with or without renal failure. About three-fourths of our patients with renal failure had a high tumor mass.

Pathogenesis of azotemia

The major laboratory features contributing to renal failure were examined

Table 1. Pathogenesis of renal failure in multiple myeloma.

	Serum creatinine (mg/100 ml)			
		< 1.7	1.8–3.0	> 3.0
	No.	(% of patients)		
Tumor Mass				
Low	110	93	5	2
Intermediate	155	87	8	5
High	124	56	27	17
High + intermediate				
Hypercalcemia* (% > 12 mg/100 ml)	279	14	44	54 ($p < 0.01$)
Bence Jones protein (BJP) (% > 2 g/day)	279	19	44	43 ($p < 0.01$)
Only BJP (%)	279	14	15	40 ($p < 0.01$)

* Corrected calcium (mg/100 ml) = serum calcium (mg/100 ml) − serum albumin (g/100 ml) + 4.0.

Table 2. Prognosis in 279 patients with high or intermediate tumor mass according to renal function.

	Serum creatinine (mg/100 ml)		
	< 1.7	1.8–3.0	> 3.0
Response rate (%)	57	46	44 (p = 0.07)
Remission (median mos)	23	24	19
Survival (median mos)	32	23	21 (p = 0.04)

in 279 patients with high or intermediate tumor mass myeloma. Hypercalcemia or Bence Jones protein excretion of more than 2.0 g/day occurred in about one half of our patients and at a similar frequency among patients with mild or severe renal failure (Table 2). De Fronzo et al. have previously stressed the importance of these features in the pathogenesis of acute renal failure [3]. In patients with serum creatinine above 3.0 mg/100 ml, 40% showed marked light chain excretion as their only protein abnormality. Either hypercalcemia or more than 2 g/day of Bence Jones protein were present in about 85% of patients. In only 4 of the 73 patients was a diagnosis of amyloidosis (AL) confirmed and only 2 patients showed albuminuria of more than 1.0 g/day. Thus, primary amyloidosis (AL) contributed rarely to the pathogenesis of renal failure in our patients with multiple myeloma.

Response to treatment

Six percent of patients with azotemia died during the first 4 weeks of treatment and were considered unresponsive. As indicated in Table 2, the frequency of response was slightly less with increasing renal failure, but the differences were not significant. Remission times were also similar in all groups. Thus, the similar response rate and remission time in patients with renal failure indicated that there was no inherent resistance to chemo therapy because of the renal status.

The survival times of patients with mild or severe azotemia were similar (median 23 months), and about 9 months shorter than that of patients with normal renal function ($p = 0.04$) (Table 2). The more extensive myeloma in patients with renal failure was considered a major factor that contributed to the shorter lifespan.

Reversible renal failure

The frequency of reversible renal failure, defined by creatinine reduction of at least 0.5 mg to less than 1.5 mg/100 ml, was examined. The median time to such improvement was 1.4 months, with all responders showing a normal creatinine within 4 months. Such rapid reversibility was also described by Rota et al. [4]. Normalization occurred in 51% of all patients, but was more frequent in patients with slight creatinine elevation (60%) or whose myeloma had responded to chemotherapy (Table 3). Bernstein and Humes reported the reversibility of renal insufficiency in 55% of patients, including 6 of 7 patients with creatinine above 5 mg/100 ml [5]. In only 4 patients did the creatinine remain above 5 mg/100 ml, testifying to the infrequency of severe and irreversible renal failure in newly diagnosed patients referred to our center. Control of azotemia was attributed primarily to the reversibility of hypercalcemia and/or Bence Jones proteinuria (prerequisites for remission), but sometimes occurred without myeloma control with the attainment of normocalcemia or a slight reduction of Bence Jones protein.

As a result, the survival of patients with reversible azotemia that included many patients responding to chemotherapy was similar to that of similarly staged, previously untreated patients without azotemia. Irreversible renal failure was associated with a low response rate (33%) and short median survival (15 months). Patients whose myeloma and azotemia both failed to respond lived a median of only 8 months. Thus, renal failure was not inherently a harmful prognostic factor. More important features among our patients were the advanced stage of the myeloma and/or the resistance of the myeloma to chemotherapy. Multivariate analyses of the major factors affecting survival in patients with renal failure should clarify this question.

Our findings were compared with those of S. Rota et al. who studied 34 patients with severe renal failure diagnosed in various phases of multiple myeloma [4]. All of the French patients, but only about one-third of our patients showed a creatinine above 3.4 mg/100 ml. Among comparable patients in both studies, only about 30% achieved a normal level. While

Table 3. Reversibility of renal failure.

	No. evaluable	% reversible to < 1.5 mg/100 ml	
Serum creatinine (mg/100 ml)			
1.8–3.0	43	60	$p = 0.02$
> 3.0	24	33	
Response of myeloma			
Yes	30	63	$p = 0.10$
No	37	41	

the utility of chronic hemodialysis was highlighted in the Paris report, very few of our patients qualified for such a program.

Acknowledgement

This work was supported by grants CA 28771 and CA 37161 from the National Cancer Institute.

References

1. Alexanian R, Dreicer R. Chemotherapy for multiple myeloma. Cancer 1984; 53: 583–8.
2. McLaughlin P, Alexanian R. Myeloma protein kinetics following chemotherapy. Blood 1982; 60: 851–5.
3. De Fronzo R, Humphrey R, Wright J, Cooke C. Acute renal failure in multiple myeloma. Medicine 1975; 54: 209–23.
4. Rota S, Mougenot B, Baudouin B, et al. Multiple myeloma and severe renal failure. Medicine 1987; 66: 126–37.
5. Bernstein S, Humes H. Reversible renal insufficiency in multiple myeloma. Arch Int Med 1982; 142: 2083–6.

4. Uraemia in myeloma: management and prognosis

N. P. MALLICK

The median survival for myeloma is 30—36 months. This is 3—4 times that recorded before the introduction of Cyclophosphamide and Melphalan, but has remained consistent since then. Infection and renal failure dominate mortality.

Over 50% of patients have severe renal impairment at presentation [1] and at post-mortem up to 70% have tubular casts, tubular damage or atrophy and interstitial scarring — 'the myeloma kidney' [2]. In earlier reports, the median survival of patients with renal impairment was very poor; for example, in the first MRC trial [3], it was only 2 months if the blood urea exceeded 80 mg/dl, compared to 37 months for patients presenting with blood urea < 40 mg/dl.

There is greater awareness now that myeloma patients tend to be fluid depleted at presentation, because of salt and water loss caused by vomiting, and water loss due to impaired renal conservation by the damaged kidney, aggravated by hypercalcaemia, and that radiographic contrast dyes should be avoided in such circumstances. Prompt fluid repletion has a beneficial effect as demonstrated in the latest MRC study [4]. The value of such repletion and of prompt management of hypercalcaemia was emphasized by Bernstein and Humes [5], in whose retrospective series the serum creatinine was lowered from its peak value in 55% of cases, with improvement in outlook.

The principal cause of myeloma kidney is nephrotoxic light chains. These have the capacity to inhibit tubular function and to destroy tubular cells. Cast formation results from the aggregation of urinary light chains with Tamm-Horsfall protein and the casts may, by obstructing urinary flow, precipitate or aggravate renal impairment. Salt and water depletion also will make worse any prevailing renal impairment by adding a prerenal element to it and by rendering cast formation more likely in a decreased urine flow.

Both hyperuricaemia and hypercalcaemia occur in myeloma, the former

Minetti et al. (eds.), The kidney in plasma cell dyscrasias. ISBN 978-94-010-7085-0

especially during a phase of tumour cell destruction, the latter insidiously in over 50% of patients at some time in the illness. It is due both to increased bone osteoclasis and to impaired calcium excretion by the kidney, an important contributing factor, especially if GFR is reduced. Urinary tract infection with involvement of the renal parenchyma occurs in myeloma and so does severe systemic infection or septicaemia. These too, add to any renal impairment.

Together one or more such complication is present frequently when a patient with myeloma presents in severe renal failure, and this has been so in series recorded over past decades. More recently, the use of drugs with nephrotoxic side-effects has been a more prominent feature, especially the non-steroidal anti-inflammatory drugs which are prescribed frequently for the non-specific or skeletal pains which are common in myeloma.

The presence of such aggravating factors in the uraemic patient is important because, if each is dealt with (see Table 1) and the patient supported, even by dialysis if necessary, renal function may recover.

A major problem is that uraemia may be the presenting feature of myeloma or may 'develop' suddenly in its course, yet in either case the underlying renal pathology cannot be predicted. Nor can the renal biopsy appearances do more than indicate the likely outcome.

In recent series [6, 7] severe tubulo-interstitial changes have been associated with a poorer outcome, while complete and substantial recovery of renal function has occurred only in the absence of such changes. Cast formation has been a common but not a prognostic feature. Extensive amyloid deposition may be found, and will limit the extent of renal recovery.

Overall, however, with prompt management there can be substantial

Table 1. Causes of renal damage in myeloma. Fluid depletion (bracketed) may aggravate any pre-existing renal impairment. Commonly in uraemia, several of these factors operate simultaneously.

Nephrotoxic light chains
Cast formation
Amyloid deposition
Cryoglobulin deposition
Parenchymal infection
Contrast dyes
Drugs
Hyperuricaemia
Hypercalcaemia
(Fluid depletion)

Table 2. Acute renal failure in myeloma. Adapted from Cohen et al. Am J Med 1984; 76: 247—56.

Rapid rise in serum creatinine
from normal to > 2.5 mg/dl in the
absence of pre or post renal factors
recovery to serum creatinine < 2.5 mg/dl.
To 1987 at least 56 such cases reported.
In almost 50% no prior diagnosis of myeloma.

---

improvement in renal function. Using strict criteria (Table 2), Cohen et al. [8] found recovery to serum creatinine < 2.5 mg/dl or blood urea nitrogen < 40 mg/dl in 46 cases reported up to 1984; in 18/46 there was no prior knowledge of myeloma. Severe hyperuricaemia (> 12 mg/dl) was present in 14 cases. Severe hypercalcaemia (> 12 mg/dl) occurred concurrently in 5 and independently in 2 cases. Septicaemia, pneumonia, urinary tract infection and the intercurrent use of nephrotoxic drugs were the commonest precipitants.

By very similar criteria Rota et al. [7] had 7 further cases in their recent series of 34 patients; two points in this study require emphasis. Recovery took up to 210 days (median more than 50 days) and while 5/7 patients survived for at least a year only one was alive 3 years from the episode, reflecting the remorseless toll of the underlying tumour.

These results underscore the finding in earlier work (for example De Fronzo et al. [9]) that uraemia in myeloma may be totally reversible and also make clear that recovery to a less impaired, stable level of renal function can be obtained, rendering a patient eventually independent of dialysis — but there is a real price to pay in terms of the time and expense involved. Rota et al. [7] point out that it may take months to achieve stable renal function independent of dialysis. Coward presented evidence of the high cost of treating such patients because of the intensive, prolonged in-patient care required. And even if renal failure is irreversible, dialysis or transplantation is technically successful (if costly) and tumour progression slowed by chemotherapy, this elderly group of patients remains vulnerable to cardiovascular and respiratory complications [6].

Some guidelines seem clear. The patient presenting with uraemia should be treated vigorously. Predisposing factors should be removed or corrected. Dialysis should be employed but not before fluid repletion is completed. Unless there are technical contraindications renal biopsy should be undertaken; it may reveal an unsuspected glomerular lesion, the degree of tubulo-interstitial damage and occasionally suggest a super-added, drug-associated nephropathy. Typical myeloma casts will be present in many but not in all cases.

Equally important is an assessment of the tumour load [10]. Evidence from all reports, considered together, leads to the conclusions that true uraemia and advanced myeloma kidney in a patient with a heavy tumour load is unlikely to recover well, and that unless the tumour has a rapid and sustained response to chemotherapy, regular dialysis treatment for end-stage renal failure will not prolong life significantly.

On the other hand, in a patient with a small tumour load and a good response to chemotherapy, biopsy appearances suggesting mild light chain nephrotoxicity should encourage vigorous therapy with the expectation of good recovery of renal function.

The principal difficulty is the management of the majority those of myeloma patients with uraemia, who are intermediate between these two categories in terms of tumour load and the degree of renal damage. In them, dialysis therapy might be required over months, might be rewarded by eventual recovery to independent but impaired renal function, or may remain necessary indefinitely. Chemotherapy and/or plasmapheresis might have reduced greatly the secretion of free light chains by the tumour, whatever the degree of improvement in renal function. What is the outlook for these patients and is dialysis treatment for the renal failure beneficial or intrusive?

Cosio et al. [11] state "if we prevent death from uraemia, the prognosis is similar to that of myeloma patients without renal insufficiency".

However, this is probably not the case. Consider the evidence presented by the MRC Working Party, using a classification for prognosis said to be a comparable discriminator to that of Durie and Salmon (Table 3).

Table 3. MRC criteria for prognosis in myeloma. Adapted from Brit J Canc 1980; 42: 831–40.

	Prognosis	
	Good	Poor
Blood urea	< 8 mmol/l	> 10 mmol/l or
Hb.	> 100 g/l	< 75 g/l
Symptoms	Minimal	Restrict activity
Survival at 2 yrs	c 65%	c 10%
Survival at 4 yrs	c 55%	c 7%

Overall, after correction of fluid depletion, even a modestly raised blood urea level remains as an indicator of poor prognosis, with survival at 2 years of ca 10% and at 4 years of ca 7%, whereas survival for the 'good prognosis' group was ca 65% and ca 55% at these times.

Whilst there are reports of much longer survival on dialysis, it seems probable that few myeloma patients with established end-stage renal disease will survive longer than the present median of 36 months, for myeloma as a whole — a point that is emphasized by Rota et al. [6], from their review of the literature. Support for the majority of such patients is essentially short-term and death will supervene from infection, cardiovascular or respiratory complications, or directly as a result of the tumour mass and its haematological or skeletal consequences, rather than from uraemia.

The value of up to three years of relatively active life is not to be denied, but equally the cost/benefit analysis cannot be ignored (see Coward p 00). Each myeloma patient treated for end-stage renal failure must be assessed regularly with this in mind.

With regard to treatment modality, there is no good evidence that either haemodialysis or continuous ambulatory peritoneal dialysis (CAPD) is superior. On CAPD infection may be troublesome while cardiovascular complications may interfere with haemodialysis especially if there is cardiac or haematological involvement by amyloid tissue.

Successful transplantation has been reported (see for example [11]). This raises further problems of the correctness of using cadaver kidneys when long-term survival is improbable and of advising, or agreeing to undertake, live donation in such circumstances.

It should be remembered that at the better end of the spectrum, patients with myeloma may respond promptly and for prolonged periods to effective chemotherapy; if irreversible renal damage by light chains has occurred during an earlier phase of active tumour development then the long-term outlook may greatly exceed the median. In such, admittedly uncommon cases, transplantation might be the optimal therapy.

The prediction of so favourable a response to chemotherapy is not within the scope of this report, and is not yet possible prespectively, on the basis of any combination of tumour load, immunoglobulin class or subclass, light chain secretion, or clinical parameters. However, ex-vivo analysis of tumour cells for their growth kinetics, colony forming potential and DNA content are being pursued. In time these, and other approaches will make the response to therapy more predictable, so making easier the decision as to whether, and for how long, to treat established renal failure by dialysis, or whether to proceed to transplantation.

References

1. Kyle RA. Multiple Myeloma: Review of 869 cases. Mayo Clin Proc 1975; 50: 29—40.
2. Kapadia S. Multiple Myeloma; a clinico-pathological study of 62 consecutive autopsied cases. Medicine 1980; 59: 380—92.
3. Medical Research Council Working Party on Leukaemia in Adults. Br J Haematol 1973; 24: 123—39.
4. Medical Research Council Working Party on Leukaemia in Adults. Analysis and management of renal failure in IVth M. R. C. myelomatosis trial. Br Med J 1984; 288: 1411—6.
5. Bernstein SP, Humes HD. Reversible renal insufficiency in multiple myeloma. Arch Intern Med 1982; 142: 2083—6.
6. Coward RA, Mallick NP, Delamore IW. Should patients with renal failure associated with myeloma be dialysed? Br Med J 1983; 287: 1575—8.
7. Rota S, Mougenot B, Baudouin B, et al. Multiple myeloma and severe renal failure. A clinico-pathologic study of outcome and prognosis in 34 patients. Medicine 1987; 66: 126—37.
8. Cohen DS, Sherman WH, Osserman EF, Appel GB. Acute renal failure in patients with multiple myeloma. Amer J Med 1984; 76: 247—56.
9. De Fronzo RA, Hymphrey RL, Wright JR, Cooke CR. Acute renal failure in multiple myeloma. Medicine 1975; 54: 209—23.
10. Durie BGM, Salmon SE. A clinical staging system for multiple myeloma. Cancer 1975; 36: 842—54.
11. Cosio FG, Pence TV, Shapiro FL, Kjellstrand CM. Severe renal failure in multiple myeloma. Clin Nephrol 1981; 15: 206—10.

5. Therapeutic prospects in amyloidosis

J. B. NATVIG, BJØRN SKOGEN & EGIL AMUNDSEN

Introduction

Although the existence of amyloid has been known for about 150 years, the specific amyloid proteins have only been characterised during the last 20 years [see 1—5]. The precursor proteins and some aspects of their synthesis and catabolism have also been described [1—5], but despite this new knowledge, the treatment of amyloidosis is very difficult and usually inefficient [6]. In this review we shall point out some of the main principles for the present and future treatment of amyloidosis.

Amyloidosis is generally a progressive disease that leads to serious organ deterioration within months or years and eventually death. The major causes of death in primary and secondary amyloidosis are cardiovascular and renal affection. The latter is more predominant in secondary amyloidosis. Patients with renal amyloidosis usually develop proteinuria, nephrotic syndrome and progressive renal insufficiency with uraemia. Although the treatment results so far have been very modest, we shall inject a slight rate of optimism by describing three major approaches to therapy in amyloidosis: (a) prevention of amyloid precursor synthesis, (b) removal or dissolution of amyloid fibrils, and (c) prevention of deposition of amyloid fibrils.

Prevention of amyloid precursor synthesis

Prevention of precursor synthesis can be achieved in three different ways.

The first method is by curing the underlying disease in cases where the disease process represents a constant stimulation to precursor synthesis, for example active treatment of rheumatoid arthritis [7], removal of a tumour, or successful treatment of an infection [8—10]. It is possible that active interference with the underlying disease may eventually also prove

Minetti et al. (eds.), The kidney in plasma cell dyscrasias. ISBN 978-94-010-7085-0

to be so positive that therapeutic irradiation and subsequent bone marrow transplantation could be considered in some of the lymphoproliferative diseases underlying myeloma or macroglobulinemia associated amyloidosis or primary amyloidosis. Selected patients with the progressive form of primary amyloidosis associated with the extremely amyloidogenic variable light chain, V*6, would lend themselves to such a trial, since in this type of light chain-associated amyloidosis several patients have shown a fairly rapidly developing disease and death [11—13]. We are not aware, however, of any such therapeutic attempts.

Another method is prevention of precursor synthesis by intervention with the serum amyloid A protein (SAA) or amyloid light chain (AL) precursors. The most successful results in preventing amyloidosis in familial Mediterranean fever (FMF) have been obtained with colchicine [2, 14, 15], which has been shown to be quite effective. A similar approach is therefore probably justifiable in other disease groups that are frequently complicated with amyloidosis, particularly if specific risk patients within the group can be identified, e.g. by continuously high SAA levels.

Another approach to the prevention of precursor synthesis would be to block IL-1, which is an SAA inducer, or to interfere with the amyloid enhancing factor (AEF) [16]. Although it is possible that the AEF primarily acts on the deposition phase and not on the synthesis phase [16] attempts to neutralise it might be rewarding. The possibility of immunotargeting against precursor synthesis is also worth exploring.

Finally, the prevention of precursor synthesis can be attempted by representing the genes coding for SAA, particularly the human equivalent of SAA_2 [18], which is the most amyloidogenic component of the precursor substances.

Removal or dissolution the amyloid fibrils

The removal or dissolution of amyloid fibrils has been tried by dimethylsulphoxide (DMSO) [19—23]. However, this is a socially unacceptable solution because of the strong odour, and for this reason it is practically never used. Other therapeutic approaches have been tried particularly with cytostatic drugs, both in secondary and primary amyloidosis, and in several instances a positive effect was obtained after years of treatment [2, 24—27].

A second method is the surgical removal of the amyloid organ and subsequent transplantation, which is particularly used in severe kidney affections, where other organ involvement is moderate. A combination of kidney transplantation and active treatment of the underlying disease causing the amyloid deposition has given fairly good results [28].

Finally, a potential approach is the use of local proteolytic enzymes. The effect of this may be enhanced by immunotargeting through coupling of active enzymes to antibodies. One of the difficulties of using enzymes, however, is the abundance of enzyme inhibitors in serum and tissues. It may be easier to catabolize the precursor protein than to dissolve already deposited fibrils. We have made some experimental attempts along these lines [29—30].

Prevention of deposition of amyloid fibrils

It is possible that interference with AEF would inhibit fibril formation [16]. Much more work is needed, however, to clarify the mechanism of action of the AEF before it can be used in a therapeutic approach.

An attractive approach to amyloid therapy would be to directly remove the precursor. This could be done by plasmapheresis or direct immunoadsorbent techniques, but this will have to be explored more fully [6].

Another interesting approach is to attempt to influence the metabolic pathway of SAA and to try to enhance the proteolysis of the amyloid precursor.

In vitro enhancing experiments

Enhance the proteolysis of the amyloid precursor may be a rewarding approach since it has been found that serine proteases on monocyte surfaces [31], in supernatants from monocyte cultures [31, 32] and in serum [33], are capable of degrading SAA.

Enzymatic degradation of the protein by these enzymes creates an intermediate fragment that resembles AA in antigenicity and molecular weight. This fragment is then further degraded to smaller peptides (Fig. 1). One of the enzymes with SAA degrading capacity is plasmin. This is the activated form of plasminogen, and it is a fibrinolytic enzyme in the circulation. Plasmin can be activated artificially by infusion of streptokinase or urokinase, which increases the fibrinolytic activity in plasma for the removal of thrombin. Our experimental approach has been to activate this proteolytic system to increase the SAA degrading activity in plasma. We have shown that the proteolytic activity against protein AA in the serum fraction corresponding to plasminogen can considerably be increased after activation of the enzyme with streptokinase (Fig. 2) [29]. The increase was not so pronounced when activation was done in whole plasma, probably because of the presence of enzyme inhibitors.

Brinase (protease I from *Aspergillus oryzae*) is a serine protease that has been proved to be effective in thrombolytic therapy in both animals and

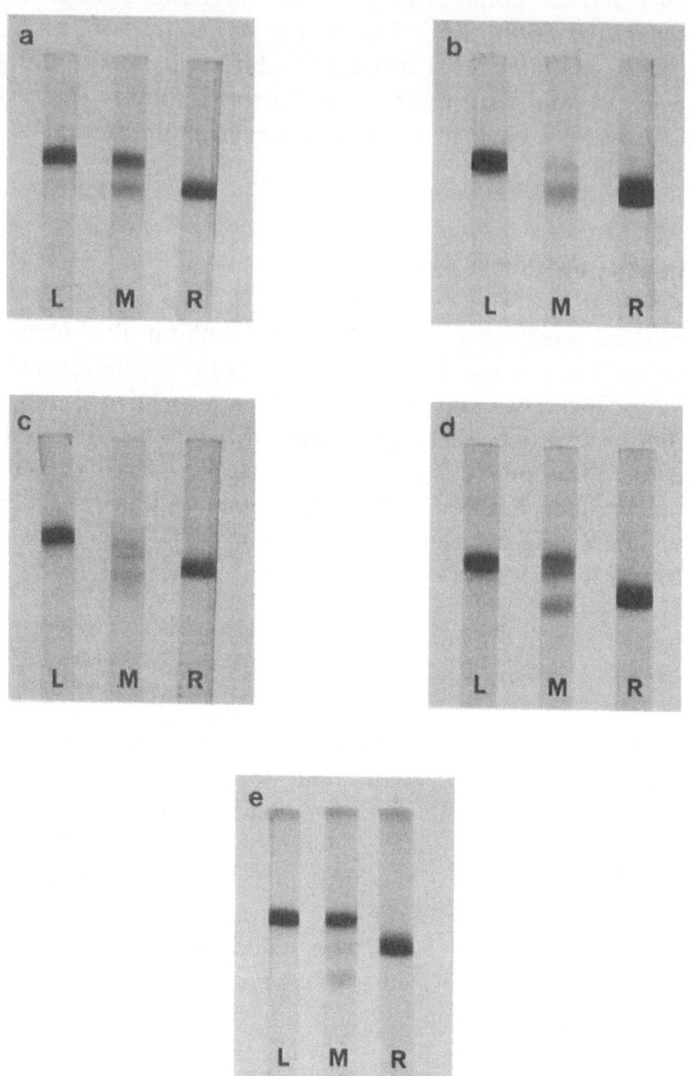

Fig. 1. Polyacrylamide gel electrophoresis (in Sodium dodecyl sulphate) of purified protein SAA incubated at 37°C in the presence of (a) elastase (20 min), (b) kallikrein (20 min), (c) collagenase (20 min), (d) thrombin (60 min) and (e) plasmin (60 min). Gel L shows protein SAA, gel M the incubated sample and gel R protein AA. The amount of SAA in sample M was equal to L before the start of the proteolysis [34].

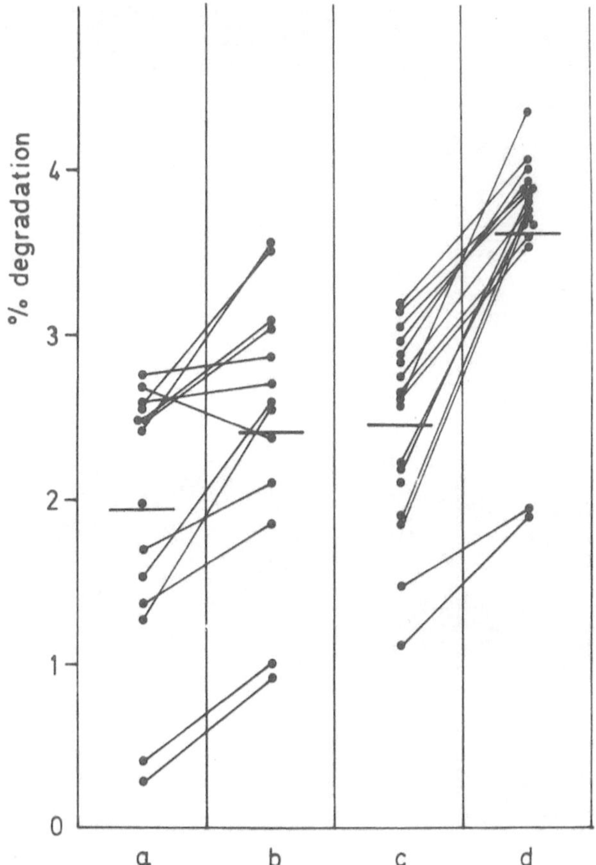

Fig. 2. Determination of AA degrading activity in human plasma in the absence and presence of streptokinase. (a) = plasma alone without streptokinase, 30 min, (b) = plasma and streptokinase, 30 min, (c) = plasma alone without streptokinase, 60 min, (d) = plasma and streptokinase, 60 min. The results from parallel experiments are connected by lines. The bars represent the mean values of each set of experiments.

humans. The enzyme was found to be proteolytically effective against SAA, AA and amyloid fibrils of the corresponding type [30].

To test the enzyme activity on native amyloid fibrils, sections of amyloidotic organs were incubated in enzyme solutions. The enzyme was able to remove most of the fibrils from the tissue leaving the original structure more or less unaffected (Fig. 3).

In vivo enhancing experiments

We also showed by in vivo experiments in rabbits that the plasma clear-

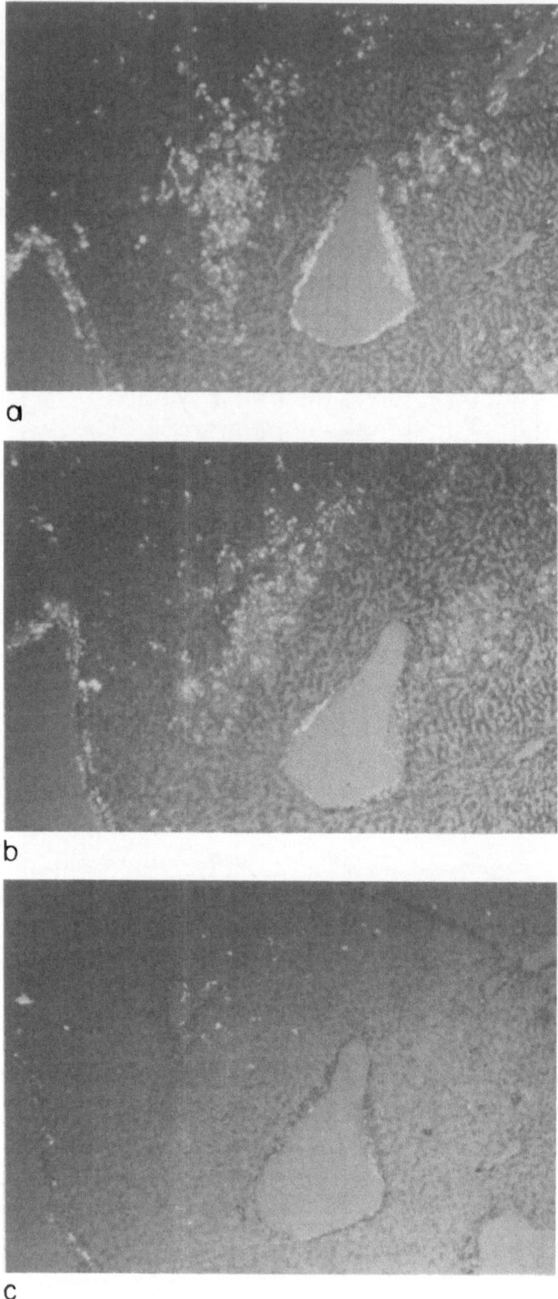

Fig. 3. Sections of an amyloidotic liver stained with Congo red and examined in polarized light, (a) unincubated, (b) incubated at 37°C for 18 h in PBS, (c) incubated at 37°C for 18 h in PBS containing 0.1 mg/ml brinase.

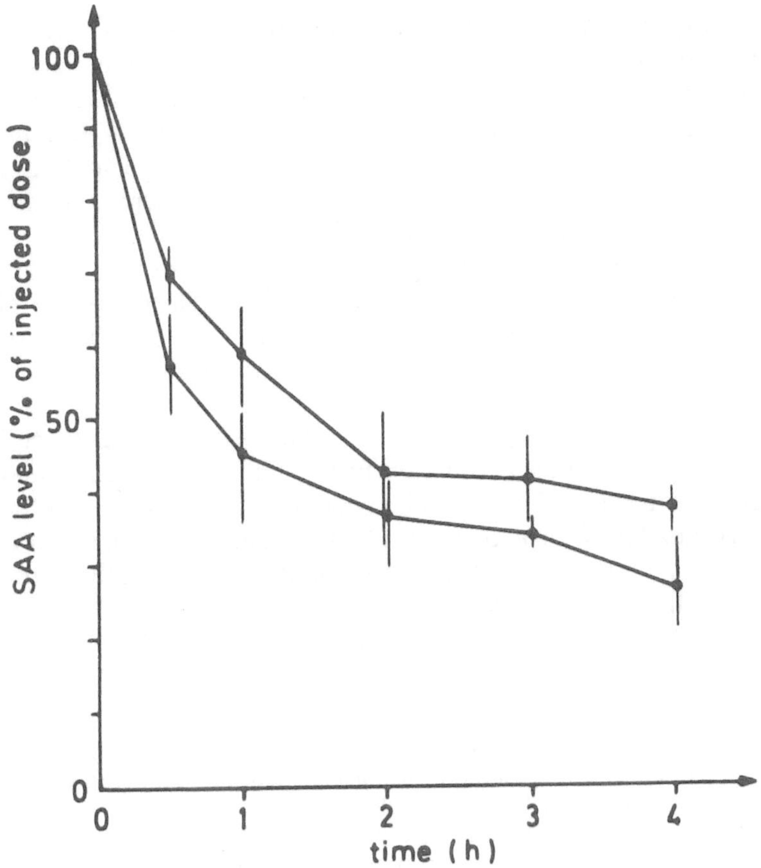

Fig. 4. Plasma clearance rate of ^{125}I-SAA in normal rabbits (000) and in rabbits treated with brinase (000). The vertical bars show the range. Levels of significance: 30 min, $P < 0.01$; 1 h, $P < 0.01$; 2 h, $P > 0.05$; 3 h, $P < 0.05$; 4 h, $P < 0.01$.

ance rate of radioactively labelled SAA could be significantly increased by the addition of brinase to the animals in vivo (Fig. 4).

Discussion

Our in vitro and in vivo enhancing experiments show that by manipulating a physiological system or by introducing an external enzyme into the circulation, we can influence the metabolic rate of the amyloid precursor SAA. It is also possible that the balance between amyloid fibril formation and fibril resolution can be influenced in the desired direction by increasing the proteolytic activity of plasma. It has been shown that treatment with proteolytic enzyme can remove or prevent the formation of glomerular immune complex deposits and decrease the proteinuria in rats with passive Heyman nephritis [35]. This is therefore a potential therapeutic approach which deserves further attention. Studies of the enzymatic degradation of SAA seem to indicate that the cleavage takes place in the C-terminal part of the protein, favouring the formation of the amyloidogenic AA protein. Amino acid sequence studies have revealed that the N-terminal part of the protein is essential for fibril formation [2—4].

Thus the search for agents that can attach the protein in the NH_2-terminus should be stepped up. Although amyloid fibrils can be created artificially by single, pure proteins such as β_2-microglobulin and immunoglobulin light chains, there is a growing consciousness that other factors may also participate in the assembly of the fibrils. The fact that so many and so different proteins can form fibrils with a similar appearance [2—4], raises the possibility that a common factor may be involved. Candidates for such a factor are the amyloid P component [2—4], the still poorly characterised AEF or proteoglycans [2—4]. If there is such a factor in fibril formation, a possible method of disrupting the fibrils would be to attack and destroy it.

References

1. Wegelius O, Pasternack A. Amyloidosis. London: Academic Press, 1976: 605 pp.
2. Glenner GG, Osserman EF, Benditt EP, Calkins E, Cohen AS, Zucker-Franklin D. Amyloidosis. New York: Plenum Press, 1986: 857 pp.
3. Glenner GG, Costa PP, Freitas AF. Amyloid and amyloidosis. Amsterdam: Excerpta Medica, 1980: 630 pp.
4. Marrink J, Van Rijswijk MH. Amyloidosis. Dordrecht: Martinus Nijhoff, 1986: 378 pp.
5. Tribe CR, Bacon PA. Amyloidosis E. A. R. S. Bristol: John Wright and Sons Limited, 1981: 214 pp.
6. Glenner GG. Future Directions in Amyloid Research. In: Marrink J, Van Rijswijk MH, eds. Amyloidosis. Dordrecht: Martinus Nijhoff, 1986: 357—63.
7. Falck HM, Törnroth T, Skrifvars B, Wegelius O. Resolution of Renal Amyloidosis Secondary to Rheumatoid Arthritis. Acta Med Scand 1979; 205: 651—6.
8. Dikman SH, Kahn T, Gribetz D, Churg J. Resolution of Renal Amyloidosis. American J Med 1977; 63: 430—3.
9. Waldenström H. On the Formation and Disappearance of Amyloid in Man. Acta chir Scand 1928; 63: 479—529.
10. Lowenstein J, Gallo G. Remission of the Nephrotic Syndrome in Renal Amyloidosis. New England Journal of Medicine. 1970; 282: 128—32.
11. Natvig JB, Westermark P, Sletten K, Husby G, Michaelsen TE. Further structural and antigenic studies of light-chain amyloid proteins. Scand J Immunol 1981; 14: 89—94.
12. Natvig JB, Westermark P, Sletten K, Husby G, Michaelsen T. Structure and Antigen Analysis of Light Chain Amyloid Proteins. In: Glenner GG, Costa PP, Freitas AF, eds. Amyloid and amyloidosis. Amsterdam: Excerpta Medica, 257—65.

13. Solomon A, Kyle RA, Frangione B. Light Chain Variable Region Subgroups of Monoclonal Immunoglobulins Amyloidosis AL. In: Glenner GG, Osserman ES, Benditt EP, Kalkin E, Cohen AS, Zucker-Franklin D, eds. Amyloidosis. New York: Plenum Press, 1986.
14. Ravid M, Robson M, Kedar I. Prolonged Colchicine Treatment in Four Patients with Amyloidosis. Annals of Internal Medicine 1977; 87: 568—70.
15. Walker F, Bear RA. Long-term Colchicine Therapy for Renal Amyloidosis in Familial Mediterranean Fever. CMA Journal 1982; 127: 1163—4.
16. Brandwin SR, Sipe JD, Skinner M, Cohen AS. Effect of Colchicine on the Acute Phase Serum Amyloid A Protein Response and Splenic Amyloid Deposition during Experimental Murine Inflammation. In: Glenner GG, Osserman EF, Benditt EP, Calkins E, Cohen AS, Zucker-Franklin D, eds. Amyloidosis. New York: Plenum Press, 1986: 129—37.
17. Kisilevsky R. Biology of Disease. Amyloidosis: A familiar problem in the light of current pathogenetic developments. Lab Invest 1983; 49: 381—90.
18. Meek RL, Hoffman JS, Benditt EP. Amyloidogenesis. One Serum Amyloid A Isotype is Selectively Removed from the Circulation. J Exp Med 1986; 163: 499.
19. Ravid M, Shapira J, Lang R, Kedar I. Prolonged Dimenthylsulphoxide Treatment in 13 Patients with Systemic Amyloidosis. Annals of Rheumatic Diseases 1982; 41: 587—92.
20. Kisilevsky R, Boudreau L, Foster D. II. The Effects of Dimethylsulphoxide and Colchicine Therapy. Lab Invest 1983; 48: 60—7.
21. Hanai N, Ishihara T, Uchino F, Imada N, Fujihara S, Ikegami J. Effects of Dimethyl Sulphoxide and Colchicine on the Resorption of Experimental Amyloid. Virchows Arch A Path Anat and Histol 1979; 384: 45—52.
22. Kedar I, Greenwald M, Ravid M. Treatment of Experimental Murine Amyloidosis with Dimethyl Sulphoxide, 1976; 7: 149—50.
23. Van Rijswijk MH, Donker Ab. JM, Ruinen L. Dimethysulphoxide in Amyloidosis. Lancet 1979; i 207—8.
24. Kyle RA, Wagoner RD, Holly KE. Primary Systemic Amyloidosis. Resolution of the Nephrotic Syndrome with Melphalan and Prednisone. Arch Intern Med 1982; 142: 1445—7.
25. Corkery J, Bern MM, Tullis JL. Resolution of Amyloidosis and Plasma-Cell Dyscrasia with Combination Chemotherapy. Lancet 1978; 425—6.
26. Cohen HJ. Combination Chemotherapy for Primary Amyloidosis Reconsidered. Annals of Internal Medicine 1978; 89: 572.
27. Kyle RA, Greipp PR. Primary Systemic Amyloidosis: Comparison of Melphalan and Prednisone versus Placebo. Blood 1978; 52: 818—27.
28. Jacob ET, Bar-Nathan N, Shapira Z, Gafni J. Renal Transplantation in the Amyloidosis of Familial Mediterranean Fever. Arch Intern Med 1979; 139: 1135—8.
29. Skogen B, Natvig JB. In Vitro Enhancement of AA-degrading Activity in Human Plasma with the Plasminogen Activator Streptokinase. Scand J Immunol 1981; 14: 637—41.
30. Skogen B, Amundsen E. Degradation of Amyloid Proteins with Protease I from Aspergillus Oryzae. In Vivo Increase in SAA Clearance Rate after Enzyme Infusion. Scand J Immunol 1982; 16: 509—14.
31. Lavie G, Zucker-Franklin D, Franklin EC. Degradation of Serum Amyloid A Protein by Surface-associated Enzymes of Human Blood Monocytes. J Exp Med 1978; 148: 1020.
32. Skogen B, Thorsteinsson L, Natvig JB. Degradation of Protein SAA to an AA-like Fragment by Enzymes of Monocytic Origin. Scand J Immunol 1980; 11: 533—40.

33. Skogen B, Natvig JB, Børresen AL, Berg K. Degradation of Amyloid-related Serum Protein SAA by a Component Present in Rabbit and Human Serum. Scand J Immunol 1980; 11: 643–8.
34. Skogen B, Natvig JB. Degradation of Amyloid Proteins by Different Serine Proteases. Scand J Immunol 1981; 14: 389–96.
35. Nakazawa M, Emancipator SN, Lamm ME. Proteolytic Enzyme Treatment Reduces Glomerular Immune Deposits and Proteinuria in Passive Heymann Nephritis. J Exp Med 1986; 164: 1973–87.

6. Sundries on therapy of multiple myeloma and amyloidosis and their renal consequences: A forum

A. SOLOMON, B. BARLOGIE, J. N. BUXBAUM, R. A. KYLE, J. B. NATVIG, G. WILLIAMS, N. IGGO, R. ALEXANIAN, Y. PIRSON, R.A. COWARD

SOLOMON: I have reported several years ago in the Journal of Clinical Investigation the effect of prednisone on Bence Jones protein excretion in patients with multiple myeloma. There were essentially three types of response as determined by measuring the amount of the Bence Jones proteins excreted daily. Patients received prednisone 75 mg/day for 7 days. The daily urine protein was measured during this period and for the succeeding 3 weeks. In one group of patients, no change in Bence Jones protein excretion occurred during this period. In a second group, there was a dramatic decrease in proteinuria within the first days. In some patients subsequently the Bence Jones proteinuria recurred and by day 28 the proteinuria reached pretreatment levels. A third group of patients had a gradual decrease in Bence Jones proteinuria. In those patients who had marked decrease in Bence Jones proteinuria by day 1, we found that in three a fragment of the Bence Jones protein could be detected in the urine. These were constant region half fragments. Although half fragments could not be found in the urine, it is possible that subfragments were deposited (as crystals?) in the kidney. Thus prednisone can induce alterations in Bence Jones protein synthesis and catabolism.
BARLOGIE: Since patients with low RNA content plasma cells have a poor prognosis there are some practical implications regarding the therapy. We do switch very quickly to other chemotherapy in our front line program, as these patients have such a low response rate. We move on to high dose melphalan-containing programs where these prognostic features are no longer relevant.
BUXBAUM: Dr Preud'Homme and I some years ago showed that melphalan is a very potent mutagen in cultural mouse myeloma cells causing a variety of changes in immunoglobulin synthesis. We have reported a case of long survival of a patient with AL amyloidosis who had been treated initially with melphalan and prednisone. His cells initially produced a lambda L-chain fragment and high molecular weight polymers.

Minetti et al. (eds.), The kidney in plasma cell dyscrasias. ISBN 978-94-010-7085-0

This pattern disappeared in the course of therapy and he developed an IgG kappa monoclonal protein. We switched his therapy from melphalan to cyclophosphamide and the IgGK went away. He then survived for approximately ten years, subsequent to that therapy, prior to death. He died from a renal cell carcinoma, but he developed hypogammaglobulinemia and had a small amount of lambda monoclonal protein in his serum with no fragments and no polymers. He thus displayed the evolution of a tri-clonal disease, in which each of the clones was marked by a different protein product. Nonetheless, without therapy he probably would have died in 18 months, whereas with therapy he lived for 11 years.

SOLOMON: Monitoring of the efficacy of chemotherapy is based on the tumor product, namely, the monoclonal immunoglobulin (Bence Jones protein, etc.). Multiple myeloma is one of the few human malignancies that has a biomarker, the immunoglobulin, which is directly related to the tumor mass, and easy to measure.

KYLE: Even though we had a large series of patients who survived ten years with this disease, and one patient whose multiple myeloma was confirmed by autopsy had survived twentyone years, I am afraid the truth is really that we do not have good treatment for multiple myeloma.

SOLOMON: As to the question of how 'much' to treat, I answer to the extent required to eliminate the synthesis of the monoclonal light chain. This can be determined by (1) serial analyses of urine specimens; (2) bone marrow examinations by immunofluorescence to determine if the normal kappa/lambda ratio among the plasma cells has been restored, and (3) bone marrow biosynthetic patterns.

We have found that chemotherapy, even of short duration, will eliminate completely Bence Jones proteinuria in patients with light chain deposition disease or amyloidosis AL. This is in contrast to patients with myeloma where chemotherapy even given over protracted periods does not eliminate completely the monoclonal protein.

NATVIG: As to the treatment of amyloid with proteolytic enzymes if we could direct the enzyme to a local site and make a local treatment we might still be able to get something that will work on the amyloid. We are also surprised to see for example that we got a difference in the in vivo rabbit model also. There was a distinct difference in the degrading time and capacity of SAA in pronase-treated and control animals. After treatment tissue sections definitely did not take up Congo red, but, as we did not test the tissue with the antiamyloid antiserum, I cannot tell whether the enzyme removed amyloid fibrils or protein or both. I do not think that we can use such a system as a long term therapy yet in man, but the therapeutic situation in amyloidosis is so difficult that we should try different approaches.

WILLIAMS: At the experimental level there is a whole series of possible models which can be used to create amyloid in the assay form, whether it is based on casein serially administered or parabiosis or what have you. We used several of those models some years ago to produce pretty extensive secondary SAA amyloids in the various organs, and naturally the spleen became an early and fairly severe victim of the system, along with the renal apparatus as well. Now we found that you could produce a spectrum or range of involvement with amyloid both in the RE system, particularly in the spleen and liver. Once this was established, if you removed the regime or disentangled the parabiosis, a fair degree of spontaneous resorption would proceed, provided that the RE system was not entirely swamped, and quite extensive, massive removal of amyloid, with replacement by giant cell occurred throughout the spleen, whereas in relation to the kidney we found that the amyloid, once formed, despite the presence of the mesangial cell, remained pretty well indefinitely. So it supports the lytic approach to the removal of the insoluble protein.

KYLE: As far as amyloidosis is concerned Dr Osserman and I treated 13 patients with DMSO. None of the patients had objective response to the agent and the major limiting factor was the very bad odor from the patient's breath. We have had a long interest in the treatment of primary systemic amyloidosis. Our initial study consisted of 60 patients who were randomized to melphalan and prednisone or to placebo. Patients who had progression of their disease stopped the treatment, and then, if they were on placebo, melphalan and prednisone were given to them. We could not demonstrate a superiority of survival for melphalan and prednisone because of the cross-over. There were patients who did not show objective response. Approximately 50% of those with nephrotic syndrome had a 50% or greater reduction in proteinuria without progressive renal insufficiency. We went on to a second study in which 101 patients with primary systemic amyloidosis were randomized to melphalan and prednisone or to colchicine; if these patients showed progression of disease they were given the other regimen. We did this because we felt that the patients would go on and take the other regimen in an uncontrolled fashion. We found that the medium survival for patients with melphalan and prednisone was 25 months; the survival for patients with colchicine was 18 months. This difference is not statistically significant. However when we reanalyzed the data and looked at the duration of time from the onset of treatment to either progression of the disease or death of the patient there was a statistically significant difference favoring melphalan and prednisone (16 versus 6 months). When we looked at the patients who had received only melphalan and prednisone and the patients who had received only conchicine there was also a statistically significant difference still favouring the melphalan-prednisone regime.

We are currently conducting a prospective randomized study in which patients are assigned to melphalan and prednisone or to colchicine or to a combination of the three agents. We have about 120 patients on study and do not have survival data yet. There is no provision of cross-over in this study.

NATVIG: I would like to point out that in some patients with light chain related amyloidosis the disease can be very fulminating and appears as a therapy resistant nephrotic syndrome. Some of the lambda-IV proteins, that we first found and described, were from such patients with a nephrotic syndrome.

IGGO: The figure of 50% of myeloma patients developing renal failure puzzled me for a little while; I suspect a lot of that was mild to moderate and reversible renal impairment. The published MRC (Medical Research Council) trial had around 80 patients who developed renal failure, but looking at the figures only two of those required long term replacement hemodialysis.

ALEXANIAN: You have to be cautious in comparing different groups of patients. The incidence of renal failure, and irreversible renal failure, in myeloma patients is quite different among the centers, the hematological ones having (markedly) lower percentage of renal failure cases than the nephrological ones.

Renal failure in myeloma provides three items almost simultaneously at the time of diagnosis: the clue to the diagnosis in an individual patient whose problem is that renal disease causes are known; it must be managed simultaneously with diagnostic studies and attempts to stage the myeloma and plan therapy; most centers have considered this to be an ominous prognostic factor but my opinion is that prognostic implications of renal failure are probably due to other factors than the renal disease itself. By performing multivariate regression type analysis you can dissect really the independence of the various factors. You could look whether marked renal insufficiency does come in as an independent factor after accounting for tumor mass, and whether the regression of renal failure is depending on a post-treatment factor such as a response of the myeloma to chemotherapy.

BARLOGIE: I think that in patients who present an acute renal failure, due to high tumor mass myeloma, the VAD (vincristine, adriamycine, dexamethasone) regimen is particularly useful because it is so very fast. In our experience untreated patients showed a response by a time of 10 to 14 days, whereas with melphalan and prednisone it takes one and a half month on the average.

So I think that in a newly diagnosed patient, who presents a renal failure, if a treatment with full dosages of all drugs can be immediately instituted and the patient is responsive, one does have a fairly high chance of reversing the renal failure.

ALEXANIAN: When treating patients with renal involvement there is to face the problem of interpreting the response of the myeloma separately from the response of the renal failure. By measuring the serum level of β_2-microglobulin at once with that of creatinine you could reveal disproportionate increases of β_2-microglobulin in beyond the expected range for renal failure, and then be able to distinguish the contribution of renal failure from tumor load in patients with myeloma. Another mean, that is an old traditional way, is also to monitor bone marrow plasmacytosis.

SOLOMON: The question whether to treat or not to treat with chemotherapy patients with multiple myeloma who have advanced renal failure is very difficult because of the very variable clinical circumstances. For the most part treatment is indicated. Patients with myeloma have many other problems, bone pain, etc. that rely to the neoplastic process, and chemotherapy is often helpful. Supportive therapy (transfusion, fluids, electrolytes) if necessary is a first step, and when the chemotherapy is given, it must be cautious. Aggressive chemotherapy can be exceedingly dangerous, and appropriate reduction in drug dosage is wanted because of the renal failure.

BUXBAUM: I think that the therapy of the AL disease, and the therapy of light chain deposition disease is pretty much in the same stage. Dr Kyle probably has the most experience with AL disease, and I think it is very clear to all of us who have tried cytostatic therapy that some patients respond and they respond in terms of improved organ function. The difficulty is that we do not know which patients are going to respond earlier. The minimum requirement for an effective response is the demonstration of the elimination of the synthesis of the abnormal protein. If that is successfully accomplished it will probably stop the accumulation of the protein. The prognosis from that point is determined by how much organ damage has already been done.

We have not systematically looked at all our patients because they have not all been treated in the same way. We have seen long survival in some patients who have responded by the cessation of their abnormal immunoglobulin synthesis. We have seen some patients who in fact presented with severe heart disease secondary to AL deposition, and while we eliminated the production of the abnormal protein, I suspect that the patient's course was unaffected since he went on to die in 2 or 3 years. With respect to transplantation, we now know of 3 patients. One of these was the first patient we reported in 1980, who has since been transplanted after we demonstrated the cessation of synthesis of abnormal light chain, and is doing very well. A patient was also transplanted with a good result after 2 years. The patient with the alpha heavy chain deposition who has been studied several times during the course of chemotherapy and clearly demonstrated a reduction and then the elimination of the abnormal protein, has been transplanted and doing very well. While this is not a prospective controlled study which would be desirable, these cases make the point that untreated deposition disease with or without the diagnosis of myeloma is ultimately fatal, with a mean survival in light chain amyloid between a year and two years. We don't know what the overall statistic is for monoclonal deposition diseases. There are some patients who clearly exceed that in terms of survival without therapy but we do not know how to recognize them. Dr Solomon is probably correct when he says that these patients respond to smaller doses of therapy. They have smaller plasma cells clones than do patients with myeloma. We feel that if you can turn off the aberrant synthesis the patients have a good crack at survival.

PIRSON: I would like to briefly report a case of renal transplantation in light chain nephropathy. It illustrates that long-term survival is possible despite renal death from light chain nephropathy, but also that recurrence of the disease in the graft must be expected.

This 37 year old man was admitted 10 years ago for rapidly progressive renal failure. The biopsy showed glomerular deposits of PAS positive material in the mesangium, resulting in typical nodular glomerular sclerosis. The TBM was considerably thickened and splitted. The bone marrow showed plasmacytosis of 30%, staining for kappa light chain, whereas light chain at that time was not detected either in urine or serum. The patient had a severe hypogammaglobulinemia. Diagnosis of light chain nephropathy was made. Two months later, the renal failure was irreversible and hemodialysis was started. No other therapy was given.

Six years later the patient was transplanted; one of the kidneys was removed and stained for kappa light chain. After the third episode of acute rejection, he was switched from azathioprine to cyclosporine and the renal function after that was stable. Four years after transplantation we noted a deterioration of the graft function with a slight proteinuria (500mg/day); kappa light chain was then detected both in urine and in serum. Graft biopsy showed, as in the native kidney, a marked thickening of the tubule walls and on immunofluorescence, a very nice linear deposit of kappa light chain on the TBM, demonstrating the recurrence of the disease in the graft. Melphalan was then given for the first time. Currently, the graft function is stable, with a serum creatinine of about 3mg/dl. We have found in the literature seven other cases of renal transplantation for light chain nephropathy; recurrence was observed in six of them.

KYLE: We have a patient with light chain deposition disease who presented severe renal insufficiency six years ago. He had a renal transplant and was treated with melphalan and prednisone for two years. The monoclonal light chain disappeared and currently the patient has no monoclonal kappa protein in his serum or urine and has normal renal function. We have not rebiopsied the kidney.

COWARD: Over the past six years I have dialyzed more than 20 patients of myeloma, most of whom have been acute patients. The data over the few patients in our chronic dialysis program show that they have quite a lot of admissions, especially during the start of their illness. They have been treated with different chemotherapies, at least for six months. In certain patients prolonged periods of well-being are possible, but the total days in hospital per year are very high. I calculated that these patients are between forty to sixty per cent more expensive to treat, not because of the chemotherapy but basically because of the hospital admissions. Infection has the major percentage of the admission time. Most of them were chest infections due to the pneumococci. We observed also six infections of subclavian lines, our frequent route of dialysis. Only 25% of the infections were related to neutropenia.

KYLE: Hemodialysis goes very well, but we run into trouble when the patient becomes resistant to chemotherapy. The patient dies usually of infection and not for renal failure. We only transplanted one patient with multiple myeloma, who did well for approximately 4 years and then died of fungal infection.

IGGO: We have collected almost 20 patients on chronic dialysis who have had myeloma, the majority of whose were treated with prednisone and melphalan or cyclophosphamide with very little problems. There were two who had more aggressive chemotherapy, one was an elderly gentleman who within a month died from a sepsis, but the other was a young patient with about 50% of plasma cells in the bone marrow who was elected for a treatment in full doses of VAD, from the start. She had a good effect but some problems from peripheral neuropathy despite the very low dose of vincristine.

Part V. Conclusions

Conclusions

J. S. CAMERON

A very clear indication of two things is given by the papers in this book: the first is that plasma cell dyscrasias are very serious diseases, and our treatment and management of them are inadequate; and second, that all of us see them as a single group of diseases expressing varying degrees of malignancy, in terms of both clinical behaviour and of cellular biology. Some of the points that emerged, particularly from Dr Barlogie's presentation and also from Dr Solomon were that we know that these B cells are very abnormal (Table 1). The B cells are characterized by the persistence of primitive markers such as the cALLA (CD 10) epitope which continues to be expressed on mature cells producing immunoglobulin fragments. Interestingly there is increased expression of *Cmyc* and *ras* genes in quite a high proportion (70%) of patients, which is of prognostic significance as well. I was interested to read, because I did not know this, that there are rearrangements of the T cell-receptor gene as well. We didn't really deal with the relationship of B cell dyscrasias to the disintegration of immune-regulation, which we know is part of normal aging, from say 25 years onwards; perhaps we should have, and this is something we may need to return to in the future.

We like to have classifications, because this is the way we make order

Table 1. Overproduction of light chains involves.

- A very early event in B cell maturation
- Persistence of primitive markers such as cALLA (CD 10) on mature plasma cell producing an abnormal product
- Increased expression of *Cmyc* and *ras* genes in 70% of cases
- An abnormal karyotype in 50% of cases (chromosomes 8 and 14, IgA)
- Rearrangement of the T receptor (CD 3) gene
- Light chain overproduction is then neoplastic, the result of somatic mutation(s) and is not antigen-driven
- Light chain overproduction increases with age ('benign' monoclonal gammopathy)

Minetti et al. (eds.), The kidney in plasma cell dyscrasias. ISBN 978-94-010-7085-0

Table 2. Origin of light chains.

- Light chains are products of complex and numerous gene rearrangements on several different chromosomes (V, J, D)
- These are rearranged to create mRNA for the complete chain
- Enormous product diversity is characteristic of the system
- No two tumours produce exactly the same product (idiotypes)

out of chaos in our universe. This, however, is one area (Table 2) in which we are *never* going to get a simple classification because we are dealing with a group of cells, part of a system, whose function *is* the generation of diversity; and as Dr Preud'Homme pointed out, there is a huge variety of products which are the result of the overproduction of the B cells in this group of diseases. Light chains are the product of numerous genes; there is an extensive rearrangement before the messenger RNA is finally assembled, and there is an enormous product diversity which is characteristic of the system. As Dr Solomon emphasized, no two tumors we are dealing with produce exactly the same product. So, we cannot expect simple classification to emerge from this system, and we must try and live with the complexity which is inevitable.

One of the central points of the second part of the book is the renal toxicity of light chains (Table 3) and we have been through, in detail, the factors which might contribute to this toxicity. These factors break down into first, factors intrinsic to the B cell product, and second, host factors. Perhaps the most important factor in the B cell product itself, which we dismiss quite frequently because it is so easy to understand, is simply the

Table 3. Renal toxicity of light chains.

This might depend upon:

(a) Factors intrinsic to the B cell product
- Amount (concentration × time)
- Amino acid composition
  - → Tertiary structure
  - → Hydrophobicity
  - → Solubility
- Subtype
- Glycosylation
- Polymerization
- pI?

(b) Host factors:
- Hypercalcaemia
- Hydration
- Contrast agents?

amount of the product in the circulation — its concentration in the blood, and also the time over which the kidney is exposed to this concentration. Dr Solomon reminds us that we really know very little about the tertiary structure of the proteins that we are dealing with, particularly when we come to look at amyloidosis. It seems that the pI, having been extensively investigated, is not giving us any useful message in terms of why some light chain are toxic, and some are not.

As far as host factors are concerned, Dr Smolens pointed out very elegantly in his model how modest hypercalcemia could increase the toxicity of light chains. There is a clear clinical message here. We have all, I think, taken on board the other clear clinical message which is the importance of hydration. Especially with the new low osmolarity contrast agents, it seems, on the other hand, that contrast medium toxicity is not a major problem. *Mechanisms* of renal toxicity are dealt with *in extenso* above, and I don't want to go into detail on this (Table 4). There is good evidence that light chains are reabsorbed mainly by pinocytosis, a high

Table 4. Mechanisms of renal damage.

Dysfunction:

- Direct proximal tubular damage by pinocytosis of toxic light chains → Prox. tubule

- Cast formation from insolubility — ? co-precipitation with Tamm-Horsfall protein

Tubular obstruction → Dist. tubule

Interstitial inflammation

- Vascular lesions

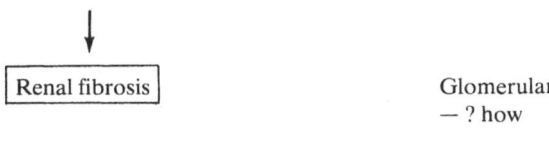

capacity and low affinity system, and that some light chains are toxic, because of properties we don't yet understand, and some are not. The major question is light chain solubility and cast formation, and the rôle of Tamm-Horsfall protein, either as a co-precipitant or as itself a toxic inflammation-inducing agent was debated also. Tubular obstruction clearly is an important event, and Dr Ronco and others reviewed evidence that tubular obstruction is indeed present. From work that Dr Colussi reviewed, it is evident also that *proximal* tubular defects are relatively common, although clinically they may not be significant in most patients, despite the increased delivery of sodium to the distal tubule and risk of desalination. Distal tubular damage really only results when there is global damage to the kidney, and an extensive fibrosis.

Little attention was given to interstitial inflammation, and Corrado Pirani mentioned vascular lesions, of which we perhaps should be more aware; I wonder whether this is in fact an insudation of some of the B cell product into the vascular walls. Finally the end-stage of all the mechanisms is renal fibrosis, and fibrogenesis was not discussed at all. We never do. We forget that inflammation is (at least to begin with) potentially completely reversible, and that the major event of all tissue damage, including the kidney, which finally leads to organ destruction is fibrogenesis. This is a whole area which we need to get into, not only in the area of B cell dyscrasias, but in all renal diseases, because we are so ignorant of how fibrogenesis arises. We do not know anything about injury in interstitial diseases, although there are many exciting new ideas emerging some of which we have touched on.

Turning to amyloid now (Table 5) we are given above several definitions of amyloids, which center around the formation of insoluble, poorly degradable — but still degradable — 10 nanometer fibrils in beta-pleated conformation, arising from a variety of proteins. In the B cell dyscrasias, it

Table 5. Amyloidogenesis (1).

- Formation of insoluble, poorly degradable 10 nm fibrils in β pleated conformation from proteins
- Dependent on subtype (λ VI), but K and λ°
- Formed from V region only, not C
- May depend on proteolysis (monocyte surface elastase, SAA — AA)
- Microenvironment important
  - Locally high concentration
  - Physico-chemical effects
- Dependent on concentration

°? Aminoacid substitutions.
? Tertiary structure.

seems that the λVI subgroup of proteins is particularly amyloidogenic. But other K and λ chains can be amyloidogenic also, and maybe their toxicity depends upon minor aminoacid substitutions. Our lack of knowledge of the tertiary structure of these proteins, which maybe determines their physical properties and therefore their propensity to get into tissues and form amyloid, is relevant. Amyloidogenic L proteins are part of the V-region, which we have known for some time. The old question of proteolysis, and in particular whether the monocyte surface elastase — which is clearly implicated (as Dr Zucker-Franklin reminded us from her work) in the genesis of amyloid A (AA) protein from serum amyloid-A (SAA) — may also be involved in the genesis of amyloid from the V-region is not yet clear. Another area of ignorance here was touched on several times: that the microenvironment in which the fibrils form may be crucial, and that there may be locally very high concentrations of protein, so it may simply be a matter of exceeding solubility limits. There may be physico-chemical effects and interactions as well, of which we know very little, in particular parts of the kidney or in particular parts of other organs.

Table 6 is almost a repeat of Dr Shirahama's diagram, just to remind us that there are many ways of getting to amyloid fibrils. I put this table in to remind us, as Dr Zucker-Franklin did, that we talk a lot about amyloido-*genesis* and we don't talk nearly enough about amyloido*lysis*, as Dr Natvig also points out. Perhaps this is where we should be looking at, in seeking to

Table 6. Amyloidogenesis (2).

Stimulus	Site of origin	Product	Processing	Fibril
?	plasma cell	LC	? macrophage degradation	AL
IL-1	hepatocyte	SAA	macrophage degradation	AA
genetic abnormality	amino-acid substitution	pre-Alb. (*normal* conc)	—	pre-Alb
renal failure, bioincompatibility	mononu-clear cells	β_2m ↑	—	β_2m

Amyloidolysis

- Monocytes have serine proteases which degrade AA in vitro
- Are resident monocytes important in limiting renal amyloid?
- Does monocyte dysfunction contribute to amyloid formation?
- What is 'amyloid accelerating factor'?

prevent amyloid or at least to treat it. Table 6 reminds us that the primary stimulus to the primitive B cell, a series of 'hits' on the gene (although we don't know what they are) leads to overproduction and high plasma concentration of light chains. Macrophages may be involved in processing these, and the fibril is formed from AL. Turning to amyloid A, the stimulus for the hepatocyte to produce serum amyloid A (SAA) is interleukin 1. Amyloid A (SAA) protein is very definitely degraded by the macrophage to AA. As Dr Shirahama reminded us, you can have substances which are present in *normal* concentrations such as abnormal pre-albumin, but which because amino-acid substitutions are insoluble, and can form amyloid. Beta-2-m-amyloidosis, which is of great interest to nephrologists because of its so far unique association with hemodialysis and chronic renal failure, is of course the product of shedding of beta-2-microglobulin from cells and its retention in renal failure, since it is a microprotein normally pinocytosed and degraded in the proximal tubule.

As far as amyloido*lysis* is concerned, there are serine proteases which, according to Dr Natvig, will, given the right conditions, degrade at least amyloid AA. We do not know whether they are able to degrade amyloid AL as well. The resident monocytes in the kidney, within the mesangium, small in number but perhaps very significant in function, may be important — as Dr Zucker-Franklin hinted. Does monocyte dysfunction contribute to amyloid formation in the kidney in renal disease, and what is the role of 'amyloid-accelerating factor' — and indeed what is it? There are lots of questions still on amyloid.

Turning to clinical aspects (Table 7) it is quite clear that clinicians looking after nephrotic patients must be aware of, and have a strong clinical suspicion of, AL amyloidosis in all nephrotics over the age of 40. If they look in the serum and in the urine with appropriate techniques such as immunofixation, the reward is that they will get at a very high positive diagnostic rate (94%). Renal biopsy, despite fear of bleeds after amyloid infiltrated organs have been punctured by sharp needles, appears to be safe. Abdominal fat biopsy was mentioned, and I think everyone who has

Table 7. Nephrotic syndrome and AL amyloid.

- — Maintain clinical suspicion of AL in all NS > 40y
- — Serum, or urine (immunofixation) will give positive in 94%
- — Renal biopsy appears safe (fat biopsy easy, but difficult to interpret, 80% positive)
- — Examine *all* biopsies for Congo Red and EM
- — Prognosis poor (mean survival 20/12) but a minority do well
- — Cardiac problems common, may be fatal
- — Prognosis the same ± evident myeloma

done it, finds it easy. However I think also many pathologists find that equally the specimen is difficult to interpret after Congo red staining, but is around 80% positive, a good deal less than renal biopsy, which maybe is 95% specific. We need to examine routinely all biopsies with Congo red, and by electronmicroscopy, to make sure we don't miss the odd patient whose protein abnormalities we can't pick up, perhaps because not all renal units have access to good enough laboratory facilities.

The terrible prognosis of this disease, with a mean survival of only 12 months or so, was pointed out from the Italian collaborative study. Also, the fact emerged that there are a minority of patients who do very well year after year; we have a couple of them in our own unit. The cardiac problem impresses on all this group of patients, and can be fatal. One thing I did not realize until this meeting is that the prognosis of a patient with amyloid AL is essentially the same, whether or not there is an evident myeloma; which emphasizes the poor prognosis of the 'primary' disease.

Light chain deposit disease (LCDD) (Table 8) from having been undescribed or unrecognized until ten years ago, is now part of our knowledge both in haematology and nephrology. As Dr Gallo and Dr Ganeval remind us, these patients are usually middle aged or elderly, more commonly males and in 20% (in contrast to AL amyloid), there are no detectable abnormal protein in urines or sera despite careful search with immunofixation techniques. There is often concomitant clinical myeloma, or these patients may evolve into myeloma, suggesting again that we are dealing with a spectrum of plasma cell dyscrasias. K chains are much more common than lambda deposits in this disease, and we would like to know why they deposit along the tubular and glomerular and vascular basement membrane. Again we come up against our ignorance of what exactly these products arc, in terms of structure, and since they are often around in very small quantities it is not always easy to do the analyses requires. The question of whether or not they may be cationic and bind to the fixed polyanion has been raised as a speculation, but there is very little evidence as yet that this is the case.

Table 8. L.C.D.D.

- — 40—80y, m:f 2:1, 20% no abnormal protein in urine serum
- — Concomitant myeloma, or prelude to myeloma
- — K $\gg$ λ in deposits ?? cationic
- — Heterogeneous clinical presentation
- — Heterogeneous biopsy appearances 'nodules' ↓, 'normal' ↑ with increasing recognition
- — Concomitant amyloid in 10%
- — Usually affects other organs
- — Regular recurrence in allografts

As nephrologists, we have to remember that patients with LCDD can present in almost any fashion. Hitherto they presented to us rather late, we having only realized what was going on, usually after the pathologist had told us that the patient has the disease. But as we have got better at remembering light chain disease, it's interesting that the number of patients with severe, advanced changes has decreased, and a number with relatively normal glomeruli on biopsy has increased. There is sometimes concomitant amyloid, again emphasizing that this is part of a spectrum. As Dr Ganeval reminded us, LCDD often affects other organs, sometimes with serious dysfunction, and as Dr Pirson reported there has been recurrence in renal allografts. This is something we have to be worried about and possibly plan ahead in relation to treatment.

Which brings me to my last subject, treatment (Table 9). I think one thing we should emphasize is that these are an appalling set of diseases. From a nephrologist's point of view, dealing as he does with relatively 'benign' disorders, in a setting where nobody dies of renal failure anymore — at least we hope they don't — we have to realize that, as Dr Kyle reported, cure is extremely rare in myeloma and the mean survival is only 30—36 months. I won't go through the various treatments but I must remind you that the effect of renal function on the excretion of some of the drugs used has not been mentioned here. All mustard-like drugs are, of course, cleared through the kidney, and thus patients with renal failure are much more liable if you use mustard-like drugs, to get leucopenia. The question of dialysis was extensively treated as well by Dr Mallick.

Table 9. Treatment.

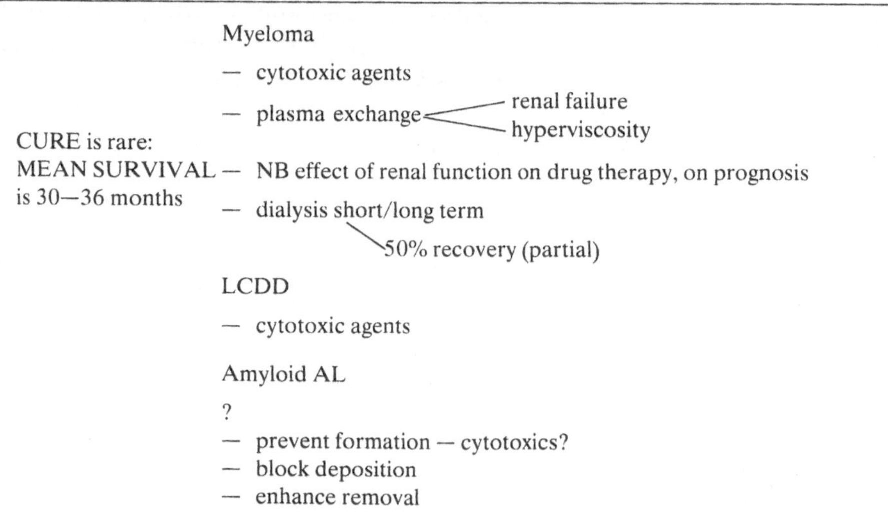

Myeloma

— cytotoxic agents

— plasma exchange — renal failure / hyperviscosity

CURE is rare:
MEAN SURVIVAL is 30—36 months

— NB effect of renal function on drug therapy, on prognosis

— dialysis short/long term — 50% recovery (partial)

LCDD

— cytotoxic agents

Amyloid AL

?

— prevent formation — cytotoxics?
— block deposition
— enhance removal

In light chain deposit disease, there seems to be a mood of optimism that this can be and should be treated by cytotoxic agents, justified by the good results in some of those caught with disease early, and also the rather frequent evolution into more aggressive forms of B cell dyscrasia.

Dr Natvig dealt with possible ways of preventing the formation, blocking the deposition or enhancing the removal of amyloid AL. We have learnt from Dr Kyle about the use of cytotoxics in his studies, on really very large numbers of patients; and certainly after an initial period of scepticism, I must say one message I am taking home is that we should probably go back to treating our patients with primary amyloid. There is one thing absolutely sure, and that is that we cannot be doing worse than we are at the moment, because these patients are doing very badly indeed.

Index

Developments in Nephrology

1. Cheigh, J.S., Stenzel, K.H. and Rubin, A.L. (eds.): Manual of Clinical Nephrology of the Rogosin Kidney Center. 1981 ISBN 90-247-2397-3
2. Nolph, K.D. (ed.): Peritoneal Dialysis. 1981 ed.: out of print
   3rd revised and enlarged ed. 1988 (not in this series) ISBN 0-89838-406-0
3. Gruskin, A.B. and Norman, M.E. (eds.): Pediatric Nephrology. 1981 ISBN 90-247-2514-3
4. Schück, O.: Examination of the Kidney Function. 1981 ISBN 0-89838-565-2
5. Strauss, J. (ed.): Hypertension, Fluid-electrolytes and Tubulopathies in Pediatric Nephrology. 1982 ISBN 90-247-2633-6
6. Strauss, J. (ed.): Neonatal Kidney and Fluid-electrolytes. 1983 ISBN 0-89838-575-X
7. Strauss, J. (ed.): Acute Renal Disorders and Renal Emergencies. 1984 ISBN 0-89838-663-2
8. Didio, L.J.A. and Motta, P.M. (eds.): Basic, Clinical, and Surgical Nephrology. 1985 ISBN 0-89838-698-5
9. Friedman, E.A. and Peterson, C.M. (eds.): Diabetic Nephropathy: Strategy for Therapy. 1985 ISBN 0-89838-735-3
10. Dzúrik, R., Lichardus, B. and Guder, W. (eds.): Kidney Metabolism and Function. 1985 ISBN 0-89838-749-3
11. Strauss, J. (ed.): Homeostasis, Nephrotoxicity, and Renal Anomalies in the Newborn. 1986 ISBN 0-89838-766-3
12. Oreopoulos, D.G. (ed.): Geriatric Nephrology. 1986 ISBN 0-89838-781-7
13. Paganini, E.P. (ed.): Acute Continuous Renal Replacement Therapy. 1986 ISBN 0-89838-793-0
14. Cheigh, J.S., Stenzel, K.H. and Rubin, A.L. (eds.): Hypertension in Kidney Disease. 1986 ISBN 0-89838-797-3
15. Deane, N., Wineman, R.J. and Benis, G.A. (eds.): Guide to Reprocessing of Hemodialyzers. 1986 ISBN 0-89838-798-1
16. Ponticelli, C., Minetti, L. and D'Amico, G. (eds.): Antiglobulins, Cryoglobulins and Glomerulonephritis. 1986 ISBN 0-89838-810-4
17. Strauss, J. (ed.), with the assistance of L. Strauss: Persistent Renal-genitourinary Disorders. 1987 ISBN 0-89838-845-7
18. Andreucci, V.E. and Dal Canton, A. (eds.): Diuretics: Basic, Pharmacological, and Clinical Aspects. 1987 ISBN 0-89838-885-6
19. Bach, P.H. and Lock, E.H. (eds.): Nephrotoxicity in the Experimental and Clinical Situation, Part 1. 1987 ISBN 0-89838-977-1

20. Bach, P.H. and Lock, E.H. (eds.): Nephrotoxicity in the Experimental and Clinical Situation, Part 2. 1987 ISBN 0-89838-980-2
21. Gore, S.M. and Bradley, B.A. (eds.): Renal Transplantation: Sense and Sensitization. 1988 ISBN 0-89838-370-6
22. Minetti, L., D'Amico, G. and Ponticelli, C. (eds.): The Kidney in Plasma Cell Dyscrasias. 1988 ISBN 0-89838-385-4